Principles and Practice of Ophthalmology

Principles and Practice of Ophthalmology

Edited by **Abigail Gipe**

hayle
medical

New York

Published by Hayle Medical,
30 West, 37th Street, Suite 612,
New York, NY 10018, USA
www.haylemedical.com

Principles and Practice of Ophthalmology
Edited by Abigail Gipe

International Standard Book Number: 978-1-63241-414-4 (Hardback)

Printed in the United States of America.

Contents

Preface

Ophthalmology is a branch of medical science which deals with the study of eyes, treatment of disorders and diseases related to eyes and visual system. Ophthalmologists treat various diseases like myopia, farsightedness, astigmatism, presbyopia, cataract, glaucoma, etc. This branch of science has many sub-fields namely medical retina, ophthalmic pathology, refractive surgery, vitreo-retinal surgery, ocular oncology, etc. This book provides comprehensive insights into the field of ophthalmology. It will provide interesting topics for research which readers can take up. This text presents researches and case studies performed by experts across the globe. It will serve as a reference guide to a broad spectrum of readers. Students, doctors, ophthalmologists, scientists, researchers and all associated with this field will benefit alike from this book.

After months of intensive research and writing, this book is the end result of all who devoted their time and efforts in the initiation and progress of this book. It will surely be a source of reference in enhancing the required knowledge of the new developments in the area. During the course of developing this book, certain measures such as accuracy, authenticity and research focused analytical studies were given preference in order to produce a comprehensive book in the area of study.

This book would not have been possible without the efforts of the authors and the publisher. I extend my sincere thanks to them. Secondly, I express my gratitude to my family and well-wishers. And most importantly, I thank my students for constantly expressing their willingness and curiosity in enhancing their knowledge in the field, which encourages me to take up further research projects for the advancement of the area.

Editor

Phlyctenulosis-Like Presentation Secondary to Embedded Corneal Foreign Body

Valliammai Muthappan[1], Jared G. Smedley[2], Carlton R. Fenzl[1], Majid Moshirfar[3*]

[1]John A. Moran Eye Center, University of Utah, Salt Lake City, USA
[2]College of Human Medicine, Michigan State University, Lansing, USA
[3]Department of Ophthalmology, Francis I. Proctor Foundation, University of California San Francisco, San Francisco, USA
Email: [*]Majid.Moshirfar@ucsf.edu

Abstract

Case Presentation: A nine-year-old boy presented to the general ophthalmologist with a several weeks history of redness, photophobia and intermittent foreign body sensation in the right eye. A pigmented lesion with anterior chamber inflammation was noted on examination. B-scan ultrasound was performed and revealed no foreign body. The patient was diagnosed with anterior uveitis, which did not completely respond to treatment. The differential diagnosis was expanded to include peripheral ulcerative keratitis, phlyctenulosis, pigmented neoplasm, and corneal foreign body. Upon referral to a cornea specialist, an exam under anesthesia revealed a large foreign body consistent with a rock fragment in the peripheral cornea, which was subsequently removed without complication. Conclusion: This case highlights an atypical presentation of foreign body as well as a differential diagnosis of pigmented peripheral corneal lesions. Foreign bodies represent the most common cause of urgent ophthalmic evaluation. When evaluating lesions of the cornea, it is imperative to keep an extensive differential diagnosis, giving the potential for severe and rapid development of visually threatening complications.

Keywords

Corneal Foreign Body, Phlyctenulosis, Pigmented Corneal Lesion, Anterior Uveitis

1. Introduction

Peripheral corneal inflammatory lesions are a group of conditions with similar signs and symptoms. Limbal and

---
[*]Corresponding author.

perilimbal injection, corneal neovascularization, corneal infiltrate, and anterior chamber inflammation are all findings commonly seen. The identification of a correct diagnosis begins with a complete history and physical exam along with necessary medical and/or surgical therapies. We report a case of unilateral peripheral corneal foreign body accompanied by injection, corneal neovascularization, and intraocular inflammation.

2. Case Presentation

A nine-year-old boy presented to the general ophthalmologist with a several week history of redness, photophobia and occasional foreign body sensation in the right eye. The patient's history was significant for playing outside on a windy day a few days prior to symptom development. Upon evaluation, uncorrected visual acuity (UCVA) was 20/25 in the right eye and 20/20 in the left. Slit lamp examination revealed anterior chamber inflammation with a dark brown lesion in the superotemporal cornea of the right eye. B-scan ultrasound was performed and revealed no foreign body. The patient was diagnosed with acute anterior uveitis with peripheral anterior synechiae. He was treated with prednisolone acetate 1% ophthalmic drops four times a day; cyclopentolate 1% ophthalmic drops twice a day and erythromycin ointment.

One week later, the patient noticed some improvement of his symptoms. Visual acuity was unchanged and gonioscopy revealed a pigmented lesion within the temporal corneal stroma, not extending beyond the endothelium. The pigmented area was no longer considered to be a peripheral anterior synechiae, and the differential diagnosis was expanded to include peripheral ulcerative keratitis, phlyctenulosis, and pigmented neoplasm, in addition to corneal foreign body. The patient was referred to a corneal specialist for further evaluation and treatment.

The patient was seen in our clinic two days later. Right UCVA was 20/20-2 and left UCVA was 20/15-2. Slit lamp examination of the right cornea revealed a 1.4 mm by 2 mm lesion at the ten o'clock position just inside the limbus (**Figure 1(a)**). The lesion had surrounding neovascular pannus and lipid deposition (**Figure 1(b)**). The anterior chamber was deep and quiet, and the iris was round and reactive. Given the patient's age, wind exposure and incomplete response to treatment, a foreign body was suspected and evaluation under anesthesia (EUA) was scheduled.

Eight days later, the patient underwent EUA and a foreign body was identified in the peripheral cornea in the area of the pigmented lesion. The foreign body was estimated to extend 90% through the cornea. It was removed without complication and identified by pathology as a fragment of rock (**Figure 2(a)**). The patient was started

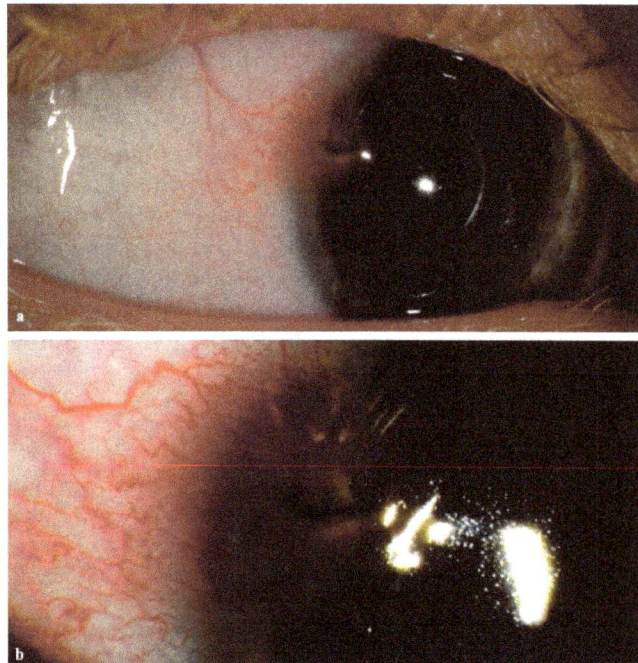

Figure 1. (a) Slit-lamp photograph showing corneal lesion with surrounding neovascular pannus and lipid deposition; (b) Higher magnification slit-lamp photograph of the right eye showing neovascularization and pannus formation.

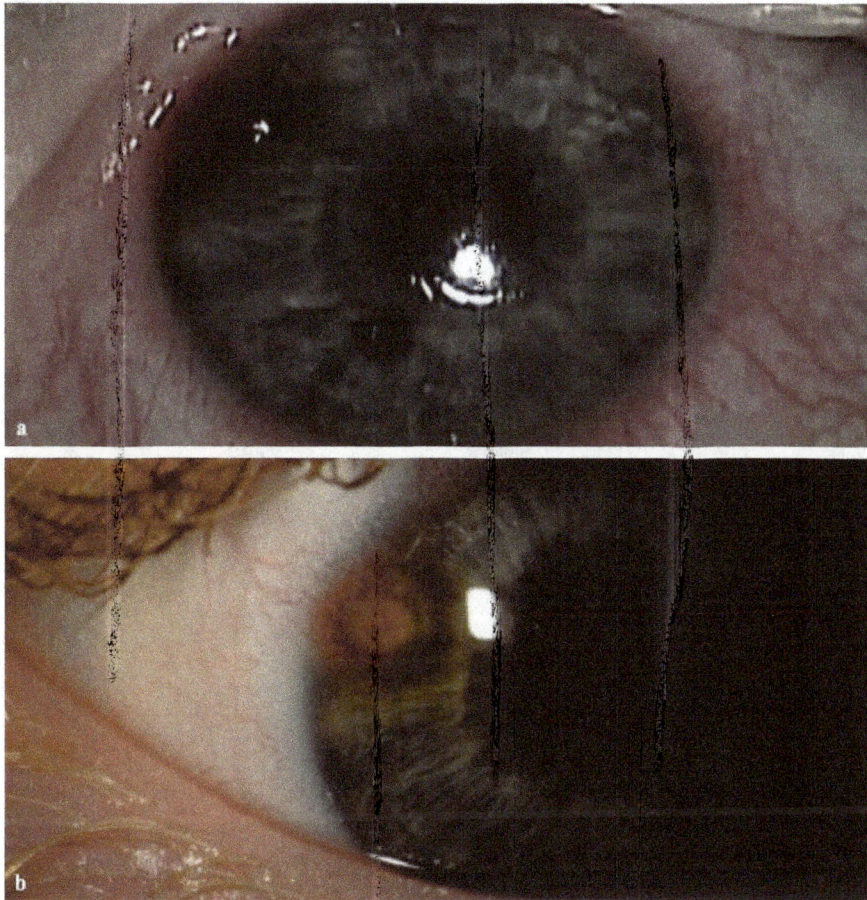

Figure 2. (a) Intraoperative photo of the corneal foreign body (yellow arrow) removed and placed on the inferior cornea at the seven o'clock position for size comparison. Surgical wound (white arrow) is visible in right superotemporal position; (b) One-week post-operative photo depicting a resolving lesion (white arrow) with a persistent peripheral lipid deposition.

on gatifloxacin 0.5% ophthalmic drops four times a day. Prednisolone acetate 1% was continued four times a day and cyclopentolate was discontinued. At one week post-operatively, the redness and irritation of the right eye had resolved and UCVA was 20/20. A healing corneal wound is visible in the superotemporal cornea (**Figure 2(b)**).

3. Discussion

We present a case of a pigmented peripheral corneal lesion associated with redness, irritation and foreign body sensation in a pediatric patient with history of sandstorm exposure. The diagnosis was confounded by the negative ultrasound. Ultrasound biomicroscopy has greater sensitivity than basic ultrasound for detecting ocular foreign bodies [1] [2]; however, this could not be performed due to patient's age and compliance. In this case, the diagnosis was not apparent until the fragment of rock was surgically identified and removed. This case illustrates an unusual presentation of a common ophthalmologic problem. This patient's corneal lesion on slit-lamp examination appeared similar to several other ocular disorders, with which the patient was diagnosed and briefly treated for, prior to the EUA.

Initially, this patient was diagnosed with peripheral anterior synechiae secondary to acute anterior iritis, which is somewhat uncommon in the pediatric population. Inflammatory causes of anterior uveitis include juvenile idiopathic arthritis (JIA), psoriatic arthritis, and tubulointerstitial nephritis and uveitis syndrome (TINU). Infectious causes such as herpetic uveitis and lyme disease are also important to consider [3]. **Figure 3(b)** shows a slit-lamp image of an unrelated patient with peripheral anterior synechiae secondary to inflammation, with iris

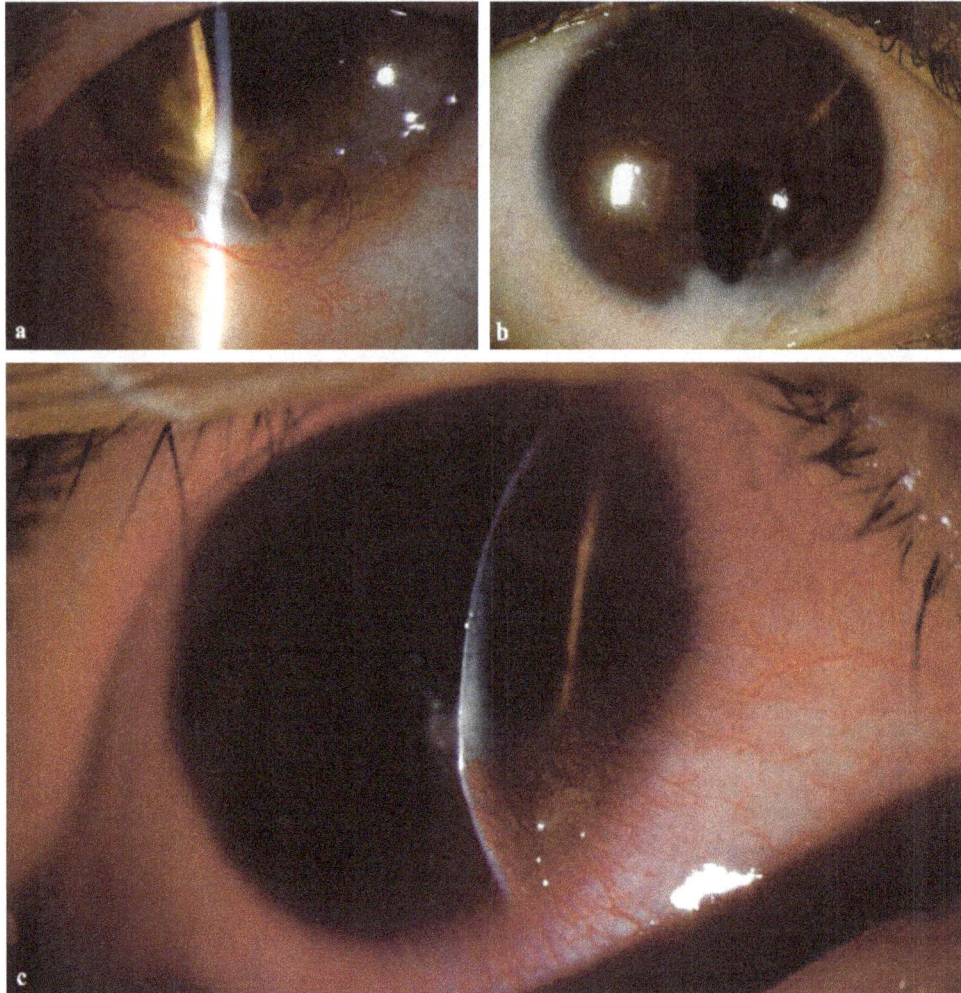

Figure 3. (a) Peripheral ulcerative keratitis. Ulcerations and stromal thinning are seen in the inferotemporal limbus. Conjunctival vasodilation and surrounding neovascularization are also seen; (b) Peripheral anterior synechiae with inflammation secondary to trauma. Irregularities of the iris are often seen with anterior synechiae; (c) Phlyctenulosis due to staphylococcus hypersensitivity. Wedge shaped neovascularization with pannus formation is visible on the inferonasal peripheral cornea. A white nodule is seen at leading edge of lesion centrally.

irregularities, somewhat resembling the peripheral corneal lesion in our patient (**Figure 1(a)**). Peripheral ulcerative keratitis (PUK) was also entertained as a diagnosis, due to the presence of a peripheral corneal lesion associated with redness, irritation and photophobia. It is extremely rare in children, but classically manifests as peripheral corneal infiltrates that lead to epithelial breakdown and frank ulceration [4] [5]. A slit-lamp image of a true peripheral ulcerative keratitis (**Figure 3(a)**) showing limbal ulceration, conjunctival injection and pannus, is shown for comparison to our patient's corneal foreign body slit-lamp image (**Figure 1(a)**). Both anterior uveitis and PUK were unlikely because of no previous history of systemic or infectious disease.

This patient was ultimately referred to us for a peripheral corneal lesion resembling phlyctenulosis. Phlyctenulosis is typically caused by a delayed (type IV) hypersensitivity reaction to staphylococcal blepharitis or tuberculosis (TB) [6]. Patients often have a history of chronic blepharitis and/or recurrent chalazia or TB exposure [7]. Corneal phlyctenules appear as white nodules at the limbus with surrounding dilated conjunctival blood vessels. Severe forms may present more centrally with accompanied corneal neovascularization. **Figure 3(c)** shows an example of a patient with phlyctenulosis to exemplify the similarities between this presentation and our patient's corneal lesion. This patient had no history of blepharitis or risk factors for TB exposure, which makes phlyctenulosis a less likely cause of the corneal lesion in our patient.

4. Conclusion

In the end, the patient was found to have a corneal foreign body, likely acquired due to flying debris in the sandstorm. Corneal foreign body is consistent with this patient's history of foreign body sensation, redness and irritation, and the examination findings of a pigmented corneal lesion. It is also consistent with the patient demographics, as 47% of emergency eye consults in children involve injuries that increase the risk for foreign body [8]. The foreign body was removed and the patient has recovered nicely. This case provides an interesting differential diagnosis of similarly appearing peripheral corneal lesions in a pediatric patient.

References

[1] Wang, Z., Jiang, H., Kang, Y. and Chen, X. (1999) The Use of Ultrasound Biomicroscope in the Diagnosis of Anterior Segment Intraocular Foreign Bodies. *Yan Ke Xue Bao*, **15**, 236-237.

[2] Kaushik, S., Ichhpujani, P., Ramasubramanian, A. and Pandav, S.S. (2008) Occult Intraocular Foreign Body: Ultrasound Biomicroscopy Holds the Key. *International Ophthalmology*, **28**, 71-73. http://dx.doi.org/10.1007/s10792-007-9110-5

[3] American Academy of Ophthalmology (2011) Pediatric Ophthalmology and Strabismus. Basic and Clinical Science Course, Section 6. American Academy of Ophthalmology, 267-272.

[4] Leung, A.K., Mireskandari, K. and Ali, A. (2011) Peripheral Ulcerative Keratitis in a Child. *Journal of AAPOS*, **15**, 486-488. http://dx.doi.org/10.1016/j.jaapos.2011.06.009

[5] Krachmer, J.H., Mannis, M.J. and Holland, E.J. (2011) Cornea: Fundamentals, Diagnosis and Management. 3rd Edition, Elsevier Inc., New York, 1121-1122.

[6] Gerstenblith, A. and Rabinowitz, M. (2012) Cornea: Phlyctenulosis. The Wills Eye Manuel: Office and Emergency Room Diagnosis and Treatment of Eye Disease. 6th Edition, Lippincott, Williams and Wilkins, Philadelphia, 17-19, 89-90.

[7] Zaidman, G.W. (2011) The Pediatric Corneal Infiltrate. *Current Opinion in Ophthalmology*, **22**, 261-266. http://dx.doi.org/10.1097/ICU.0b013e3283479ffc

[8] Upshaw, J.E., Brenkert, T.E. and Losek, J.D. (2008) Ocular Foreign Bodies in Children. *Pediatric Emergency Care*, **24**, 409-414. http://dx.doi.org/10.1097/PEC.0b013e318177a806

Transmittance Spectrum of Unbranded Sunglasses Using Spectrophotometer

Huseyin Gursoy[1]*, Hikmet Basmak[1], Hamza Esen[2], Ferhan Esen[2]

[1]Eskisehir Osmangazi University Medical Faculty, Department of Ophthalmology, Eskisehir, Turkey
[2]Eskisehir Osmangazi University Medical Faculty, Department of Biophysics, Eskisehir, Turkey
Email: *hhgursoy@hotmail.com

Abstract

Background: The sunglass standards are not strictly implemented in many countries except Australia. The purpose of the study was to evaluate the optical properties of unbranded sunglasses for light transmittance. Methods: Unbranded sunglasses with no information about their specifications were included. They were allocated to two groups based on their prices; the ones > 25 US\$ (Group A) and the cheaper ones (Group B). Their transmittance spectrum was measured between 190 nm and 900 nm using a double beam scanning spectrophotometer. The European standard for sunglasses was used to evaluate their compliance regarding ultraviolet radiation (UVR) transmittance and minimum requirement for wearing when driving. Results: Thirty-eight sunglasses (Group A = 20 and Group B = 18) were evaluated. Four sunglasses in each group were non-compliant. Percentage transmittance of visible light was <8% in five sunglasses of Group A and in three of Group B, so these were not appropriate to wear when driving. Totally six sunglasses of Group A and five of Group B were non-compliant and/or inappropriate to wear when driving. Conclusions: Based on our findings about their UVR protection and visible light transmittance %, eye care professionals must warn people against the use of unbranded sunglasses without any information about their specifications.

Keywords

Sunglass, Spectrophotometer, Transmittance Spectrum, Ultraviolet Radiation, Visible Light

1. Introduction

Ultraviolet (UV) radiation (UVR) is defined as invisible light rays with a wavelength of less than approximately 400 nm. Three types of UVR based on their wavelengths: UV-A (315 to 400 nm), UV-B (280 to 315 nm), and

---

*Corresponding author.

UV-C (<280 nm) exist [1]. UV-C radiation does not penetrate the atmosphere's ozone layer, while some UV-A and UV-B reach the earth [2]. Both UV-A and UV-B may cause many dermatologic and ocular disorders [1] [3]-[6].

Although many people consider sunglasses as a symbol of style and trend, they are mainly produced to protect our eyes and the skin around the eyes from the harmful effects of the UVR. In our opinion the majority of people, including many eye care professionals are not aware of these regulations and just prefer the cheaper and more fashionable sunglasses. Over the counter sunglasses without any information about their specifications are being sold all over the world. Our aim was to evaluate the optical properties of unbranded sunglasses for light transmittance.

2. Material and Methods

The study was conducted at our University Medical Faculty, Department of Biophysics. Unbranded brown sunglasses that were purchased in optical shops or supermarkets in the city centre were included. Only the sunglasses with no information about their specifications were studied. They were allocated into two groups based on their prices; the ones over 25 US$ (Group A) and the cheaper ones less than 25 US$ (Group B).

Absorbance is the measure of the quantity of light that a sample neither transmits nor reflects, whereas the transmittance is the ratio of the intensity of the light that has passed through the sample to the intensity of the light when it entered it. The transmittance of a sample is given as a percentage. In the current study, the transmittance spectrum of the sunglasses was measured between 190 and 900 nm using a double beam scanning spectrophotometer (ATI Unicam, Cambridge and model UV2-100) with a 1.5 nm spectral bandwidth. The instrument measured the absorbance spectrum through the sunglasses (test sample) relative to air (reference sample). The measurements are sent to a computer interface for graphical analysis. Percentage transmittance was plotted on the y axis against the wavelength in nm on the x axis. The % of luminous transmittance (LT) at visible spectral range and the % of UV-A and UV-B transmittance were recorded.

The sunglasses were categorized according to their range of LT at visible spectral range based on the European standard for sunglasses [7]. Category 4 includes the sunglasses with <8% LT, Category 3 the ones with 8% - 18%, Category 2 the ones with 18% - 43%, Category 1 the ones with 43% - 80% and Category 0 with 80% - 100%. The European standard for sunglasses allows UV-B transmittance to reach 10% of all LT in all sunglasses categories [7]. UV-A transmittance has to be no more than the LT for the categories 0, 1 and 2, while it should not exceed 50% of all the LT for the categories 3 and 4 [7]. The sunglasses that did not meet the criteria for compliance with these standards were recorded.

Statistical analysis was performed using SPSS 15.0 (SPSS Inc., Chicago, IL, USA). The results of two groups were compared by the independent samples t-test or chi-square test. Significance was attributed when $p < 0.05$.

3. Results

Group A included twenty brown unbranded sun glasses with a price of >25 US$ and Group B eighteen brown unbranded sun glasses with a price of <25 US$.

The graph of the % transmittances of Group B in the wavelength range of 250 - 600 nm was shown in **Figure 1**.

The mean % of LT was 15.8 ± 8.3 and 16.6 ± 6.9 for Group A and B, respectively (range 3.1% - 32% in Group A vs. 4.5% - 31.2% in Group B) ($p = 0.2$). The categories of sunglasses based on their LT were shown in **Table 1**. Five sunglasses of Group A and three of Group B had LT of <8%, so fell in Category 4 ($p = 0.4$). These were not appropriate to wear when driving.

UV-B radiation was blocked appropriately according to the European standard in all sun glasses [7]. However, four sun glasses in each group was non-compliant with the European standard regarding the UV-A blockage ($p = 0.6$) [7]. The categories for each non-compliant sun glasses were shown in **Table 2**. Eleven out of thirty-eight sunglasses (29%); six sunglasses in Group A and five sunglasses in Group B were non-compliant with the European standard and/or lacking the necessary warning against wearing when driving ($p = 0.5$).

4. Discussion

In the current study including unbranded sunglasses, we found that four out of twenty sunglasses in Group A and

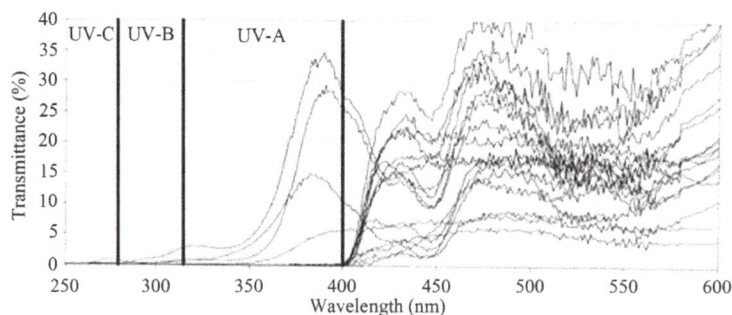

Figure 1. Transmittances of Group B in the wavelength range of 250 - 600 nm.

Table 1. The categories of sunglasses based on their luminous transmittance.

Category for the sun glasses	Group A (n = 20)	Group B (18)
4 (Luminous transmittance < 8%)	5	3
3 (Luminous transmittance 8% - 18%)	7	9
2 (Luminous transmittance 18% - 43%)	8	6

Table 2. The categories for each non-compliant sun glasses.

Category of the sun glasses	Group A (n = 20)	Group B (18)
4	0	1
3	3	1
2	1	2

four out of eighteen in group B were non-compliant with the European standard for sunglasses. In addition to this finding, % transmittance of visible light was less than 8% in five sunglasses in Group A and three in Group B. Regardless of their prices, 29% (11/38) of the sunglasses were not appropriate to protect the eyes from UVR hazards and/or were not appropriate to use when driving.

UV radiation is invariably damaging to eye tissues by the formation of free radicals [8]. Both UV-A and UV-B may cause skin disorders, skin cancers and many diverse ocular disorders including senile cataract, pterygium, photokeratitis, photoconjunctivitis, and ocular melanoma [1] [3]-[6]. Many epidemiologic studies showed that latitude and sunlight hours are positively correlated with the incidence of various ocular diseases such as pterygium, cataract, and ocular surface squamous neoplasia [6] [9] [10]. Each individual is exposed to a variable amount of UVR, which is dependent on many environmental factors such as latitude and altitude and personal behaviours such as the use of protective clothing and sunglasses. Out of these factors, the personal protection measures, including the use of brimmed hats and sunglasses were shown to be the most modifiable ones. They can effectuate up to an 18-fold difference in ocular UVR exposure [11].

There are three main standards for sunglasses in the world. These are the Australian, United Stated, and European standards [12]. Ideally sunglasses should absorb the entire UV spectrum including UV-A and UV-B [11]. Sunglasses are classified according to the LT based on the European standard for sunglasses. The ones with the LT % < 18 are classified in Category 3 and 4. These should satisfy the requirements for UVR transmittance to provide good protection from UVR. Category 2 provides some UVR protection, if meets the criteria, while the other 2 categories are fashion spectacles without providing adequate UVR protection. In the current study, none of the sunglasses were fashion spectacles based on their LT and all of them satisfied the requirements for the UV-B transmittance regardless of their prices. However, three Category 3 and one Category 2 sunglasses of Group A and one Category 4, one Category 3 and two Category 2 sunglasses of Group B were non-compliant with the European standard based on their UV-A transmittance %. Among UVR types, all of the UV-C and 90% of UV-B radiations are filtered by the ozone layer, so UV-A is the most prevalent one in nature [13]. Although, both UV-A and B have harmful effects on human eye and skin, UV-B radiation was shown to be more damaging on human lenses, cornea, conjunctiva and skin than UV-A radiation [1] [3]-[6] [14]. The link between age related macular degeneration and UVR is controversial [15] [16]. It is proposed that visible light, especially blue light, is one of the etiologic factors for the development of AMD [17]. According to our findings, some of the sunglasses did not meet the criteria for their categories regarding UV-A transmittance, so should be labelled as fashion spectacles.

Australia is the only country where the sunglass standards are directly enacted in law [18]. All sunglasses sold in Australia must be labelled indicating the % of UVR protection and 100% protection is considered a good level [12]. There is no mandatory testing in other countries. There are several studies in which the sunglasses are evaluated for their compliance with the standards [18]-[20]. In a study conducted by the "Optics and Radiometry Laboratory" 20% noncompliance was reported with the European standards [18]. Ultraviolet radiation protection was not satisfactory in another study performed in India [19]. On the other hand UVR protection was shown to be satisfactory in a study from Poland [20].

In the current study, % transmittance of visible light was also evaluated. Some of the sunglasses were shown to transmit less than 8% of the visible light regardless of their prices. This had to be indicated, because the minimum visible light transmittance requirement for driving is 8% according to the sunglass standards [7]. Besides the UVR protection the sunglasses should meet other requirements to be certified. These additional requirements are related to the refractive power, prismatic power, and polarization [12] [18]. These properties enable higher visual acuity while providing UVR protection. We did not evaluate these properties, but some noncompliance with the regulations regarding the transmittance spectrum was detected.

Based on our findings, regardless of their prices, some of the unbranded sunglasses were non-compliant with the European standard for sunglasses and some of them were not appropriate to wear when driving. Therefore, optometrists and ophthalmologists should warn the consumers against wearing unbranded sunglasses without any specifications, to provide protection from UVR and also when driving.

According to our findings some of the sunglasses did not meet the criteria for their categories regarding UV-A transmittance, so should be labelled as fashion spectacles. Also the visible light transmittance was less than 8%. This had to be indicated, because the minimum visible light transmittance requirement for driving is 8% according to the sunglass standards. Two things can be done to solve the problem: enact laws like in Australia, or publicize the findings and enhance customer knowledge about the need to have details specifications about UV and visible light transmission and customers should not wear except glasses with certificates that meet the safety standards.

References

[1]   Weinstock, M.A. (1995) Overview of Ultraviolet Radiation and Cancer: What Is the Link? How Are We Doing? *Environmental Health Perspectives*, **103**, 251-54. http://dx.doi.org/10.1289/ehp.95103s8251

[2]   Fioletov, V., Kerr, J.B. and Fergusson, A. (2010) The UV Index: Definition, Distribution and Factors Affecting It. *Canadian Journal of Public Health*, **101**, 15-19.

[3]   Boettner, E.A. and Wolter, J.R. (1962) Transmission of the Ocular Media. *Investigative Ophthalmology & Visual Science*, **1**, 776-83.

[4]   Ambach, W., Blumthaler, M., Schopf, T., Ambach, E., Katzgraber, F., Daxecker, F., *et al.* (1994) Spectral Transmission of the Optical Media of the Human Eye with Respect to Keratitis and Cataract Formation. *Documenta Ophthalmologica*, **88**, 165-73. http://dx.doi.org/10.1007/BF01204614

[5]   Gallagher, R.P. and Lee, T.K. (2006) Adverse Effects of Ultraviolet Radiation: A Brief Review. *Progress in Biophysics and Molecular Biology*, **92**, 119-31. http://dx.doi.org/10.1016/j.pbiomolbio.2006.02.011

[6]   Moran, D.J. and Hollows, F.C. (1984) Pterygium and Ultraviolet Radiation: A Positive Correlation. *British Journal of Ophthalmology*, **68**, 343-346. http://dx.doi.org/10.1136/bjo.68.5.343

[7]   European Standards Organisation (CEN) 2005 EN 1836 Personal Eye Protection: Sunglasses and Sunglare Filters for General Use and Filters for Direct Observation of the Sun: EN 1836:2005. CEN, Brussels.

[8]   Kulms, D. and Schwarz, T. (2002) Molecular Mechanisms Involved in UV-Induced Apoptotic Cell Death. *Skin Pharmacology and Physiology*, **15**, 342-47. http://dx.doi.org/10.1159/000064539

[9]   Schein, O.D., West, S., Munoz, B., *et al.* (1994) Cortical Lenticular Opacification: Distribution and Location in a Longitudinal Study. *Investigative Ophthalmology & Visual Science*, **35**, 363-66.

[10]   Newton, R. (1996) A Review of the Aetiology of Squamous Cell Carcinoma of the Conjunctiva. *British Journal of Cancer*, **74**, 1511-513. http://dx.doi.org/10.1038/bjc.1996.581

[11] Rosenthal, F.S., West, S.K., Munoz, B., Emmett, E.A., Strickland, P.T. and Taylor, H.R. (1991) Ocular and Facial Skin Exposure to Ultraviolet Radiation in Sunlight: A Personal Exposure Model with Application to a Worker Population. *Health Physics*, **61**, 77-86. http://dx.doi.org/10.1097/00004032-199107000-00008

[12] Dain, S.J. (2003) Sunglasses and Sunglass Standards. *Clinical and Experimental Optometry*, **86**, 77-90. http://dx.doi.org/10.1111/j.1444-0938.2003.tb03066.x

[13] WMO (1995) Scientific Assessment of Ozone Depletion: 1994. World Meteorlogical Organization, Global Ozone Research and Monitoring Project, Report No. 37, Geneva.

[14] Kessel, L., Eskildsen, L., Lundeman, J.H., Jensen, O.B. and Larsen, M. (2011) Optical Effects of Exposing Intact Human Lenses to Ultraviolet Radiation and Visible Light. *BMC Ophthalmology*, **11**, 41. http://dx.doi.org/10.1186/1471-2415-11-41

[15] Darzins, P., Mitchell, P. and Heller, R.F. (1997) Sun Exposure and Age-Related Macular Degeneration. An Australian Case-Control Study. *Ophthalmology*, **104**, 770-776. http://dx.doi.org/10.1016/S0161-6420(97)30235-8

[16] Cruickshanks, K.J., Klein, R. and Klein, B.E. (1993) Sunlight and Age-Related Macular Degeneration. The Beaver Dam Eye Study. *Archives of Ophthalmology*, **111**, 514-518. http://dx.doi.org/10.1001/archopht.1993.01090040106042

[17] Taylor, H.R., Munoz, B., West, S., Bressler, N.M., Bressler, S.B. and Rosenthal, F.S. (1990) Visible Light and Risk of Age-Related Macular Degeneration. *Transactions of the American Ophthalmological Society*, **88**, 163-173.

[18] Dain, S.J., Ngo, T.P., Cheng, B.B., Hu, A., Teh, A.G.B., Tseng, J. and Vu, N. (2010) Sunglasses, the European Directive and the European Standard. *Ophthalmic and Physiological Optics*, **30**, 253-256. http://dx.doi.org/10.1111/j.1475-1313.2010.00711.x

[19] Dongre, A.M., Pai, G.G. and Khopkar, U.S. (2007) Ultraviolet Protective Properties of Branded and Unbranded Sunglasses Available in the Indian Market in UV Phototherapy Chambers. *Indian Journal of Dermatology, Venereology and Leprology*, **73**, 26-28. http://dx.doi.org/10.4103/0378-6323.30647

[20] Cader, A. and Jankowski, J. (1996) Evaluation of Protective Properties of Sunglasses Commonly Available in the Marketplace. *Medycyna Pracy*, **47**, 365-371.

3

Functional PET Scan in Four Patients with Higher Order Neglect-Like Cognitive Dysfunction Associated to Chiasm Related Pathology

Hans Callø Fledelius[1*], Kirsten Korsholm[2], Ian Law[2]

[1]Copenhagen University Eye Clinics, Rigshospitalet and Glostrup Hospital, Capital Region, Denmark
[2]Department of Clinical Physiology, Nuclear Medicine and PET, Rigshospitalet, Capital Region, Denmark
Email: [*]hcfled@mail.dk

Abstract

Cognitive disturbances with neglect-like features have been reported occasionally in patients with chiasmal disorders, so far however with no obvious substrate by conventional brain imaging. Thus, there were no right hemisphere lesions that could explain the lateralised visual inattention as observed in particular during monocular visual acuity testing. On this background, we further examined four adult patients who consented to functional ^{18}F-fluoro-deoxyglucose (FDG) positron emission tomography (PET) scan. In three there were no significant findings. The fourth patient, a 26-year-old male with cognitive defects after surgery for craniopharyngioma, will be discussed in more detail. His PET scan demonstrated a widespread reduction of regional metabolic activity in left hemisphere primary visual cortex and higher order visual areas, despite absence of explanatory pathological signal changes on MRI. As present in only one out of four patients, however, the findings do not allow specific pathogenetic mechanisms to be suggested, nor generally to substantiate involvement of higher cerebral circuits. Obviously, even developed imaging has its limits, and in the very theory the visual dysfunctions observed might still depend on higher brain centres' faulty adaptation to loss of pre-geniculate visual information.

Keywords

Chiasmal Lesions, Visual Field Defects, Neglect-Like Behaviour, Cognitive Disturbances, Functional PET Scan (FDG) of Brain

---

[*]Corresponding author.

1. Introduction

Reading can be disturbed out of proportion to visual acuity findings in patients with lesions of the chiasm, and some patients cannot mobilize the search saccades as usually triggered during monocular visual acuity testing. Accordingly they show neglect-like visual inattention to the temporal part of the visual chart [1]-[4]. Various neuro-psychological tests have confirmed the occurrence of cognitive disturbances [5], but patho-physiologic mechanisms are not clear. MRI scan had given no clue in such cases, and after written and oral information and patients' consent ^{18}F-fluoro-deoxyglucose (FDG) PET scanning of the brain was performed, in a search for deviating metabolic patterns. Four adult patients were studied, however with significant deviation from normal in only one, a young male aged 26 who suffered from sequels after surgery for an extensive craniopharyngioma.

To stress the clinical similarities, all four case stories are given below, though with more detail regarding the young male patient who has shown positive findings on the functional PET scan (Case No. 4).

In respect of the tenets of the Helsinki Declaration, all had given informed consent to the study.

2. Case Reports

2.1. Case 1

A 53-year-old female laboratory technician with well controlled diabetes type 2 had visual disturbances of the left eye over 2 months, when first seen. Best corrected visual acuities (BCVA) were 1.0 and 0.4, and the left eye further had dyschromatopsia (Ishiharas plates). Initial tangent screen examinations (white 5/1000) indicated normal visual fields, but Octopus static perimetry subsequently suggested relative bitemporal loss of sensitivity, and CT scan demonstrated a $3 \times 3 \times 3.5$ cm suprasellar tumour. Visual complaints worsened after extirpation of a pituitary adenoma, visual acuities fell to 0.8 and 0.16, and both eyes showed neglect-like temporal blocking on the visual chart when tested monocularly. She further presented temporal hemianopia for all isoptres, and the absolute losses of the left eye even crossed the mid-vertical. Binocular reading was hampered due to "loosing words", and cognition in space presented misinterpretations. Optic disc atrophy developed.

By neuro-psychological testing her left eye showed substantial losses by Gothenburg test, BIT star test, and chimeric faces. The right eye only had slight losses, but cofunction was poor when binocular.

Only slight improvement over 11 years follow-up. A functional FDG PET scan was added in 2012, however without indicative findings.

She is on a pension.

2.2. Case 2

A 39-year-old locksmith with headache and visual loss over a month, BCVA at admission 0.1 and 1.0. Tangent screen showed inferior temporal defect of right eye, left eye normal. His orientation and navigation in space became severely impaired after extirpation of a $2.5 \times 2.5 \times 2.5$ cm pituitary tumour, despite a maintained BCVA of the left eye of 1.0. Visual testing, however, demanded extra time, and the right eye had not improved. Massive bitemporal visual field losses were demonstrated, to midline of the better eye and above midline for the right eye. Both optic discs were pale, and a 6 pd horisontal diplopia could not be relieved by prisms. By monocular visual acuity testing the right eye kept the pattern of catching only the nasal column on the chart, whereas eventually the left eye could compensate for the initial neglect-like temporal ignorance and, letter by letter, deliver the full line. Reading a text has remained slow and fragmented.

At most neuropsychological tests, his right eye could not cope with the demands. The Gothenburg test, BIT star test, chimeric faces and line division were passed close to normal for the left eye, provided he was allowed to choose a skew gaze direction.

Only slight functional improvement over 10 years follow up, when he had functional FDG PET scan performed, in 2013, without explanatory findings.

He is on a pension.

2.3. Case 3

A 42-year-old female office clerk was referred for bilateral loss of visual acuity and field. At admission right eye BCVA was 0.25 and left eye 0.7. Colour sense was normal, but reading a text was slow. Surgery for craniopharyngioma appeared uneventful, but four days later malaise and loss of vision occurred. Monocular testing of vision was not feasible, and binocularly she could hardly catch the visual chart at a distance of 1 meter. The right eye however soon improved, to 0.9 BCVA, though with full ignorance of the temporally located test symbols on the chart. The left eye had dropped to visual acuity 0.03, but conceived only on and off, nasally on the chart. A massive bitemporal hemianopia tended to incorporate the vertical midline in the defect. Poor reading ability (easier vertically!) and spatial disorientation were also noted. Optic discs pale, partly atrophic.

Neuropsychological testing: Only moderate drop out by all tests, provided lots of time allowed; reading slow with loss of words. In the binocular situation trouble regarding eye-hand coordination.

Still severely incapacitated in everyday functions, over 10 years, and no explanatory findings at the FDG PET scan performed in 2012.

She is on a pension.

2.4. Case 4

A 26-year-old otherwise healthy male IT technician had a large parasellar tumour diagnosed on MRI scan of the brain. The exam was prompted by general loss of concentration, headache, and fainting episodes over 2 - 3 weeks, and ophthalmic evaluation was not carried out prior to the first neurosurgical approach, in December 2009. This had the character of an emergency decompression, a large cystic craniopharyngioma being partially removed transnasally. Immediately after surgery he had best corrected visual acuities of 0.6 right eye and 0.4 left eye, and bitemporal hemianopia was recorded.

Transcranial extirpation of residual tumour was performed one year later, based mainly on poor capacity in his job and a considerable weight gain. A 9 mm suprasellar cyst formation on MRI led to stereotactic radiotherapy (July 2012).

Reading a text had become increasingly difficult, sometimes also cognition in space, and he is currently followed in the University Clinic for Brain Damage. He is under hormone substitution for pituitary insufficiency and has had a single episode with convulsions.

His post-radiation ophthalmic state has been stable. Each eye can yield a slow 0.4 decimal visual acuity, however with an obvious nasal preference on the chart, manifesting as visual ignorance and "blocking" of the search saccades to the temporal side. Using both eyes, he can compensate for the lateral attention deficit and also read a medium size text (N8), though slowly and without natural rhythm. There is a left eye relative afferent pupil defect.

Both eyes had complete loss of colour sense, whereas contrast sensitivity was reduced only slightly (Pelli-Robson). Kinetic Goldmann and static Octopus perimetry both indicated bitemporal hemianopia (**Figure 1**). Pursuit eye movements appeared normal and alternate cover test indicated a slight exophoria. A hemifield slide disturbance could not be demonstrated by Schober's test (red-green dissociation), where the left eye image was ignored or suppressed most of the time. Except slight pallor of both optic discs fundus examination was normal, and MRI scan in 2013 has given no indication of tumour recurrence.

The *FDG PET scan* was performed in 2013. In addition to visual analysis, a quantitative 3-dimensional stereotactic surface projection analysis (Scenium (v 3.0), Siemens) was employed that allowed direct visualization of the extent and the topography of FDG uptake abnormalities. In addition, the PET images were co-registered to T1 and T2 weighted cerebral MRI scanning performed 7 months before, for identification of structural pathology and identification of anatomical structures. Significant metabolic reduction compared to a database of healthy subjects were found in the orbitofrontal cortex corresponding to treatment related damage after surgery, but also in multiple left posterior cortical areas known from extensive clinical studies and brain mapping experiments to subserve functions in the computation of visual input [6] [7]: the medial occipital region in the posterior part of the calcarine fissure, the inferior parietal lobe, and the inferior temporal lobe, starting from the occipito-temporal junction and extending into the temporal pole (**Figure 2** and **Figure 3**). Corresponding to these areas MRI had shown no explanatory pathological signal changes.

3. Discussion

As for the clinical features, emphasis is on the neglect-like attentional deficits as evident in all four patients when testing the visual acuity for each eye. Clinically, they all belong to the heavy tail of the chiasmal spectrum, here factually to include cognitive dysfunction. The patient thus knows there is a full line of optotypes, but

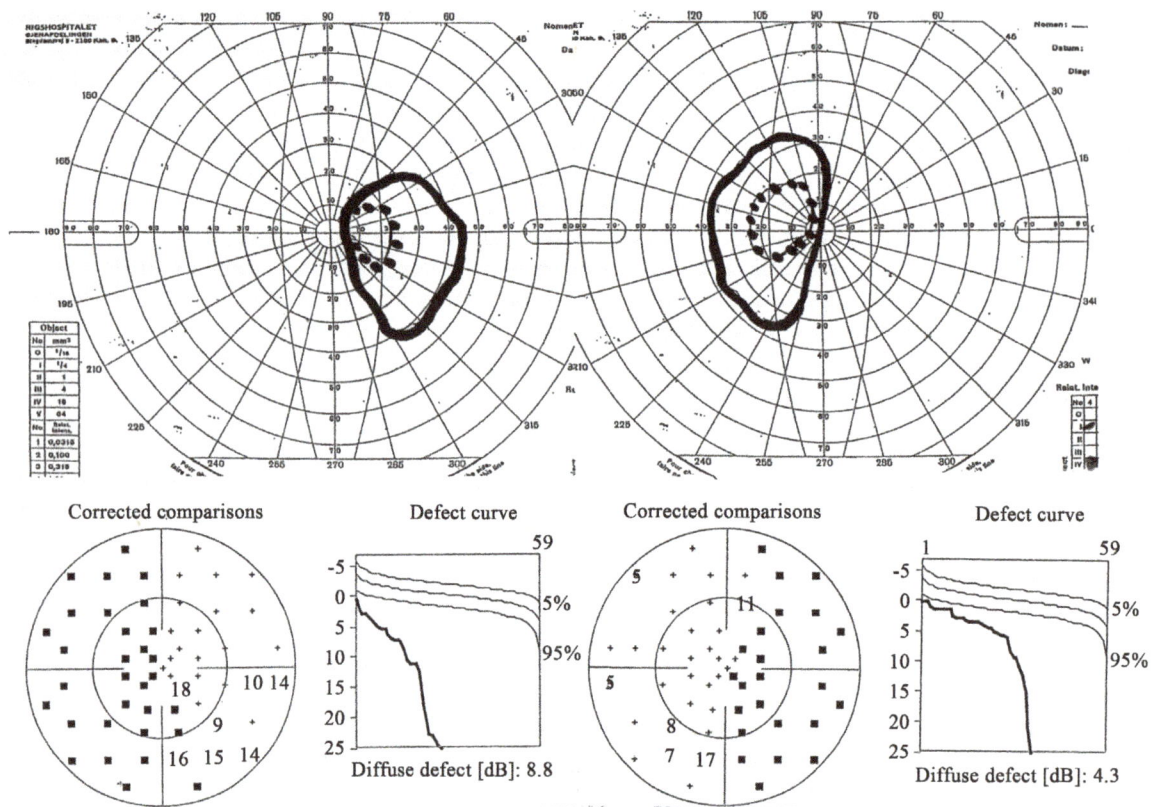

Figure 1. On top, kinetic Goldmann perimetry, white objects IV, 4 and I, 4, showing the borders of preserved nasal fields, apparently leaving a vertical midline bar of non-attention. Bottom: static octopus G standard programme, central 30° field, black squares indicating bitemporal absolute scotoma test points; cumulated decibel loss of sensitivity is further demonstrated.

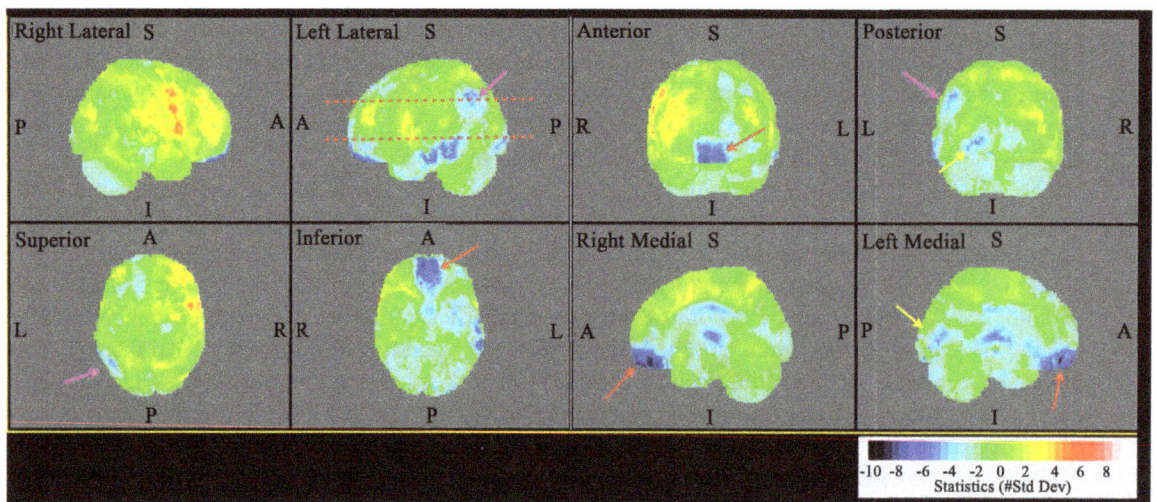

Figure 2. Statistical surface projection comparing the patient's regional metabolic activity to a database of healthy age matched subjects showing right and left lateral, and anterior and posterior projections (top), and superior, inferior, and right and left medial projections (bottom). There are significant reductions in the orbitofrontal cortex (red arrow) corresponding to the neurosurgical route of entrance, and to remote locations in left hemisphere visual areas, such as the primary visual cortex (yellow arrow), inferior parietal lobe (pink arrow), and inferior temporal lobe. The scale refers to standard deviations. A Z-score of <3 is considered significant. The two dotted lines denote approximate levels of the slices in **Figure 3**.

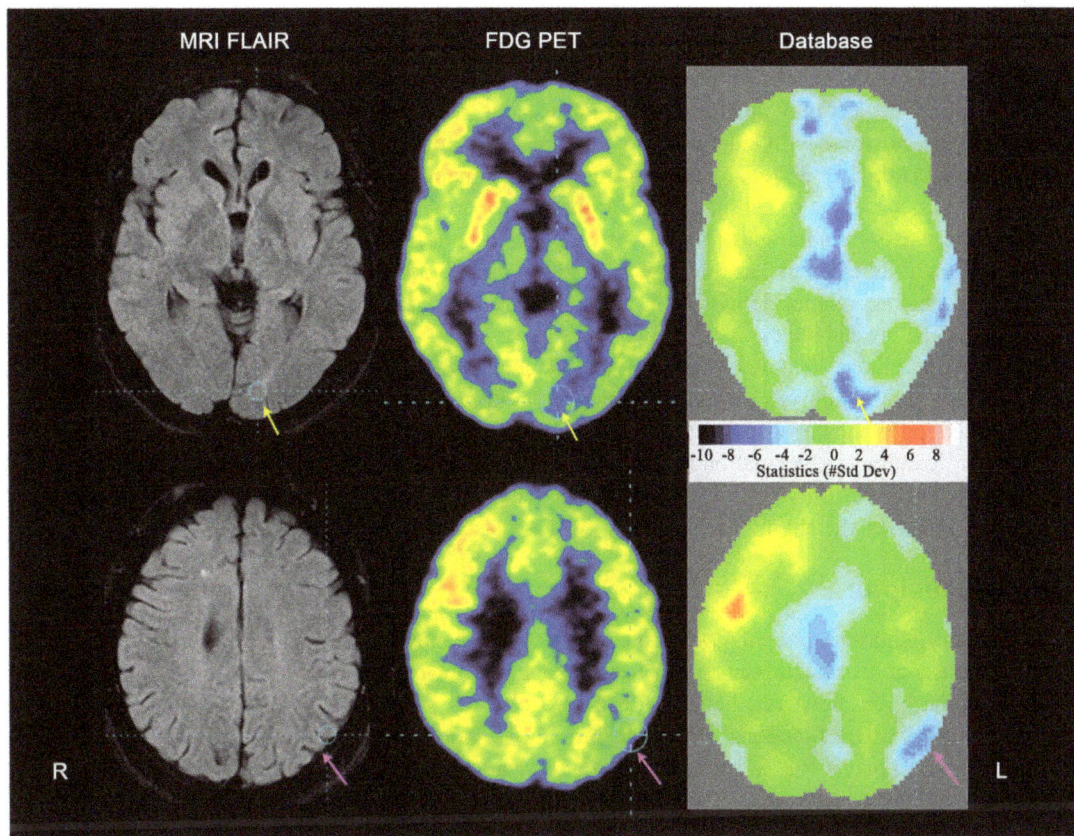

Figure 3. Two trans-axial brain imaging slices corresponding to the levels denoted in **Figure 2** showing MRI FLAIR, FDG PET, and a statistical comparison of FDG PET to a database of healthy subjects. Significant metabolic reductions are seen in left hemisphere in the primary visual area close to the calcarine fissure (yellow arrow), and in the inferior parietal lobe (pink arrow). There is an impression of diffusely reduced metabolism in the whole left hemisphere, which increases the right pre-frontal cortex relatively. A Z-score of <3 (p < 0.001) is considered significant.

appears functionally blocked to what is located on the temporal side of the chart and reads only what is nasal [1] [3] [4]. Obviously, the usual search saccades cannot be triggered. The patients further presented loss of former abilities also when binocular, for instance when confronted with a simple text, in print or on screen [5].

The left eye Goldmann perimetry isoptres shown in **Figure 1** illustrate an apparent paradox, as evident also in the worse eye of the other patients under study: fixation is maintained and centred in the bottom of the Goldmann globe despite the apparent position of the fixation mark in the recorded scotoma zone. Goldmann recordings might further suggest a blind central bar along the mid-vertical in binocular visual space, but this is refuted by hand movements (testing by bimanual confrontation) and likewise by targeted small object (white 5/1000) binocular tangent screen examination. This seems in accord with many chiasmal patients' lack of noticing visual field trouble, in part obviously by virtue of the two mainly undisturbed nasal half-fields. An element of neglect may further contribute to ignorance, and the apparent absence of complaints may explain clinicians' occasional omission of early visual field testing. However, the striking performance at customary unilateral visual acuity testing should alert the medical staff and trigger the essential evaluation of the visual field. The specific neglect-like behaviour of nasal reading/temporal blocking is only sporadically emphasised in textbooks [1] [2]. In earlier clinical series we gave lengthy consideration to the clinical variety. It may range from solid evidence to discreet hints only, it can be uni- or bilateral, and complaints may be minimal [3]-[5].

The distribution of relative regional cerebral glucose metabolic rate (rCMRglc) is recognized as an indirect imaging biomarker of neural activity, as assessed here by FDG PET scanning [6] [7]) The expectations were that the PET scanning of the brain might suggest compensatory functional pathways in the brain of relevance for the deviant visual behaviour under study, possibly to indicate dysfunction of higher order visual areas. For instance, this could be through a coupled functional deactivation or disconnection syndrome known as diaschisis, either by the loss of afferent neural input via connecting white matter tracts from the primary cortex (V1), or through the lateral geniculate body [8]-[10]. Diaschisis is a frequent clinical functional neuroimaging finding in other contexts, e.g. crossed cerebellar diaschisis in patients with frontal lobe damage.

Attentional neglect may include disordered saccades. Most often it is associated to lesions in the right inferior parietal lobe, however with a definite role also for the frontal lobe, as based on frontoparietal and other network associations [11]-[16]. Splenial interhemispheric disconnection has further been reported, with the authors' suggestion that deprivation of sensory inputs to intact parietal and frontal areas can also yield spatial neglect limited to specific sensory modalities or sectors of space [17]. Imaging in our feature case (patient No. 4) presented extensive frontal lobe defects, as direct sequels to the open brain surgery performed. Possibly this was a co-factor underlying his attentional deficits [18], but similar lesions of a frontal location were not disclosed in the other patients of the present series.

Comparing clinical features in general, another item should be mentioned: Typical neglect is on a proven lesional basis, with emphasis on macroscopic gray and white matter pathology, usually in the right hemisphere and presenting binocular visuo-spatial neglect in the left hemifield. In contrast, the characteristic single eye neglect-like features in chiasmal patients may lateralise to either side, and damage to the optic pathways usually appears the main or only lesion to brain tissue. Thus there is no obvious structural link to the pathology that typically underlies the attentional deficits known as classical visual neglect.

4. Conclusions

In summary, chiasmal patients' occasional neglect-like behaviour at single eye vision testing, sometimes combined with cognitive disturbances, has been recognized for decades. Neuro-psychological evaluations and MRI scans of the brain, however, have not disclosed obvious pathophysiological mechanisms. This motivated the present study, where functional PET scan presented evidence of suprageniculate functional deficits in cortical areas known to play a role in primary visual and visuo-spatial analysis, though only in one of the four chiasmal patients actually under study. Accordingly, more specific generalisations are not allowed regarding abnormal brain processing as possibly associated to pre-geniculate visual pathway disorders. In the theory, however, such pathology might have curtailed information to suprageniculate networks usually considered of importance for cognition in free space [12]-[16].

Our second aim with the presentation was to direct the attention of ophthalmic colleagues when confronted with reading trouble out of proportion to visual acuity findings in young patients—and/or the striking monocular lateralising behaviour on a visual chart—as potential early markers of chiasmal pathology.

References

[1]   Glaser, J.S. (1990) Neuro-Ophthalmology. 2nd Edition, Lippincott, Philadelphia, 12, 172.

[2]   Miller, N.R. and Newman, N.J. (1999) Topical Diagnosis of Chiasmal and Retrochiasmal Lesions. In: Walsh, F.B. and Hoyt, W.F., Eds., *Clinical Neurophthalmology*, 5th Edition, Lippincott, Philadelphia, 326-335.

[3]   Fledelius, H.C. (2004) Chiasmal Pathology Causing Inability to Access Information in the Temporal Visual Field. *Neuro-Ophthalmology*, **28**, 77-85. http://dx.doi.org/10.1076/noph.28.2.77.23740

[4]   Fledelius, H.C. (2009) Temporal Visual Field Defects Are Associated with Monocular Inattention in Chiasmal Pathology. *Acta Ophthalmologica*, **87**, 769-775. http://dx.doi.org/10.1111/j.1755-3768.2008.01328.x

[5]   Fledelius, H.C. (2014) Neuropsychological Testing in Chiasmal Patients Exhibiting Inattention in the Temporal Visual Space during Monocular Testing. *Neuro-Ophthalmology*, Accepted for Publication.

[6]   Gerlach, G., Law, I.A., Gade, A. and Paulson, O.B. (1999) Perceptual Differentiation and Category Effects in Normal Object Recognition: A PET Study. *Brain*, **122**, 2159-2170. http://dx.doi.org/10.1093/brain/122.11.2159

[7]   Nobre, A.C., Sebestyen, G.N., Gitelman, D.R., Mesulam, M.M., Frankowiak, R.S. and Frith, C.D. (1997) Functional Localisation of the System for Visuospatial Attention Using Positron Emission Tomography. *Brain*, **120**, 515-533. http://dx.doi.org/10.1093/brain/120.3.515

[8]   Von Monakow, C. (1914) Die Lokalisation in Grosshirn unter dem Abbau der Funktion durch kortikale Herde. JF Bergmann, Wiesbaden.

[9]   Finger, S., Koehler, J. and Jagella, C. (2004) The Monakow Concept of Diaschisis. Origin and Perspectives. *Archives of Neurology*, **61**, 283-288. http://dx.doi.org/10.1001/archneur.61.2.283

[10]   Baron, J.C., Bousser, M.G., Comar, D., Sousaline, F. and Castaigne, P. (1981) Non-Invasive Tomographic Study of

Cerebral Bloodflow and Oxygen Metabolism *in Vivo*. Potentials, Limitations, and Clinical Applications in Cerebral Ischemic Disorders. *European Neurology*, **20**, 273-284. http://dx.doi.org/10.1159/000115247

[11] Ringman, J.M., Saver, J.L., Woolson, R.E., Clarke, S.W.R. and Adams, H.P. (2004) Frequency, Risk Factors, Anatomy, and Course of Unilateral Neglect in an Acute Stroke Cohort. *Neurology*, **63**, 468-474. http://dx.doi.org/10.1212/01.WNL.0000133011.10689.CE

[12] Swan, L. (2001) Unilateral Spatial Neglect. *Physical Therapy*, **81**, 1572-1580.

[13] Bartolomeo, P., Thiebaut de Schotten, M. and Chica, A.B. (2012) Brain Networks of Visuospatial Attention and Their Disruption in Visual Neglect. *Frontiers in Human Neuroscience*, **6**, Article 110. http://dx.doi.org/10.3389/fnhum.2012.00110

[14] Ptak, R. and Fellrath, J. (2013) Spatial Neglect and the Neural Coding of Attentional Priority. *Neuroscience and Biobehavioral Reviews*, **37**, 705-722. http://dx.doi.org/10.1016/j.neubiorev.2013.01.026

[15] Balslev, D., Odoj, B. and Karnath, H.O. (2013) Role of Somatosensory Cortex in Visuospatial Attention. *Journal of Neuroscience*, **33**, 1311-1318. http://dx.doi.org/10.1523/JNEUROSCI.1112-13.2013

[16] Mesulam, M.M. (1981) A Cortical Network for Directed Attention and Unilateral Neglect. *Annals of Neurology*, **10**, 309-325. http://dx.doi.org/10.1002/ana.410100402

[17] Tomaiulolo, F., Voci, L., Bresci, M., Cozza, A., Posterano, F., *et al.* (2010) Selective Visual Neglect in Right Brain Damaged Patients with Splenial Interhemispheric Disconnection. *Experimental Brain Research*, **206**, 209-217. http://dx.doi.org/10.1007/s00221-010-2230-6

[18] Stone, J., Renolds, M.R. and Leuthardt, E.C. (2011) Transient Hemispatial Neglect after Surgical Resection of a Right Frontal Lobe Mass. *World Neurosurgery*, **76**, 361. http://dx.doi.org/10.1016/j.wneu.2010.03.018

4

The Emerging Role of Statins in Glaucoma Pathological Mechanisms and Therapeutics

O. Pokrovskaya[1], D. Wallace[1,2], C. O'Brien[1,2]

[1]School of Medicine and Medical Science, University College Dublin, Dublin, Ireland
[2]Department of Ophthalmology, Mater Misericordiae University Hospital, Dublin, Ireland
Email: olya.pokrovskaya@gmail.com

Abstract

Statins inhibit the enzyme 3-hydroxy-3-methylglutaryl-coenzyme A (HMG-CoA) reductase, and hence have a profound effect in lowering serum cholesterol. Their predominant clinical use to date is in primary and secondary prevention of cardiovascular disease. However recently interest has developed regarding the so-called "pleiotropic" effects of statins—these drugs have significant anti-fibrotic, anti-inflammatory, and immunomodulatory properties. Such effects of statins have already been shown to be beneficial in modulating the pathological mechanisms involved in pulmonary fibrosis, renal disease, non-ischaemic cardiac failure, and tissue scarring. Many of these actions are mediated by inhibition of the Rho kinase pathway. Epidemiological studies suggest that patients who take statins have a lower risk of developing glaucoma, and lower rates of glaucoma progression. Here, we review what is known about the pleiotropic effect of statins to date, and examine how these effects may modulate the molecular mechanisms involved in glaucoma pathogenesis.

Keywords

Statin, Glaucoma, Rho Kinase, Optic Nerve, Trabecular Meshwork

1. Introduction

Recent population-based studies suggest that the use of 3-hydroxy-3-methylglutaryl-coenzyme A (HMG-CoA) reductase inhibitors (commonly known as statins) may reduce the risk of glaucoma development and progression [1] [2]. Statins are already established as a first-line treatment in cardiovascular disease due to their cholesterol lowering effect. However, statins also possess important pleiotropic immunomodulatory and anti-inflammatory capabilities, which have resulted in an expansion of their indications for usage [3]. They appear to have a neuroprotective effect in several diseases of the central nervous system including Alzheimer's disease, and ischaemic stroke [3]. They also have an antifibrotic action—as seen in models of pulmonary and renal fibrosis [4]-[6]. The mechanism of action of statins in these disease processes is still the subject of much debate. Numerous molecular pathways seem to be involved, including the Rho-kinase pathway and modulation of the actin cytoskeleton [7]-[9]. We hypothesise that statins may also be protective in glaucoma. Glaucoma is a progressive optic neuropathy, with a known fibrotic and neurodegenerative component [10]. The purpose of this article is to review the emerging role of statins in primary open angle glaucoma (POAG). In order to understand the potential mechanisms of action of statins in glaucoma, it is beneficial to first review the aetiology of the disease process and current treatment options.

2. POAG

Glaucoma is the second leading cause of irreversible, but potentially preventable vision loss worldwide, affecting an estimated 60.5 million people [11]-[13]. It refers to a spectrum of clinical conditions distinguished by a progressive optic neuropathy and associated visual field loss, with raised intraocular pressure (IOP) being one of the primary risk factors [14] [15]. Two principal theories have been described for the pathophysiological mechanism for primary open angle glaucoma (POAG), but these are not mutually exclusive. The vascular theory proposes that optic neuropathy results from a compromise to the microvasculature resulting in ischaemic damage to the optic nerve head. This may be as a consequence of the raised IOP or other factors which influence ocular blood flow [16]. The mechanical theory suggests that raised IOP alters the architecture of the lamina cribrosa (LC), compromising the retinal ganglion cell (RGC) axons as they pass through this structure. The LC is a specialised series of plates of connective tissue which acts as a support for axons as they traverse the corneoscleral shell.

   The normal intraocular pressure (range 11 - 21 mmHg) is dependent upon a delicate balance of aqueous humour production, inflow and outflow [17]. Aqueous humour is produced by the ciliary body, and provides nourishment to the avascular cornea and lens (**Figure 1**). The main drainage pathway for the aqueous from the anterior chamber is the pressure-dependent conventional outflow pathway—through the trabecular meshwork (TM).

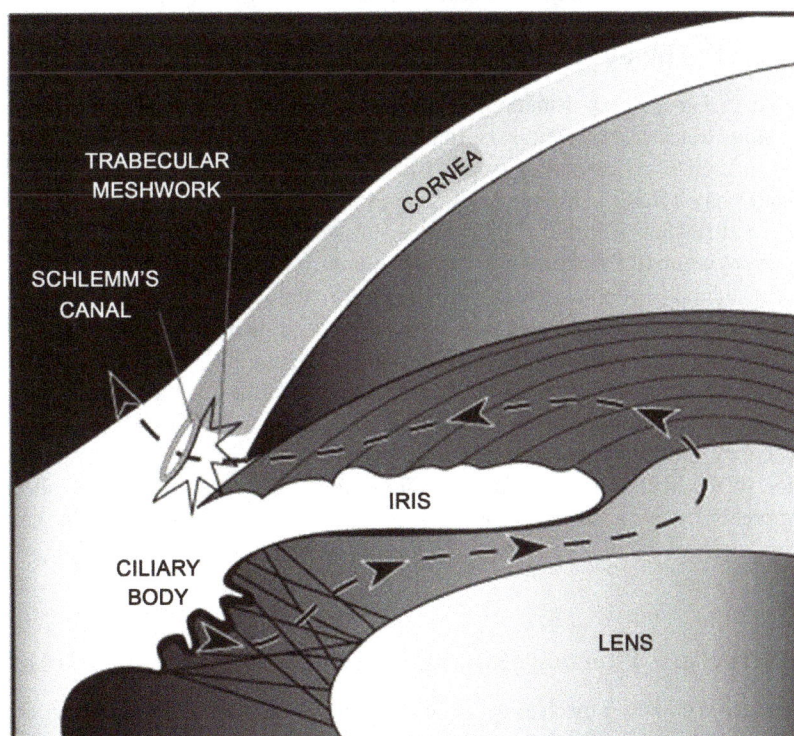

Figure 1. The aqueous outflow pathway (Goel, M., *et al.*, *Aqueous humor dynamics: a review.* Open Ophthalmol J, 2010, **4**, pp. 52-59).

This normally accounts for up to 90% of aqueous outflow. A framework of lattice-like collagen beams forms the TM, with extracellular matrix (ECM) residing in the paracellular spaces between the beams [18]. Aqueous humour drains through the TM, then the juxtacanalicular connective tissue (JCT) region, and then into Schlemm's canal (SC), from where it is returned to the systemic circulation via the episcleral veins. In order to enter SC, aqueous must diffuse through the paracellular spaces between the endothelial cells of SC, or through giant vacuoles which form as outpouchings into SC. The unconventional, or uveoscleral outflow pathway normally accounts for the remaining ~10% of aqueous outflow. However, with increasing age, up to 50% of aqueous outflow can occur by the uveoscleral pathway [18].

Extracellular matrix remodelling is at the heart of glaucomatous pathophysiology, and has been shown to be a feature of glaucomatous damage both at the TM where it impairs aqueous drainage, and at the optic nerve head—particularly the LC [19] [20]. Importantly in the LC, remodelling affects its biomechanical properties—leading to increased tissue stiffness, fibrosis, and posterior bowing of this structure [14] [16] [21] [22]. The resultant mechanical compression of the RGC in this area induces axoplasmic stasis contributing to cell death [10] [23]. Two important types of cell that populate the LC include astrocytes (glial fibrillary acidic protein (GFAP) positive) and LC cells (GFAP negative) [24]. Results of previous research in our laboratory support the profibrotic nature of LC cells when exposed to glaucomatous stimuli, suggesting they play an integral role in glaucomatous ECM remodelling [25]-[27].

Present day glaucoma therapies aim only to reduce the IOP—the only modifiable risk factor for glaucoma progression. Most agents aim to reduce aqueous production (beta-blockers, carbonic anhydrase inhibitors, alpha-agonists), and some increase outflow via the uveoscleral pathway (prostaglandin analogues). However glaucoma may progress despite apparently normal IOP, suggesting the need for novel treatments that may modulate the inflammatory and fibrotic aspects of glaucoma pathophysiology. Our own research group has investigated the role of anti-connective tissue growth factor (CTGF) as a potential anti-fibrotic agent in glaucoma. We have shown that anti-CTGF is effective in blocking extracellular matrix production in human TM and LC cells [28]. Very promising novel agents are inhibitors of the Rho pathway, which is integral to the regulation of aqueous outflow and matrix composition [29] [30]. Various Rho kinase inhibitors are already in phase 2 and 3 clinical trials, with conjunctival hyperaemia being one of the main adverse effects [31]. Clinical trials of combination therapies of Rho kinase inhibitors with prostaglandin analogues are also underway.

3. The HMG CoA Pathway

Statins are inhibitors of 3-hydroxy-3-methylglutaryl-coenzyme A (HMG-CoA) reductase—the crucial rate limiting step in hepatic cholesterol biosynthesis. Independently of the cholesterol lowering effect, the inhibition of HMG-CoA leads to reduced synthesis of isoprenoid intermediaries—farnesyl pyrophosphate (FPP) and geranylgeranyl pyrophosphate (GGPP) (**Figure 2**) [32]. These precursors of cholesterol biosynthesis are essential for post-translational modification and prenylation of certain small GTPase proteins, include the Ras and Rho superfamilies [33]. Prenylation of these proteins facilitates their intracellular trafficking and covalent attachment to the lipid membrane, which is often essential for biological function. These small GTPases cycle between an inactive GDP bound form found in the cytosol in association with guanine dissociation inhibitor (Rho GDI), and an active GTP bound form usually associated with the cell membrane (**Figure 3**). When Rho proteins are released from GDIs, they can insert into the cell membrane where they are activated by guanine nucleotide exchange factors (GEFs), and this initiates interaction with membrane effector proteins such as Rho kinase (ROCK). The Rho family of proteins is implicated in many key intracellular events and signalling pathways, including regulation of the actin cytoskeleton, cell adhesion, cell to cell interaction, and cell-cycle progression. This topic is comprehensively reviewed by Burridge and colleagues [34]. It is thought that inhibition of the Rho pathway by statins is one of the major mechanisms via which statins affect cell physiology.

4. Statins

4.1. Chemical Structure, Pharmacokinetic, and Pharmacodynamics Properties

While all statins share a common mechanism of action, they differ in the chemical structures, pharmacokinetic profiles, and lipid-modifying efficacy. Lovastatin, pravastatin, and simvastatin are fungal-derived, whereas atorvastatin, cerivastatin, fluvastatin, pravastatin, pitavastatin, and rosuvastatin are fully synthetic compounds [35]. All statins have a similar chemical structure composed of the following: an analogue of the target enzyme

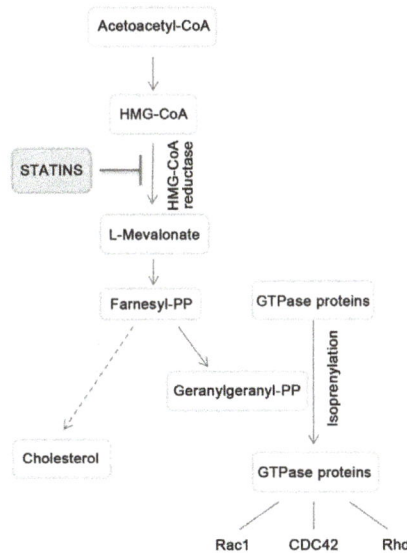

Figure 2. The HMG CoA pathway-inhibition by statins. Inhibition of HMG-CoA by statins inhibits the rate-limiting step in cholesterol biosynthesis, as well as reducing the production of isoprenoid intermediaries. The latter limits the isoprenylation of small GTPase proteins such as Rho, Rac1, and CDC42, and results in modulation of various cellular functions.

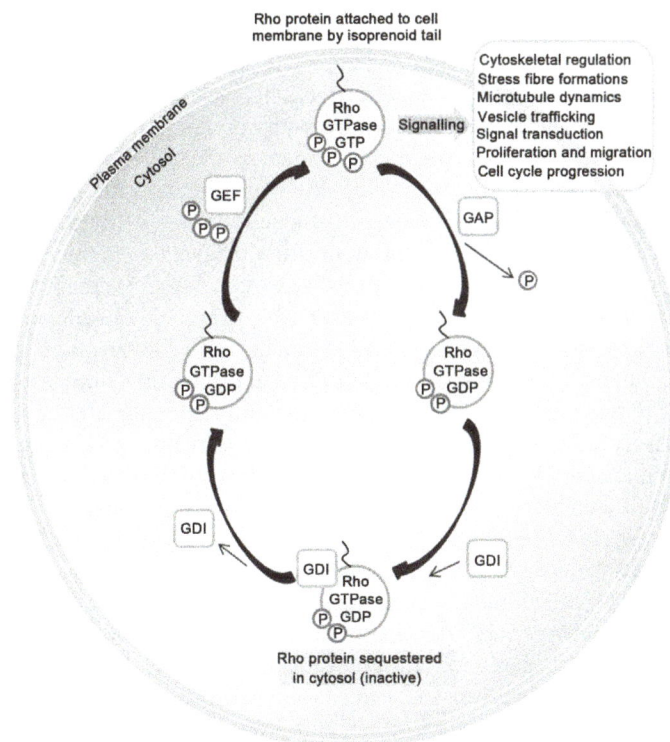

Figure 3. The Rho cycle. GEF: Guanine Exchange Factor. GAP: GTPase-Activating Protein. GDI: Guanine Dissociation Inhibitor. GEF proteins promote the exchange of GDP for GTP on Rho proteins. Binding of GTP facilitates a conformational change in Rho proteins leading to their interaction with effector molecules, and initiation of downstream signalling. GAPs facilitate GTP hydrolysis—so the Rho protein is left bound to GDP. In this state GDIs bind the inactive Rho protein. GDIs prevent membrane translocation of Rho proteins, so they are sequestered in the cytosol.

substrate HMG-CoA; a photophobic ring structure that is involved in binding of the statin to the enzyme; and side groups of the rings that define the solubility properties of the drug [35]. Through examination of this structure the mechanism of action of statins becomes evident—competitive inhibition of HMG-CoA through mimicry of the enzymes substrate.

Much of the pharmacokinetic properties of statins stem from the structure of the side groups—atorvastatin, fluvastatin, lovastatin, and simvastatin are relatively lipophilic compounds, whereas pravastatin and rosuavastatin are more hydrophilic [35]. The absorption of all statins is rapid, and peak plasma concentration is reached within 4 hours after administration [36]-[38]. All statins show great hepatoselectivity with respect to inhibition of HMG-CoA reductase, largely because of efficient first-pass uptake. The bioavailability of statins varies, from 5% for lovastatin, to 60% for pitavastatin [38] [39]. Statins are predominantly metabolised by the cytochrome P_{450} family of enzymes (CYP450) [40]. The main route for elimination for the majority of statins is via the bile after metabolism by the liver [41]. Statins are highly efficacious at lowering serum low-density lipoprotein (LDL), and can also increase serum high-density lipoprotein (HDL) by varying degrees [42] [43]. The widespread use of statins is now testament to their safety and efficacy. Generally statins are well tolerated with serious adverse effects being very rare [44]. The most serious adverse effect is myopathy, which may progress to rhabdomyolysis. The incidence of myopathy is dose-related, with an approximate incidence of 1 in 1000 patients treated [45]. The risk is increased when statins are used alongside other agents that share common metabolic pathways.

4.2. Application of Statins

The clinical application of statins is rapidly expanding. While prevention of cardiovascular disease is still the primary indication for statins, recent research in the fields of pulmonary and renal disease strongly suggests that statins would also be of benefit in these diseases. Lowering of serum cholesterol is considered to be the main mechanism responsible for the widely recognised beneficial effect of statins in cardiovascular disease [46]-[48]. As well as being of benefit in atherosclerosis and hypercholesterolaemia, statins also improve survival in non-ischaemic heart failure—which is generally unrelated to atherosclerosis [49]. This variant of heart failure has a prominent inflammatory component, and is associated with neurohormonal imbalance—for example activation of the renin-angiotensin-aldosterone and sympathetic system by the low-output state. In vascular cells, angiotensin-II is a key stimulant of reactive oxygen species (ROS) production [50]. Statins are effective in modifying these maladaptive responses, reducing angiotension-II-induced release of ROS, and improving cardiac function in non-ischaemic heart failure [50]-[52]. Recent clinical trials have also demonstrated the benefit of statins as stroke prophylactic agents—reducing the sequelae of stroke by 25% to 35% [53] [54].

The beneficial effect of statins in pulmonary diseases such as chronic obstructive pulmonary disease (COPD) and idiopathic pulmonary fibrosis (IPF) has recently come to light. Observational studies suggest that patients with COPD who take statins have reduced hospitalisation and mortality rates from COPD exacerbations [55] [56]. The prominent inflammatory and fibrotic components in these lung pathologies bear similarity to the molecular mechanisms observed in the glaucomatous trabecular meshwork and lamina cribrosa. These pathological mechanisms—including abnormal matrix remodelling secondary to enhanced matrix metalloprotease action, increased release of pro-inflammatory cytokines (including TGF-β1, IL-6 and IL-8), dysregulated apoptosis, increased reactive oxygen species—are modulated by statins in *in vitro* models of pulmonary disease [57]-[60].

A recent meta-analysis showed that statins are effective in reducing progression in chronic kidney disease [61]. In renal diseases such as renal interstitial fibrosis and diabetic nephropathy, statins have been shown to reduce fibrosis. Statins are capable of inhibiting TGF-β expression and collagen production [62], but may also reduce fibrosis via a TGF-β independent mechanism [63]. Importantly, recent laboratory evidence shows that statins are effective in inhibiting the pressure-induced fibrotic response of rat renal tubular cells—rosuvastatin reduced the expression of CTGF, TGF-β, fibronectin, and SMAD3 in cells cultured in a high pressure environment [4]. The anti-inflammatory and anti-fibrotic effect of statins was also observed in a model of diabetic nephropathy—rosuvastatin reverses the angiotensin-II-induced upregulation of TGF-β1, fibronectin, and collagen-IV [64]. These studies are very relevant to the field of glaucoma—where differential expression of genes involved in fibrosis and inflammation occurs in the setting of high intraocular pressure [19].

The anti-fibrotic effect of statins observed in pulmonary and renal disease has prompted innovative research in the area of anti-scarring therapeutics. Treatment of experimental wounds to rabbit ears with local statin injections resulted in reduced hypertrophic scar formation [65], where mRNA analysis of the tissue revealed significantly lower CTGF expression. Prevention of intra-abdominal scarring and adhesion formation is another emerging therapeutic target. Intra-peritoneal administration of losartan and atorvastatin in mice resulted in reduction of intra-peritoneal bands to a minimum [66]. Statin-containing cellulose film (statofilm) has also been shown to be superior to the established Seprafilm™ in preventing post-operative intraperitoneal adhesion in a rat model, opening up new avenues for future clinical application [67].

5. Statins and Glaucoma

5.1. Epidemiological Evidence

There are conflicting findings in the literature regarding whether statins are beneficial in patients with POAG. Stein et al conducted a retrospective longitudinal cohort analysis which found that statin use was associated with a significant reduction in the risk of POAG [1]. A dose response effect was also observed—suggesting that longer duration of statin exposure was associated with great reduction in the risk of developing glaucoma or requiring medical treatment for glaucoma. McGwin and colleagues carried out a case control study in male patients which showed that persons who had been prescribed statins for at least 2 years had a 40% reduced odds of developing glaucoma [68]. An interesting study by Leung and co-workers prospectively examined rates of visual field progression in patients who were taking statins versus those who were not. They found that statins were associated with visual field stabilisation in patients with normal tension glaucoma (NTG) [2]. The optic nerve and retinal nerve fibre layer in glaucoma suspects was examined by De Castro and colleagues using the confocal scanning laser ophthalmoscope—and findings suggested that glaucomatous progression was slowed in patients who were taking a statin medication [69]. In contrast to this, other researchers have found no support for the beneficial effect of statins in glaucoma [70] [71].

By what molecular mechanisms might statins be potentially beneficial in glaucoma? This question opens up many intriguing avenues regarding the pleiotropic effects of statins, and few studies have directly addressed this dilemma to date. Evidence from both human and animal studies has shown that statins have prominent anti-fibrotic and immune-modulating actions in several organ systems including the eye (**Table 1**), which may have useful effects in glaucoma. Let us review the known pleiotropic effects of statins and see how these may apply to glaucoma.

5.2. Rho Inhibition

Probably the most important pleiotropic effect of statins is the inhibition of small GTPases, including the Rho family of proteins [77]. The Rho pathway is responsible for various integral intracellular processes and for the interaction between cells and their environment. Three subfamilies constitute the Rho superfamily—Rho, Rac, and Cdc42. Regulation of the actin cytoskeleton, microtubule dynamics, vesicle trafficking, cell polarity and cell-cycle progression are all under the control of the Rho proteins (**Figure 4**). This topic is comprehensively reviewed by Burridge *et al.* [34]. The human trabecular meshwork expresses many components of the Rho pathway, suggesting that this is a key player in regulating the contractile tone and cellular morphology of the aqueous outflow pathway [30] [78]. The Rho proteins contain a lipophilic isoprenoid group, which permits their attachment to the cell membrane and is generally essential for biological function. By inhibiting the conversion of HMG-CoA to L-mevalonic acid, statins inhibit the synthesis of isoprenoid intermediaries, including FFP and GGPP. Hence proper subcellular localisation and trafficking of these GTPase proteins is inhibited, with significant functional consequences. Importantly, post-translationally immature forms of G-proteins may maintain partial function [79] [80], and interfere with the activity of mature membrane-anchored proteins.

By inhibiting Rho and its downstream effector proteins including Rho kinase (ROCK), statins are likely to affect the contractile properties of the conventional outflow pathway. Cells of the conventional pathway possess a contractile tone which is regulated through Rho signaling [81]. ROCK phosphorylates and inhibits the myosin-binding subunit of myosin light chain (MLC) phosphatase. This action increases MLC phosphorylation and myosin contractility, hence driving the formation of stress fibres and focal adhesion [34]. Early work on specific inhibitors of the Rho pathway has shown that Rho inhibition results in relaxation of the contractile tone of cells of the aqueous outflow pathway *in vitro* and *ex vivo* [78] [82] [83]. This increases aqueous outflow and reduces intraocular pressure. Indeed Rho kinase inhibitors have been shown to be potent agents in lowering intraocular pressure, and are undergoing phase 2 and 3 clinical trials [31] [84]. This effect of Rho inhibition in lowering the

Table 1. Summary of statin-mediated pharmacological effects on pathological mechanisms in glaucoma.

Summary of statin mediated pharmacological effects on pathological mechanisms in glaucoma			
Glaucoma mechanism	**Study type/tissue**	**Statin effect**	**Reference**
Fibrosis	Rat renal tubular cells (*in vitro*)	Inhibit pressure-induced fibrotic response (decreased CTGF, TGF-β1, fibronectin, Smad, phospho-Smad3)	[4]
	Rat renal tubular cells Human airway fibroblasts (*in vitro*)	Reduce TGF-β induced expression of fibronectin, CTGF, α-SMA	[4]-[6]
	Human airway fibroblasts (*in vitro*)	Reduced collagen gel contraction	[6]
	Murine model, rat model (*in vivo*)	Reduced post-operative adhesions (via downregulation of TGF-β1, tPA, PAI-1)	[66] [67]
	Murine model (*in vivo*)	Protect against tubulointestinal fibrosis injury via upregulation of eNOS/HSP70, and downregulation of Cav-1	[72]
	Rabbit model, skin (*in vivo*)	Reduced hypertrophic scar formation (reduced CTGF expression)	[65]
Matrix remodelling	Rat model, vascular smooth muscle cells (*in vitro, in vivo*)	Inhibit Ang-II-induced SMAD activation and related fibrosis	[64]
	Murine model (*in vivo*)	Reduced post-infarct tissue remodelling	[74]
	Human mesangial cells (*in vitro*)	Inhibit Ang-II-induced downregulation of MMP-2. Inhibit Ang-II-induced upregulation of TIMP-2 and MMP-9. Reduce TGF-β, Fibronectin, Col-IV	[64]
	Primary human TM cells	Suppress SPARC expression	[74]
Cytokine production	Human vascular smooth muscle cells (*in vitro*)	Reduced basal and Ang-II-induced IL-8 production	[58]
	Primary bronchial epithelial cells (*in vitro*)	Reduced IL-17-induced upregulation of IL-8, IL-6, VEGF. Reduced TGF-β1-induced upregulation of IL-6, MMP-2, MMP-9	[57]
	Rat primary astrocytes, microglia, macrophages (*in vitro*)	Inhibit iNOS, TNF-α, IL-1beta, IL-6	[75]
Endothelial function	Human model (*in vivo*)	Improved cardiac endothelial function Decreased serum s-ICAM1, CRP, vWF	[51]
Oxidant response	Human model (*in vivo*)	Promote systemic anti-oxidant effects, via inhibition of myeloperoxidase-derived and nitric oxide-derived oxidants	[60]
Apoptosis	Murine model (*in vivo*)	Decreased myocyte apoptosis post-infarct	[73]
Ischaemia	Murine model (*in vivo*)	Improved retinal ganglion cell survival post ischaemic injury	[76]

TGF: Transforming growth factor; CTGF: Connective tissue growth factor; IL: Interleukin; eNOS: Endothelial nitric oxide synthase; iNOS: Inducible nitric oxide synthase; HSP70: Heat shock protein-70; Cav-1: Caveolin-1; tPA: Tissue plasminogen activator; PAI-1: Plasminogen activator inhibitor-1; Ang-II: Angiotensin-II; S-ICAM1: Soluble intercellular adhesion molecule-1; vWF: Von Willibrand factor; CRP: C-reactive protein; TNF: Tumour necrosis factor; TM: Trabecular meshwork.

contractile tone of smooth muscle structures has already proven beneficial in other pathologies—including sub-arachnoid haemorrhage—where Rho inhibitors have been shown to reduce the incidence of cerebral vasospasm [85]. More recent studies in this field have demonstrated the potential beneficial effect of combination therapy with a statin plus a Rho kinase inhibitor [86].

Rho inhibitors also affect the actin cytoskeleton, and cellular morphology of the aqueous outflow pathway. *In vitro* work has shown decreases in actin stress fibres and focal adhesions in cultured porcine and human TM cells [83]. Treatment of monkey Schlemm's canal (SC) cells with a Rho inhibitor increases the number of giant vacuoles within cell, and decreases the expression of certain cytoskeletal proteins (ZO-1 and claudin-5) [87]. This leads to morphological changes—cell rounding and detachment of cells from each other, as well as wider paracellular spaces [78] [88]. In cultured cells of the SC, Rho inhibition results in increased permeation *in vitro*, which facilitates aqueous drainage [88]. *Ex vivo* perfusion experiments, where porcine, monkey, cow and ca-daver eyes are perfused with an aqueous humour substitute, have shown that perfusion with a Rho inhibitor in-creases the conventional outflow facility [78] [83] [88] [89]. To our knowledge, no such experiments have been

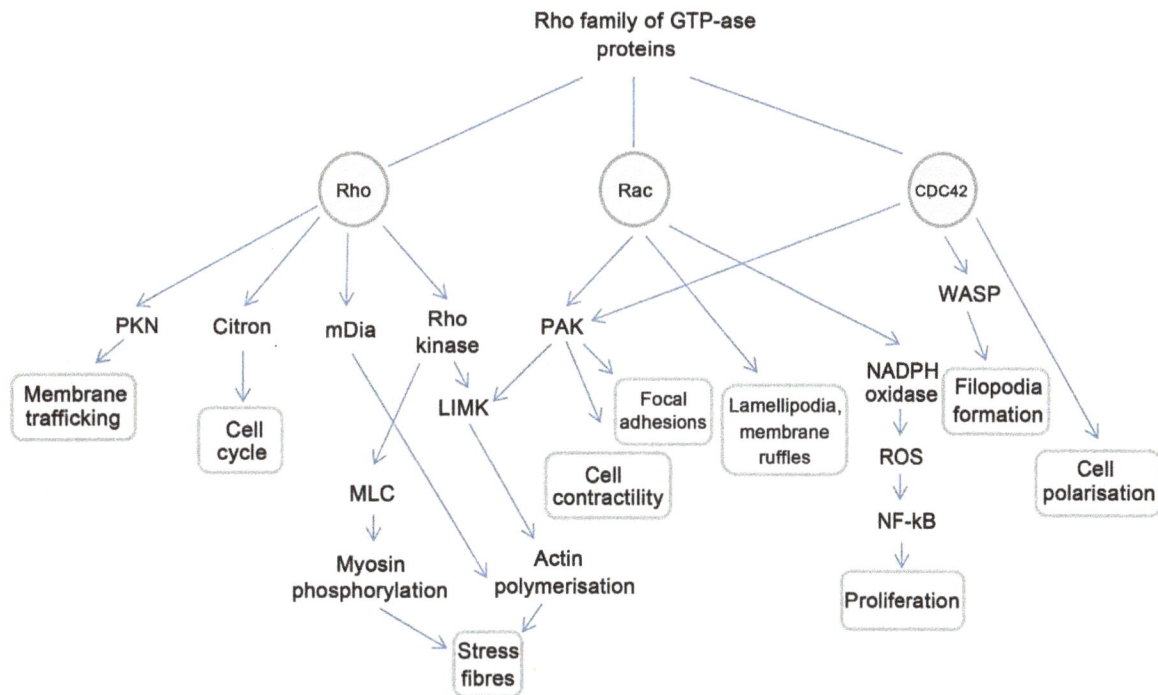

Figure 4. The Rho signalling pathway. PKN: Protein kinase N; mDia: Mammalian diaphanous protein; MLC: Myosin light chain; LIMK: LIM kinase; PAK: p21-activated kinase; NADPH: Nicotinamide adenine dinucleotide phosphate; ROS: Reactive oxygen species; NF-κB: Nuclear factor kappa-light-chain-enhancer of activated B cells; WASP: Wiskott-Aldrich syndrome protein. This diagram illustrates the major effector pathways for the Rho family of proteins (Rho, Rac and CDC-42) which are relevant to glaucoma pathogenesis.

carried out to date with statins, however considering the Rho inhibiting action of statins, it is likely that they have similar results. There is certainly potential for further studies to ascertain the effect of statins themselves on the cell morphology and contractile tone of the aqueous outflow pathway.

5.3. Rac and Reactive Oxygen Species (ROS)

One of the 3 key members of the Rho family is Rac1—this important GTPase protein is responsible for cytoskeletal remodelling—specifically the formation of lamellipodia and membrane ruffles [90]. Lamellipodia are actin-rich cellular protrusions, essential for cell migration, and play an important role in the invasion and metastases of cancer cells [91]. Furthermore, Rac1 binds to p67^{phox} which leads to activation of the NADPH oxidase system and generation of ROS [92]. The presence of high concentrations of ROS can overwhelm the cell's natural defence mechanisms and lead to programmed cell death. However the role of ROS in cell physiology is more complex thanthat and more recent studies have shown that in some scenarios, ROS (in small doses) promote cell survival—contrary to the traditional view that they are solely destructive molecules [93] [94]. ROS have also been shown to act as signalling molecules in their own right [95]. In smooth muscle and heart cells, it has been shown that by inhibiting the prenylation and subsequent activation of Rac1, statins inactivate NADPH oxidase and hence reduce angiotensin-II-induced ROS production [50] [96]. Our own research group has previously demonstrated evidence of oxidative stress and mitochondrial dysfunction in lamina cribrosa cells from the optic nerve heads of glaucoma donors, compared to normal donors [97]. Furthermore, our group has shown that up to 50% of POAG patients have a pathogenic mitochondrial DNA mutation, which may lead to mitochondrial respiratory dysfunction and subsequent predisposition to oxidative stress in TM, LC and RGC [98]. Increased levels of ROS have been found in the aqueous humour of glaucoma patients [99] [100]. Glutathione is a tripeptide found in the eye and other tissues, and is a key element of the protective mechanism of the eye against oxidative stress [101]. Altered glutathione levels have been reported in the aqueous humour of glaucoma patients [102], and abnormally low levels of glutathione have even been demonstrated in the serum of glaucoma patients [101]. ROS affect the cellularity of the trabecular meshwork, and may cause endothelial dysfunction—

which would contribute to impaired aqueous outflow and higher IOP [103]. Mitochondrial dysfunction in LC and RG cells allows the build-up of ROS, and may lead to increased susceptibility to cell death and impaired repair mechanisms [97] [104]. By reducing the production of ROS in ocular tissues, statins may help to reduce ROS-induced damage and glaucoma progression.

5.4. Endothelium-Derived Nitric Oxide

In the eye, endothelium-derived nitric oxide (NO) is an important regulator of blood flow to the choroid, optic nerve and retina [105]. Since NO is derived from the endothelium, endothelial dysfunction impairs ocular haemodynamics by reducing the production of NO and increasing the production of ROS. Endothelial dysfunction and abnormalities of the L-arginine/nitric oxide system in the vascular tree have been observed in a variety of ocular pathologies, including glaucoma [106]-[108]. Furthermore, studies in humans using laser Doppler flowmetry have demonstrated that inhibition of NO synthase leads to reduced choroidal and optic nerve head blood flow [105].

Statins influence NO levels by a number of mechanisms. Firstly—the cholesterol lowering effect. Raised serum LDL-cholesterol causes endothelial dysfunction, downregulated endothelial nitric oxide synthase (eNOS) expression, decreased receptor-mediated NO release [109], and increased ROS production which decreases NO bioavailability [110]. By reducing LDL-cholesterol, statins therefore improve endothelial function and facilitate NO production. Statins also affect NO production through cholesterol independent mechanisms. Statins increase eNOS gene expression by prolonging eNOS mRNA half-life, via a mechanism owing to inhibition of RhoA [111]. Furthermore, statins reduce the bio-availability of the membrane protein Caveolin-1. eNOS binds to Caveolin-1 in caveolae, which results in reduced NO production [112]. Genome wide association studies have suggested Caveolin-1 and -2 mutations in glaucoma [113]. Finally, statins activate the phosphatidylinositol 3-kinase (PI3K)/protein kinase Akt pathway. Akt is an important kinase involved in a number of key cellular functions including cell survival and growth, but it also serves to phosphorylate and activate eNOS—hence facilitating NO production. Statins therefore improve endothelial and vascular function via numerous cholesterol-dependent and -independent mechanisms. Such evidence suggests that statins would be of benefit in improving ocular blood flow in pathologies with compromised vasculature—including glaucoma. By improving endothelial function, statins may also mediate improved function of the endothelium-lined Schlemm's canal, which has altered biomechanical behaviour in glaucoma [114].

5.5. The Immune System

Immunomodulation is a well-known pleiotropic effect of statins. This has been shown to be beneficial in several pathologies where the immune system is upregulated, including multiple sclerosis and systemic lupus erythematosus [115]. Antigen presentation requires endocytosis of the antigen, internal processing, and presentation of major histocompatibility complex (MHC) II molecules at the cell surface. MHC II has been shown to be upregulated in a mouse model of glaucoma [116]. Furthermore, in a rat model of glaucoma microglial activation in the optic nerve correlated with the degree of axonal damage, and both MHC I and II were persistently upregulated in the microglia of optic nerves in the rat glaucoma model [117]. Gene expression of cytokines, including IL-6, have been shown to be upregulated in rat optic nerve heads subjected to raised intraocular pressure [118]. Many of the immunomodulatory effects of statins occur via the inhibition of small GTPase proteins [50] [77]. Antigen presentation and MHC II expression is related to changes in the actin cytoskeleton—which is controlled by the Rho pathway. Statins also decrease macrophage expression of tumour necrosis factor and interleukin-1β [75].

6. Effect of Statins on Ocular Tissues

Novel work by Villarreal *et al.* at the Massachusetts Eye and Ear Infirmary is one of the few to examine the molecular mechanisms involved in ocular tissues treated with statins [74]. In this project, human trabecular meshwork cells were treated with lovastatin *in vitro*, and SPARC mRNA and protein expression were determined. SPARC is a matricellular protein—and a critical mediator of aqueous outflow and IOP [119]-[121]. It is associated with increased tissue fibrosis and aberrant tissue remodelling, and it has been shown to be upregulated in TM cells following TGF-β2 treatment [122]. Statin treatment suppressed SPARC expression in TM cells—supporting the potential therapeutic role for statins in glaucoma.

The Rho signalling pathway has also been examined in TM cells treated with statins. Stubbs *et al.* showed that lovastatin increases the accumulation of unprenylated forms of RhoA and RhoB in human TM cells [123]. This may disrupt the Rho-dependent regulation of TM cell cytoskeletal organisation. Treatment of human TM cells with lovastatin resulted in disruption of filamentous actin organisation, an effect which was reversed by the supplementation of the cell cultures with GGPP.

Krempler *et al.* conducted novel research into the effect of statins on retinal ganglion cell survival and visual function following acute retinal ischaemia/reperfusion in mice [76]. Treatment of the animals with statins after the ischaemic insult resulted not only in histological evidence of improved retinal ganglion cell survival, but also improved visual function as measured behaviourally (by visual acuity and contrast sensitivity). This technique of producing acute global ischaemia represents a model of the changes observed after central retinal artery occlusion, as well as acute angle closure glaucoma [124]. This work hence supports the role for statins as a useful pharmacological tool in various ocular pathologies associated with ischaemic damage.

7. Concluding Remarks

The beneficial effect of statins extends far beyond cholesterol-lowering. Their pleiotropic effects include anti-fibrotic, anti-inflammatory, and immunomodulatory action, many of which are mediated by inhibition of the Rho pathway. These effects are evident in a multitude of human tissues, and statins as pleiotropic agents are already being studied in the fields of cardiovascular, pulmonary, and renal disease. Now, statins have caught the eye of glaucoma scholars as an intriguing new therapeutic agent, opening up many new avenues for molecular and clinical research.

References

[1]   Stein, J.D., *et al.* (2012) The Relationship between Statin Use and Open-Angle Glaucoma. *Ophthalmology*, **119**, 2074-2081. http://dx.doi.org/10.1016/j.ophtha.2012.04.029

[2]   Leung, D.Y., *et al.* (2010) Simvastatin and Disease Stabilization in Normal Tension Glaucoma: A Cohort Study. *Ophthalmology*, **117**, 471-476. http://dx.doi.org/10.1016/j.ophtha.2009.08.016

[3]   Schmeer, C., Kretz, A. and Isenmann, S. (2006) Statin-Mediated Protective Effects in the Central Nervous System: General Mechanisms and Putative Role of Stress Proteins. *Restorative Neurology and Neuroscience*, **24**, 79-95.

[4]   Chen, C.H., *et al.* (2013) Rosuvastatin Inhibits Pressure-Induced Fibrotic Responses via the Expression Regulation of Prostacyclin and Prostaglandin E2 in Rat Renal Tubular Cells. *European Journal of Pharmacology*, **700**, 65-73. http://dx.doi.org/10.1016/j.ejphar.2012.12.017

[5]   Schaafsma, D., *et al.* (2011) Simvastatin Inhibits TGFbeta1-Induced Fibronectin in Human Airway Fibroblasts. *Respiratory Research*, **12**, 113. http://dx.doi.org/10.1186/1465-9921-12-113

[6]   Watts, K.L., *et al.* (2005) Simvastatin Inhibits Growth Factor Expression and Modulates Profibrogenic Markers in Lung Fibroblasts. *American Journal of Respiratory Cell and Molecular Biology*, **32**, 290-300. http://dx.doi.org/10.1165/rcmb.2004-0127OC

[7]   Cordle, A., *et al.* (2005) Mechanisms of Statin-Mediated Inhibition of Small G-Protein Function. *Journal of Biological Chemistry*, **280**, 34202-34209. http://dx.doi.org/10.1074/jbc.M505268200

[8]   Laufs, U., *et al.* (2000) Neuroprotection Mediated by Changes in the Endothelial Actin Cytoskeleton. *Journal of Clinical Investigation*, **106**, 15-24. http://dx.doi.org/10.1172/JCI9639

[9]   Kato, T., *et al.* (2004) Statin Blocks Rho/Rho-Kinase Signalling and Disrupts the Actin Cytoskeleton: Relationship to Enhancement of LPS-Mediated Nitric Oxide Synthesis in Vascular Smooth Muscle Cells. *Biochimica et Biophysica Acta*, **1689**, 267-272. http://dx.doi.org/10.1016/j.bbadis.2004.04.006

[10]   Quigley, H.A., *et al.* (1981) Optic Nerve Damage in Human Glaucoma. II. The Site of Injury and Susceptibility to Damage. *Archives of Ophthalmology*, **99**, 635-649. http://dx.doi.org/10.1001/archopht.1981.03930010635009

[11]   Quigley, H.A. and Broman, A.T. (2006) The Number of People with Glaucoma Worldwide in 2010 and 2020. *British Journal of Ophthalmology*, **90**, 262-267. http://dx.doi.org/10.1136/bjo.2005.081224

[12]   Lambert, W., *et al.* (2001) Neurotrophin and Neurotrophin Receptor Expression by Cells of the Human Lamina Cribrosa. *Investigative Ophthalmology & Visual Science*, **42**, 2315-2323.

[13]   Cassard, S.D., *et al.* (2012) Regional Variations and Trends in the Prevalence of Diagnosed Glaucoma in the Medicare Population. *Ophthalmology*, **119**, 1342-1351. http://dx.doi.org/10.1016/j.ophtha.2012.01.032

[14]   Hernandez, M.R. and Pena, J.D. (1997) The Optic Nerve Head in Glaucomatous Optic Neuropathy. *Archives of Oph-*

thalmology, **115**, 389-395. http://dx.doi.org/10.1001/archopht.1997.01100150391013

[15]   Hernandez, M.R., Andrzejewska, W.M. and Neufeld, A.H. (1990) Changes in the Extracellular Matrix of the Human Optic Nerve Head in Primary Open-Angle Glaucoma. *American Journal of Ophthalmology*, **109**, 180-188. http://dx.doi.org/10.1016/S0002-9394(14)75984-7

[16]   Roberts, M.D., *et al.* (2010) Changes in the Biomechanical Response of the Optic Nerve Head in Early Experimental Glaucoma. *Investigative Ophthalmology & Visual Science*, **51**, 5675-5684. http://dx.doi.org/10.1167/iovs.10-5411

[17]   Fautsch, M.P. and Johnson, D.H. (2006) Aqueous Humor Outflow: What Do We Know? Where Will It Lead Us? *Investigative Ophthalmology & Visual Science*, **47**, 4181-4187. http://dx.doi.org/10.1167/iovs.06-0830

[18]   Johnson, M. (2006) What Controls Aqueous Humour Outflow Resistance? *Experimental Eye Research*, **82**, 545-557. http://dx.doi.org/10.1016/j.exer.2005.10.011

[19]   Kirwan, R.P., *et al.* (2009) Differential Global and Extra-Cellular Matrix Focused Gene Expression Patterns between Normal and Glaucomatous Human Lamina Cribrosa Cells. *Molecular Vision*, **15**, 76-88.

[20]   Liu, Y., *et al.* (2013) Gene Expression Profile in Human Trabecular Meshwork with Primary Open Angle Glaucoma. *Investigative Ophthalmology & Visual Science*, **54**, 6382-6389.

[21]   Coleman, A.L., *et al.* (1991) Displacement of the Optic Nerve Head by Acute Changes in Intraocular Pressure in Monkey Eyes. *Ophthalmology*, **98**, 35-40. http://dx.doi.org/10.1016/S0161-6420(91)32345-5

[22]   Hernandez, M.R. (1992) Ultrastructural Immunocytochemical Analysis of Elastin in the Human Lamina Cribrosa. Changes in Elastic Fibers in Primary Open-Angle Glaucoma. *Investigative Ophthalmology & Visual Science*, **33**, 2891-2903.

[23]   Quigley, H.A., *et al.* (2000) Retrograde Axonal Transport of BDNF in Retinal Ganglion Cells Is Blocked by Acute IOP Elevation in Rats. *Investigative Ophthalmology & Visual Science*, **41**, 3460-3466.

[24]   Hernandez, M.R., Igoe, F. and Neufeld, A.H. (1988) Cell Culture of the Human Lamina Cribrosa. *Investigative Ophthalmology & Visual Science*, **29**, 78-89.

[25]   Kirwan, R.P., *et al.* (2005) Influence of Cyclical Mechanical Strain on Extracellular Matrix Gene Expression in Human Lamina Cribrosa Cells *in Vitro*. *Molecular Vision*, **11**, 798-810.

[26]   Kirwan, R.P., *et al.* (2005) Transforming Growth Factor-Beta-Regulated Gene Transcription and Protein Expression in Human GFAP-Negative Lamina Cribrosa Cells. *Glia*, **52**, 309-324. http://dx.doi.org/10.1002/glia.20247

[27]   Quill, B., *et al.* (2011) The Effect of Graded Cyclic Stretching on Extracellular Matrix-Related Gene Expression Profiles in Cultured Primary Human Lamina Cribrosa Cells. *Investigative Ophthalmology & Visual Science*, **52**, 1908-1915. http://dx.doi.org/10.1167/iovs.10-5467

[28]   Wallace, D.M., *et al.* (2013) Anti-Connective Tissue Growth Factor Antibody Treatment Reduces Extracellular Matrix Production in Trabecular Meshwork and Lamina Cribrosa Cells. *Investigative Ophthalmology & Visual Science*, **54**, 7836-7848. http://dx.doi.org/10.1167/iovs.13-12494

[29]   Pattabiraman, P.P., Maddala, R. and Rao, P.V. (2014) Regulation of Plasticity and Fibrogenic Activity of Trabecular Meshwork Cells by Rho GTPase Signaling. *Journal of Cellular Physiology*, **229**, 927-942. http://dx.doi.org/10.1002/jcp.24524

[30]   Honjo, M., *et al.* (2001) Effects of Rho-Associated Protein Kinase Inhibitor Y-27632 on Intraocular Pressure and Outflow Facility. *Investigative Ophthalmology & Visual Science*, **42**, 137-144.

[31]   Tanihara, H., *et al.* (2013) Phase 2 Randomized Clinical Study of a Rho Kinase Inhibitor, K-115, in Primary Open-Angle Glaucoma and Ocular Hypertension. *American Journal of Ophthalmology*, **156**, 731-736. http://dx.doi.org/10.1016/j.ajo.2013.05.016

[32]   Goldstein, J.L. and Brown, M.S. (1990) Regulation of the Mevalonate Pathway. *Nature*, **343**, 425-430. http://dx.doi.org/10.1038/343425a0

[33]   Van Aelst, L. and D'Souza-Schorey, C. (1997) Rho GTPases and Signaling Networks. *Genes Development*, **11**, 2295-2322. http://dx.doi.org/10.1101/gad.11.18.2295

[34]   Burridge, K. and Wennerberg, K. (2004) Rho and Rac Take Center Stage. *Cell*, **116**, 167-179. http://dx.doi.org/10.1016/S0092-8674(04)00003-0

[35]   Gaw, A. (2000) Statins: The HMG CoA Reductase Inhibitors in Perspective. Martin Dunitz Ltd.

[36]   Cilla Jr., D.D., *et al.* (1996) Pharmacodynamic Effects and Pharmacokinetics of Atorvastatin after Administration to Normocholesterolemic Subjects in the Morning and Evening. *The Journal of Clinical Pharmacology*, **36**, 604-609. http://dx.doi.org/10.1002/j.1552-4604.1996.tb04224.x

[37]   Tse, F.L., Jaffe, J.M. and Troendle, A. (1992) Pharmacokinetics of Fluvastatin after Single and Multiple Doses in Normal Volunteers. *The Journal of Clinical Pharmacology*, **32**, 630-638.

http://dx.doi.org/10.1002/j.1552-4604.1992.tb05773.x

[38] Pan, H.Y., *et al.* (1990) Comparative Pharmacokinetics and Pharmacodynamics of Pravastatin and Lovastatin. *The Journal of Clinical Pharmacology*, **30**, 1128-1135. http://dx.doi.org/10.1002/j.1552-4604.1990.tb01856.x

[39] Kajinami, K., Mabuchi, H. and Saito, Y. (2000) NK-104: A Novel Synthetic HMG-CoA Reductase Inhibitor. *Expert Opinion on Investigational Drugs*, **9**, 2653-2661. http://dx.doi.org/10.1517/13543784.9.11.2653

[40] Bottorff, M. and Hansten, P. (2000) Long-Term Safety of Hepatic Hydroxymethyl Glutaryl Coenzyme A Reductase Inhibitors: The Role of Metabolism-Monograph for Physicians. *Archives of Internal Medicine*, **160**, 2273-2280. http://dx.doi.org/10.1001/archinte.160.15.2273

[41] Knopp, R.H. (1999) Drug Treatment of Lipid Disorders. *The New England Journal of Medicine*, **341**, 498-511. http://dx.doi.org/10.1056/NEJM199908123410707

[42] McKenney, J.M., *et al.* (2003) Comparison of the Efficacy of Rosuvastatin versus Atorvastatin, Simvastatin, and Pravastatin in Achieving Lipid Goals: Results from the STELLAR Trial. *Current Medical Research and Opinion*, **19**, 689-698. http://dx.doi.org/10.1185/030079903125002405

[43] Olsson, A.G., *et al.* (2001) Effect of Rosuvastatin on Low-Density Lipoprotein Cholesterol in Patients with Hypercholesterolemia. *American Journal of Cardiology*, **88**, 504-508. http://dx.doi.org/10.1016/S0002-9149(01)01727-1

[44] Black, D.M. (2002) A General Assessment of the Safety of HMG CoA Reductase Inhibitors (Statins). *Current Atherosclerosis Reports*, **4**, 34-41. http://dx.doi.org/10.1007/s11883-002-0060-0

[45] Ballantyne, C.M., *et al.* (2003) Risk for Myopathy with Statin Therapy in High-Risk Patients. *Archives of Internal Medicine*, **163**, 553-564. http://dx.doi.org/10.1001/archinte.163.5.553

[46] Scandinavian Simvastatin Survival Study Group (1994) Randomised Trial of Cholesterol Lowering in 4444 Patients with Coronary Heart Disease: The Scandinavian Simvastatin Survival Study (4S). *The Lancet*, **344**, 1383-1389.

[47] Shepherd, J., *et al.* (1995) Prevention of Coronary Heart Disease with Pravastatin in Men with Hypercholesterolemia. West of Scotland Coronary Prevention Study Group. *The New England Journal of Medicine*, **333**, 1301-1307. http://dx.doi.org/10.1056/NEJM199511163332001

[48] Heart Protection Study Collaborative Group (2002) MRC/BHF Heart Protection Study of Cholesterol Lowering with Simvastatin in 20,536 High-Risk Individuals: A Randomised Placebo-Controlled Trial. *The Lancet*, **360**, 7-22. http://dx.doi.org/10.1016/S0140-6736(02)09327-3

[49] Horwich, T.B., MacLellan, W.R. and Fonarow, G.C. (2004) Statin Therapy Is Associated with Improved Survival in Ischemic and Non-Ischemic Heart Failure. *Journal of the American College of Cardiology*, **43**, 642-648. http://dx.doi.org/10.1016/j.jacc.2003.07.049

[50] Wassmann, S., *et al.* (2001) Inhibition of Geranylgeranylation Reduces Angiotensin II-Mediated Free Radical Production in Vascular Smooth Muscle Cells: Involvement of Angiotensin AT1 Receptor Expression and Rac1 GTPase. *Molecular Pharmacology*, **59**, 646-654.

[51] Liu, M., *et al.* (2009) Atorvastatin Improves Endothelial Function and Cardiac Performance in Patients with Dilated Cardiomyopathy: The Role of Inflammation. *Cardiovascular Drugs and Therapy*, **23**, 369-376. http://dx.doi.org/10.1007/s10557-009-6186-3

[52] Landmesser, U., *et al.* (2005) Simvastatin versus Ezetimibe: Pleiotropic and Lipid-Lowering Effects on Endothelial Function in Humans. *Circulation*, **111**, 2356-2363. http://dx.doi.org/10.1161/01.CIR.0000164260.82417.3F

[53] Gil-Nunez, A.C. and Villanueva, J.A. (2001) Advantages of Lipid-Lowering Therapy in Cerebral Ischemia: Role of HMG-CoA Reductase Inhibitors. *Cerebrovascular Diseases*, **11**, 85-95. http://dx.doi.org/10.1159/000049130

[54] Vaughan, C.J., Delanty, N. and Basson, C.T. (2001) Statin Therapy and Stroke Prevention. *Current Opinion in Cardiology*, **16**, 219-224. http://dx.doi.org/10.1097/00001573-200107000-00001

[55] Mancini, G.B., *et al.* (2006) Reduction of Morbidity and Mortality by Statins, Angiotensin-Converting Enzyme Inhibitors, and Angiotensin Receptor Blockers in Patients with Chronic Obstructive Pulmonary Disease. *Journal of the American College of Cardiology*, **47**, 2554-2560. http://dx.doi.org/10.1016/j.jacc.2006.04.039

[56] Soyseth, V., *et al.* (2007) Statin Use Is Associated with Reduced Mortality in COPD. *European Respiratory Journal*, **29**, 279-283. http://dx.doi.org/10.1183/09031936.00106406

[57] Murphy, D.M., *et al.* (2008) Simvastatin Attenuates Release of Neutrophilic and Remodeling Factors from Primary Bronchial Epithelial Cells Derived from Stable Lung Transplant Recipients. *American Journal of Physiology-Lung Cellular and Molecular Physiology*, **294**, L592-L599. http://dx.doi.org/10.1152/ajplung.00386.2007

[58] Ito, T., *et al.* (2002) Regulation of Interleukin-8 Expression by HMG-CoA Reductase Inhibitors in Human Vascular Smooth Muscle Cells. *Atherosclerosis*, **165**, 51-55. http://dx.doi.org/10.1016/S0021-9150(02)00194-6

[59] Newton, C.J., *et al.* (2002) Statin-Induced Apoptosis of Vascular Endothelial Cells Is Blocked by Dexamethasone. *Journal of Endocrinology*, **174**, 7-16. http://dx.doi.org/10.1677/joe.0.1740007

[60] Shishehbor, M.H., *et al.* (2003) Statins Promote Potent Systemic Antioxidant Effects through Specific Inflammatory Pathways. *Circulation*, **108**, 426-431. http://dx.doi.org/10.1161/01.CIR.0000080895.05158.8B

[61] Geng, Q., *et al.* (2014) Meta-Analysis of the Effect of Statins on Renal Function. *American Journal of Cardiology*, **114**, 562-570. http://dx.doi.org/10.1016/j.amjcard.2014.05.033

[62] Li, Y.B., *et al.* (2011) Effect of Simvastatin on Expression of Transforming Growth Factor-Beta and Collagen Type IV in Rat Mesangial Cells. *Pharmacology*, **88**, 188-192. http://dx.doi.org/10.1159/000330739

[63] Rodrigues Diez, R., *et al.* (2010) Statins Inhibit Angiotensin II/Smad Pathway and Related Vascular Fibrosis, by a TGF-Beta-Independent Process. *PLoS ONE*, **5**, e14145. http://dx.doi.org/10.1371/journal.pone.0014145

[64] Solini, A., *et al.* (2011) Angiotensin-II and Rosuvastatin Influence Matrix Remodeling in Human Mesangial Cells via Metalloproteinase Modulation. *Journal of Hypertension*, **29**, 1930-1939. http://dx.doi.org/10.1097/HJH.0b013e32834abceb

[65] Ko, J.H., *et al.* (2012) HMG-CoA Reductase Inhibitors (Statins) Reduce Hypertrophic Scar Formation in a Rabbit Ear Wounding Model. *Plastic and Reconstructive Surgery*, **129**, 252e-261e. http://dx.doi.org/10.1097/PRS.0b013e31823aea10

[66] Dinarvand, P., *et al.* (2013) Novel Approach to Reduce Postsurgical Adhesions to a Minimum: Administration of Losartan plus Atorvastatin Intraperitoneally. *Journal of Surgical Research*, **181**, 91-98. http://dx.doi.org/10.1016/j.jss.2012.05.035

[67] Lalountas, M., *et al.* (2012) Postoperative Adhesion Prevention Using a Statin-Containing Cellulose Film in an Experimental Model. *British Journal of Surgery*, **99**, 423-429. http://dx.doi.org/10.1002/bjs.7817

[68] McGwin Jr., G., *et al.* (2004) Statins and Other Cholesterol-Lowering Medications and the Presence of Glaucoma. *Archives of Ophthalmology*, **122**, 822-826. http://dx.doi.org/10.1001/archopht.122.6.822

[69] De Castro, D.K., *et al.* (2007) Effect of Statin Drugs and Aspirin on Progression in Open-Angle Glaucoma Suspects Using Confocal Scanning Laser Ophthalmoscopy. *Clinical & Experimental Ophthalmology*, **35**, 506-513. http://dx.doi.org/10.1111/j.1442-9071.2007.01529.x

[70] Owen, C.G., *et al.* (2010) Hypotensive Medication, Statins, and the Risk of Glaucoma. *Investigative Ophthalmology & Visual Science*, **51**, 3524-3530. http://dx.doi.org/10.1167/iovs.09-4821

[71] Iskedjian, M., *et al.* (2009) Effect of Selected Antihypertensives, Antidiabetics, Statins and Diuretics on Adjunctive Medical Treatment of Glaucoma: A Population Based Study. *Current Medical Research and Opinion*, **25**, 1879-1888. http://dx.doi.org/10.1185/03007990903035083

[72] Garcia, I.M., *et al.* (2012) Caveolin-1-eNOS/Hsp70 Interactions Mediate Rosuvastatin Antifibrotic Effects in Neonatal Obstructive Nephropathy. *Nitric Oxide*, **27**, 95-105. http://dx.doi.org/10.1016/j.niox.2012.05.006

[73] Tang, X.L., *et al.* (2011) Atorvastatin Therapy during the Peri-Infarct Period Attenuates Left Ventricular Dysfunction and Remodeling after Myocardial Infarction. *PLoS ONE*, **6**, e25320. http://dx.doi.org/10.1371/journal.pone.0025320

[74] Villarreal Jr., G., *et al.* (2014) Pharmacological Regulation of SPARC by Lovastatin in Human Trabecular Meshwork Cells. *Investigative Ophthalmology & Visual Science*, **55**, 1657-1665. http://dx.doi.org/10.1167/iovs.13-12712

[75] Pahan, K., *et al.* (1997) Lovastatin and Phenylacetate Inhibit the Induction of Nitric Oxide Synthase and Cytokines in Rat Primary Astrocytes, Microglia, and Macrophages. *Journal of Clinical Investigation*, **100**, 2671-2679. http://dx.doi.org/10.1172/JCI119812

[76] Krempler, K., *et al.* (2011) Simvastatin Improves Retinal Ganglion Cell Survival and Spatial Vision after Acute Retinal Ischemia/Reperfusion in Mice. *Investigative Ophthalmology & Visual Science*, **52**, 2606-2618. http://dx.doi.org/10.1167/iovs.10-6005

[77] Tanaka, S., *et al.* (2013) Statins Exert the Pleiotropic Effects through Small GTP-Binding Protein Dissociation Stimulator Upregulation with a Resultant Rac1 Degradation. *Arteriosclerosis, Thrombosis, and Vascular Biology*, **33**, 1591-1600. http://dx.doi.org/10.1161/ATVBAHA.112.300922

[78] Rao, P.V., *et al.* (2001) Modulation of Aqueous Humor Outflow Facility by the Rho Kinase-Specific Inhibitor Y-27632. *Investigative Ophthalmology & Visual Science*, **42**, 1029-1037.

[79] Allal, C., *et al.* (2000) RhoA Prenylation Is Required for Promotion of Cell Growth and Transformation and Cytoskeleton Organization but Not for Induction of Serum Response Element Transcription. *The Journal of Biological Chemistry*, **275**, 31001-31008. http://dx.doi.org/10.1074/jbc.M005264200

[80] Lebowitz, P.F., Du, W. and Prendergast, G.C. (1997) Prenylation of RhoB Is Required for Its Cell Transforming Function but Not Its Ability to Activate Serum Response Element-Dependent Transcription. *The Journal of Biological Chemistry*, **272**, 16093-16095. http://dx.doi.org/10.1074/jbc.272.26.16093

[81] Ramos, R.F., Sumida, G.M. and Stamer, W.D. (2009) Cyclic Mechanical Stress and Trabecular Meshwork Cell Contractility. *Investigative Ophthalmology & Visual Science*, **50**, 3826-3832. http://dx.doi.org/10.1167/iovs.08-2694

[82] Honjo, M., *et al.* (2001) Effects of Protein Kinase Inhibitor, HA1077, on Intraocular Pressure and Outflow Facility in Rabbit Eyes. *Archives of Ophthalmology*, **119**, 1171-8. http://dx.doi.org/10.1001/archopht.119.8.1171

[83] Rao, P.V., *et al.* (2005) Expression of Dominant Negative Rho-Binding Domain of Rho-Kinase in Organ Cultured Human Eye Anterior Segments Increases Aqueous Humor Outflow. *Molecular Vision*, **11**, 288-297.

[84] Tanihara, H., *et al.* (2013) Phase 1 Clinical Trials of a Selective Rho Kinase Inhibitor, K-115. *JAMA Ophthalmology*, **131**, 1288-1295. http://dx.doi.org/10.1001/jamaophthalmol.2013.323

[85] Takanashi, Y., *et al.* (2001) Efficacy of Intrathecal Liposomal Fasudil for Experimental Cerebral Vasospasm after Subarachnoid Hemorrhage. *Neurosurgery*, **48**, 894-900.

[86] Naraoka, M., *et al.* (2013) Suppression of the Rho/Rho-Kinase Pathway and Prevention of Cerebral Vasospasm by Combination Treatment with Statin and Fasudil after Subarachnoid Hemorrhage in Rabbit. *Translational Stroke Research*, **4**, 368-374. http://dx.doi.org/10.1007/s12975-012-0247-9

[87] Thieme, H., *et al.* (2000) Mediation of Calcium-Independent Contraction in Trabecular Meshwork through Protein Kinase C and Rho-A. *Investigative Ophthalmology & Visual Science*, **41**, 4240-4246.

[88] Kameda, T., *et al.* (2012) The Effect of Rho-Associated Protein Kinase Inhibitor on Monkey Schlemm's Canal Endothelial Cells. *Investigative Ophthalmology & Visual Science*, **53**, 3092-3103.

[89] Lu, Z., *et al.* (2008) The Mechanism of Increasing Outflow Facility by Rho-Kinase Inhibition with Y-27632 in Bovine Eyes. *Experimental Eye Research*, **86**, 271-281. http://dx.doi.org/10.1016/j.exer.2007.10.018

[90] Nobes, C.D. and Hall, A. (1995) Rho, Rac, and Cdc42 GTPases Regulate the Assembly of Multimolecular Focal Complexes Associated with Actin Stress Fibers, Lamellipodia, and Filopodia. *Cell*, **81**, 53-62. http://dx.doi.org/10.1016/0092-8674(95)90370-4

[91] Kato, T., *et al.* (2014) Rac1-Dependent Lamellipodial Motility in Prostate Cancer PC-3 Cells Revealed by Optogenetic Control of Rac1 Activity. *PLoS ONE*, **9**, e97749. http://dx.doi.org/10.1371/journal.pone.0097749

[92] Sundaresan, M., *et al.* (1996) Regulation of Reactive-Oxygen-Species Generation in Fibroblasts by Rac1. *Biochemical Journal*, **318**, 379-382.

[93] Farrell, S.M., *et al.* (2011) bFGF-Mediated Redox Activation of the PI3K/Akt Pathway in Retinal Photoreceptor Cells. *European Journal of Neuroscience*, **33**, 632-641. http://dx.doi.org/10.1111/j.1460-9568.2010.07559.x

[94] Groeger, G., Quiney, C. and Cotter, T.G. (2009) Hydrogen Peroxide as a Cell-Survival Signaling Molecule. *Antioxidants Redox Signaling*, **11**, 2655-2671. http://dx.doi.org/10.1089/ars.2009.2728

[95] Rhee, S.G. (2006) Cell Signaling. H_2O_2, a Necessary Evil for Cell Signaling. *Science*, **312**, 1882-1883. http://dx.doi.org/10.1126/science.1130481

[96] Takemoto, M., *et al.* (2001) Statins as Antioxidant Therapy for Preventing Cardiac Myocyte Hypertrophy. *Journal of Clinical Investigation*, **108**, 1429-1437. http://dx.doi.org/10.1172/JCI13350

[97] McElnea, E.M., *et al.* (2011) Oxidative Stress, Mitochondrial Dysfunction and Calcium Overload in Human Lamina Cribrosa Cells from Glaucoma Donors. *Molecular Vision*, **17**, 1182-1191.

[98] Sundaresan, P., *et al.* (2014) Whole-Mitochondrial Genome Sequencing in Primary Open-Angle Glaucoma Using Massively Parallel Sequencing Identifies Novel and Known Pathogenic Variants. *Genetics in Medicine*, Published Online. http://dx.doi.org/10.1038/gim.2014.121

[99] Schlotzer-Schrehardt, U. (2010) Oxidative Stress and Pseudoexfoliation Glaucoma. *Klinische Monatsblätter für Augenheilkunde*, **227**, 108-113. http://dx.doi.org/10.1055/s-0028-1109977

[100] Sacca, S.C. and Izzotti, A. (2008) Oxidative Stress and Glaucoma: Injury in the Anterior Segment of the Eye. *Progress in Brain Research*, **173**, 385-407. http://dx.doi.org/10.1016/S0079-6123(08)01127-8

[101] Gherghel, D., *et al.* (2005) Systemic Reduction in Glutathione Levels Occurs in Patients with Primary Open-Angle Glaucoma. *Investigative Ophthalmology & Visual Science*, **46**, 877-883. http://dx.doi.org/10.1167/iovs.04-0777

[102] Ferreira, S.M., *et al.* (2004) Oxidative Stress Markers in Aqueous Humor of Glaucoma Patients. *American Journal of Ophthalmology*, **137**, 62-69. http://dx.doi.org/10.1016/S0002-9394(03)00788-8

[103] Sacca, S.C., *et al.* (2007) Glaucomatous Outflow Pathway and Oxidative Stress. *Experimental Eye Research*, **84**, 389-399. http://dx.doi.org/10.1016/j.exer.2006.10.008

[104] Maher, P. and Hanneken, A. (2005) The Molecular Basis of Oxidative Stress-Induced Cell Death in an Immortalized Retinal Ganglion Cell Line. *Investigative Ophthalmology & Visual Science*, **46**, 749-757. http://dx.doi.org/10.1167/iovs.04-0883

[105] Luksch, A., *et al.* (2000) Effects of Systemic NO Synthase Inhibition on Choroidal and Optic Nerve Head Blood Flow in Healthy Subjects. *Investigative Ophthalmology & Visual Science*, **41**, 3080-3084.

[106] Polak, K., *et al.* (2007) Altered Nitric Oxide System in Patients with Open-Angle Glaucoma. *Archives of Ophthalmol-*

ogy, **125**, 494-498. http://dx.doi.org/10.1001/archopht.125.4.494

[107] Henry, E., *et al.* (2006) Altered Endothelin-1 Vasoreactivity in Patients with Untreated Normal-Pressure Glaucoma. *Investigative Ophthalmology & Visual Science*, **47**, 2528-2532. http://dx.doi.org/10.1167/iovs.05-0240

[108] Henry, E., *et al.* (1999) Peripheral Endothelial Dysfunction in Normal Pressure Glaucoma. *Investigative Ophthalmology & Visual Science*, **40**, 1710-1714.

[109] Liao, J.K. (1994) Inhibition of Gi Proteins by Low Density Lipoprotein Attenuates Bradykinin-Stimulated Release of Endothelial-Derived Nitric Oxide. *The Journal of Biological Chemistry*, **269**, 12987-12992.

[110] Alderson, L.M., *et al.* (1986) LDL Enhances Monocyte Adhesion to Endothelial Cells *in Vitro*. *The American Journal of Pathology*, **123**, 334-342.

[111] Laufs, U. and Liao, J.K. (1998) Post-Transcriptional Regulation of Endothelial Nitric Oxide Synthase mRNA Stability by Rho GTPase. *The Journal of Biological Chemistry*, **273**, 24266-24271. http://dx.doi.org/10.1074/jbc.273.37.24266

[112] Plenz, G.A., Hofnagel, O. and Robenek, H. (2004) Differential Modulation of Caveolin-1 Expression in Cells of the Vasculature by Statins. *Circulation*, **109**, e7-e8.

[113] Thorleifsson, G., *et al.* (2010) Common Variants near CAV1 and CAV2 Are Associated with Primary Open-Angle Glaucoma. *Nature Genetics*, **42**, 906-909. http://dx.doi.org/10.1038/ng.661

[114] Overby, D.R., *et al.* (2014) Altered Mechanobiology of Schlemm's Canal Endothelial Cells in Glaucoma. *Proceedings of the National Academy of Sciences of the United States of America*, **111**, 13876-13881. http://dx.doi.org/10.1073/pnas.1410602111

[115] Ulivieri, C. and Baldari, C.T. (2014) Statins: From Cholesterol-Lowering Drugs to Novel Immunomodulators for the Treatment of Th17-Mediated Autoimmune Diseases. *Pharmacological Research*, **88**, 41-52. http://dx.doi.org/10.1016/j.phrs.2014.03.001

[116] Gallego, B.I., *et al.* (2012) IOP Induces Upregulation of GFAP and MHC-II and Microglia Reactivity in Mice Retina Contralateral to Experimental Glaucoma. *Journal of Neuroinflammation*, **9**, 92. http://dx.doi.org/10.1186/1742-2094-9-92

[117] Ebneter, A., *et al.* (2010) Microglial Activation in the Visual Pathway in Experimental Glaucoma: Spatiotemporal Characterization and Correlation with Axonal Injury. *Investigative Ophthalmology & Visual Science*, **51**, 6448-6460. http://dx.doi.org/10.1167/iovs.10-5284

[118] Johnson, E.C., *et al.* (2011) Cell Proliferation and Interleukin-6-Type Cytokine Signaling Are Implicated by Gene Expression Responses in Early Optic Nerve Head Injury in Rat Glaucoma. *Investigative Ophthalmology & Visual Science*, **52**, 504-518. http://dx.doi.org/10.1167/iovs.10-5317

[119] Haddadin, R.I., *et al.* (2009) SPARC-Null Mice Exhibit Lower Intraocular Pressures. *Investigative Ophthalmology & Visual Science*, **50**, 3771-3777. http://dx.doi.org/10.1167/iovs.08-2489

[120] Swaminathan, S.S., *et al.* (2013) Secreted Protein Acidic and Rich in Cysteine (SPARC)-Null Mice Exhibit More Uniform Outflow. *Investigative Ophthalmology & Visual Science*, **54**, 2035-2047. http://dx.doi.org/10.1167/iovs.12-10950

[121] Oh, D.J., *et al.* (2013) Overexpression of SPARC in Human Trabecular Meshwork Increases Intraocular Pressure and Alters Extracellular Matrix. *Investigative Ophthalmology & Visual Science*, **54**, 3309-3319. http://dx.doi.org/10.1167/iovs.12-11362

[122] Bollinger, K.E., *et al.* (2011) Quantitative Proteomics: TGFbeta(2) Signaling in Trabecular Meshwork Cells. *Investigative Ophthalmology & Visual Science*, **52**, 8287-8294. http://dx.doi.org/10.1167/iovs.11-8218

[123] Von Zee, C.L., *et al.* (2009) Increased RhoA and RhoB Protein Accumulation in Cultured Human Trabecular Meshwork Cells by Lovastatin. *Investigative Ophthalmology & Visual Science*, **50**, 2816-2823. http://dx.doi.org/10.1167/iovs.08-2466

[124] Osborne, N.N., *et al.* (2004) Retinal Ischemia: Mechanisms of Damage and Potential Therapeutic Strategies. *Progress in Retinal and Eye Research*, **23**, 91-147. http://dx.doi.org/10.1016/j.preteyeres.2003.12.001

5

Suturing Technique to Promote Graft Attachment in Challenging Cases of Descemet Stripping Endothelial Keratoplasty

Miltiadis Papathanassiou, Lamprini Papaioannou

Cornea Clinic, 2nd Ophthalmology Department, Attikon University Hospital, Athens, Greece
Email: papathanassiou1@gmail.com

Abstract

Aims: To describe a technique that uses a transcorneal fixation suture for graft attachment in endothelial keratoplasty in high-risk for graft dislocation eyes. Materials and Methods: Case series included 12 eyes of 12 patients who underwent Descemet Stripping Automated Endothelial Keratoplasty (DSAEK) in the presence of high risk for graft dislocation factors. We describe a surgical technique that uses a transcorneal fixation suture to compress the donor graft onto the back surface of the recipient cornea. Outcome measures included intraoperative and postoperative complications, graft attachment and clarity and endothelial cell count at a 12 months follow-up period. Results: No intraoperative complications were noted and 11 grafts remained attached and clear with no suture related complications at a 12-month follow-up period. Partial peripheral graft detachment due to suture related graft folds, accompanied by mild corneal edema was noticed in one patient postoperatively. Reattachment and edema resolution occurred spontaneously after suture removal. The mean endothelial cell loss was 38.21% at 12 months. Conclusions: Temporary transcorneal fixation suture can be helpful in preventing graft detachment in eyes with high risk for graft dislocation.

Keywords

Descemet Stripping Endothelial Keratoplasty, Endothelial Graft Detachment, Transcorneal Fixation Suture

1. Introduction

Descemet Stripping Automated Endothelial Keratoplasty (DSAEK) is a form of corneal transplantation in which a donor posterior corneal button, including donor corneal endothelium, Descemet's membrane, and posterior corneal stroma, is used for selective replacement of corneal endothelium in conditions characterized by corneal endothelial dysfunction. It is considered a safe technique that results in early visual recovery and refractive and tectonic stability [1]. Graft dislocation is the most common post-operative complication of DSAEK [1] [2]. Dislocations may represent either fluid in the interface of an otherwise well-positioned graft or complete dislocation into the anterior chamber and are typically evident within the first postoperative week, although reports of late dislocations exist [3]. Postoperative hypotony, maintained viscoelastic material in the interface, incomplete air fill, donor disc placed upside down, delayed endothelial pump function, primary graft failure and eye rubbing are considered as intraoperative and postoperative possible causes of dislocation [4] [5]. The presence of glaucoma drainage devices and minimal or absent iris-lens diaphragm, including aphakia, are risk factors for higher rates of graft dislocation as they can result in loss of tamponading air [6]-[9]. The presence of an anterior chamber intraocular lens (AC IOL) can also make the filling of the anterior chamber with air and maintenance of the air bubble difficult, while it also interferes with the surgical handling of the graft [10]-[13]. Prior failed penetrating keratoplasty (PK), especially in patients with irregular internal PK wound and graft-to-host disparity, can also make the DSAEK procedure challenging [14]-[16]. We report a case series of 12 patients who undergo DSAEK in the presence of high risk for graft detachment factors. We describe a technique that uses a transcorneal fixation suture to compress the donor graft onto the back surface of the recipient cornea, promoting endothelial graft attachment.

2. Materials and Methods

We present a case series including 12 eyes of 12 patients, 9 male and 3 female, whounderwent DSAEK in the presence of high risk for graft dislocation factors. Five patients underwent DSAEK under prior failed PK with irregular internal PK wound, 2 of them had AC IOL and 1 of them had also undergone primary failed DSEK. Two patients had endothelial decompensation in the presence of a glaucoma drainage device and 5 patients had pseudophakic bullous keratopathy in the presence of an AC IOL. Demographic and clinical patient data are summarized in **Table 1**. All procedures were uneventful, performed by a single surgeon. Outcome measures

Table 1. Demographic and clinical data of patients.

Patient	Age	Sex	Indication for keratoplasty	Risk factors	Preoperative BCVA	Postoperative BCVA (at 12 months)
1	71	M	Endothelialde compensation	Ahmed valve	20/160	20/50
2	68	M	Fuchs' endothelial dystrophy, primary failed DSEK	Failed PK	20/200	20/50
3	79	F	Pseudophakic bullous keratopathy	Failed PK	20/400	20/50
4	87	M	Pseudophakic bullous keratopathy	AC-IOL with large anomalous pupil (> 8 mm, larger than the AC-IOL body)	20/400	20/40
5	80	M	Pseudophakic bullous keratopathy	Failed PK, AC-IOL, broad peripheral iridectomy	20/200	20/32
6	69	F	Pseudophakic bullous keratopathy	AC-IOL	20/160	20/25
7	72	M	Endothelialde compensation	Ahmed valve	20/200	20/40
8	76	M	Pseudophakic bullous keratopathy	Failed PK, AC-IOL	20/400	20/40
9	65	M	Pseudophakic bullous keratopathy	AC-IOL	20/100	20/25
10	80	F	Pseudophakic bullous keratopathy	AC-IOL	20/100	20/32
11	79	M	Pseudophakic bullous keratopathy	Failed PK	20/200	20/50
12	75	M	Pseudophakic bullous keratopathy	AC-IOL	20/160	20/50

BCVA = best corrected visual acuity, M = male, F = female, PK = penetrating keratoplasty, DSEK = descemet stripping endothelial keratoplasty, AC-IOL = anterior chamber intraocular lens included intraoperative and postoperative complications, graft attachment and clarity and endothelial cell count at a 12 months follow-up period.

Surgical Technique

Descemet stripping was performed aiming for a diameter of 8.5 mm, using an 8.5 mm circular marker dipped in trypan blue. An anterior chamber maintainer was placed at the 6 o'clock position. Precut endothelial grafts were used in all 12 cases (1 mm larger than previous failed PK graft in 5 cases). Folded donor disc was inserted through a 4.5 mm incision using Busin glide. The graft was allowed to unfold spontaneously and the anterior chamber maintainer was removed. Gentle external cornea tapping resulted in centration of the graft. On correct positioning, air was injected into the anterior chamber (AC) to attach the graft onto the stromal bed. After all incisions being sutured airtight with 10.0 nylon sutures, air was injected with a 30-gauge needle filling the AC with air. Afterwards, 1 to 2 transcorneal sutures were used to stabilize the graft. 10.0 nylon sutures were placed full-thickness passing from the peripheral cornea inwards, and then passing through the donor tissue, and through the full thickness of the cornea stroma. Knots were buried, rotating the sutures to the periphery away from the graft. Opposite rotation could lead to graft folds. After the knots being buried, the AC was refilled with air for 10 minutes. Thereafter the air was reduced, leaving a 50% air bubble in the AC. The ensuing steps of the technique are illustrated in **Figure 1**. Sutures were removed four weeks later.

3. Results

There were no intraoperative complications. 11 grafts (91.7%) remained attached and clear at a 12-months follow-up period (**Figure 2**, **Figure 3**). Partial peripheral graft detachment due to suture related graft folds, accompanied by mild corneal edema, was noticed in one patient postoperatively. Reattachment and edema resolution occurred spontaneously after suture removal (**Figure 4**). No further suture-related complications, such as endophtalmitis and epithelial ingrowth were noted. Mean best corrected visual acuity (BCVA) was 20/40. Mean endothelial cell count measured by specular microscope (EM-3000, Tomey, Erlangen, Germany) was 1569 cells/mm² at 12 months postoperatively, representing a mean endothelial cell loss of 38.21% compared with post-cut cell count (**Table 2**).

4. Discussion

The presence of AC IOL, prior failed PK, minimal or absent iris-lens diaphragm and glaucoma drainage devices have been examined as risk factors for higher rates of graft dislocation. In cases where the AC IOL is not the cause of endothelial decompensation and the depth of the anterior chamber is adequate, an intraocular lens exchange is not required [10]-[12]. As reported, DSAEK in the presence of a well-centered AC IOL and AC IOL-to-endothelium depth greater than 3 mm, resulted in no significant difference in cell loss compared with DSAEK cases in the presence of a posterior chamber intraocular lens [10] [11]. In such cases, the DSAEK procedure becomes more challenging, as it is difficult for an adequate air bubble to remain in the anterior chamber without escaping into the vitreous cavity, while the presence of an intraocular lens in the anterior chamber interferes with surgical handlings.

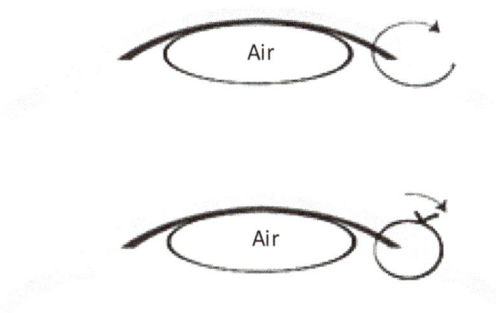

Figure 1. Fixation suture technique: 10.0 nylon sutures are placed full-thickness passing from the peripheral cornea towards the center, through the donor disc and the corneal stroma. Knots are buried, rotating the sutures to the periphery away from the graft.

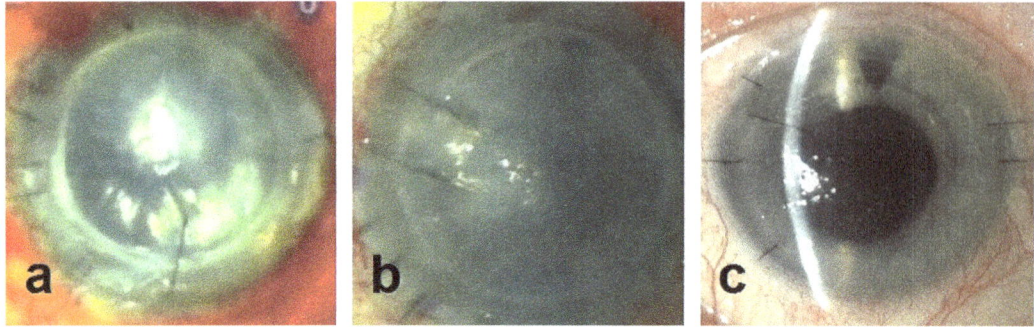

Figure 2. Intraoperative (a) (b) and postoperative (c) figures of transcorneal fixation suture in high risk patients. Two sutures were used to offer additional attachment in a patient with a prior failed PK and abnormal internal PK wound (b).

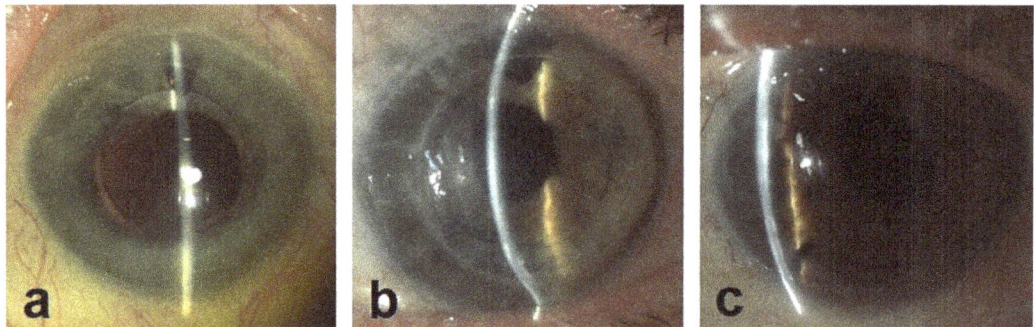

Figure 3. Attached and clear grafts at a 12-month follow-up period in a patient with AC-IOL and a large anomalous pupil (a), a case of prior failed PK in the presence of AC-IOL (b) and a patient with glaucoma drainage device (c).

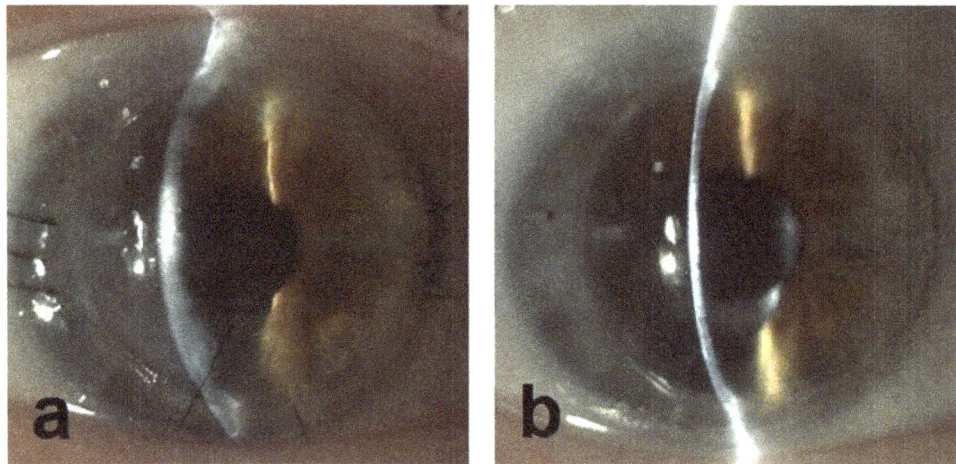

Figure 4. Postoperative partial peripheral graft detachment due to graft folds, accompanied by mild corneal edema in a second (redo) DSEK case with a history of failed DSEK and failed PK (a). Spontaneous reattachment and edema resolution after suture removal (b).

Minimal or absent lens-iris diaphragm and glaucoma drainage devices also result in difficulty for an adequate air bubble to be maintained in the anterior chamber, while the risk of posterior graft dislocation into the vitreous cavity in aphakic eyes is high [6]-[9]. Prior failed PK represents an indication for DSAEK procedure in eyes with an acceptable topography and refractive outcome before PK graft failure [15]. Endothelial graft diameter and irregular internal PK wound in prior failed PK have also been examined as risk factors for graft dislocation. Clements *et al.* have reported higher rates of graft dislocation in cases where endothelial graft diameter was smaller than the previous PK graft, as well as in cases with glaucoma drainage devices [14]. This result is consistent with Anshu *et al.* series of 60 patients, where low dislocation rates (6.6%) were noticed using

Suturing Technique to Promote Graft Attachment in Challenging Cases of Descemet...

37

Table 2. Endothelial cell count.

Patient	Post-cut cell count/mm^2	12 Months postoperatively
1	2511	1622
2	3012	1731
3	2600	1604
4	2508	1539
5	2514	1562
6	2410	1451
7	2462	1511
8	2471	1506
9	2511	1553
10	2502	1547
11	2453	1617
12	2517	1585

oversized grafts [15]. On the other hand Straiko *et al.* reported similar rates of dislocation (5.9%) using graft diameters less than or equal to the PK diameter in 17 cases [16].

Suture fixation has already been reported as an alternative management of dislocated grafts after the first reposition, aiming to engage the peripheral edge of the donor tissue and support it in place until the endothelial pump function takes over [17] [18]. "Preventive" transcorneal suturing as part of the insertion technique has also been reported [8] [19]. Patel *et al.* described a technique that uses an anchoring suture as part of the insertion technique in eyes with minimal or absent iris-lens diaphragm. This technique aims in safe delivery and fixation of donor disk while facilitating the management of graft detachment by rebubbling, as the graft remains attached at sutured edge [8]. The use of one transcorneal sutures either as a part of the insertion technique or as a separated suture has also been described by Elderkin *et al.* in eyes with AC IOL [12]. In both series one single suture was used to hold the graft in place preventing complete detachment, while partial detachment occurred in 2 out of 13 cases in Patel series and in 1 out of 11 cases in Elderkin series.

We propose the use of a full-thickness, temporary, "preventive", transcorneal suture as part of the DSAEK procedure which can fixate the graft at the posterior surface of the cornea preventing graft dislocation in high risk cases. We believe that the use of 2 transcorneal sutures when needed offers additional attachment and eliminates even partial detachment. Although more sutures could result in higher rates of suture related complications, prevention of dislocation is considered a safer approach by the authors, as reposition and rebubbling is associated with increased endothelial cell loss [4] [20]. In our series no significant suture related complication, such as endophthalmitis and epithelial ingrowth due to the full-thickness suturing was noticed. A limitation of this study is the small number of participants, but the encouraging results could suggest the use of this technique and the assessment of its efficacy in larger series.

5. Conclusion

In summary, temporary transcorneal fixation sutures as a part of the primary DSAEK procedure can be helpful in high risk for graft dislocation eyes. Although our series is small, results are encouraging, as all grafts remain attached and clear, while no significant complication is noticed.

References

[1]   Lee, W.B., Jacobs, D.S., Mush, D.C., Kaufman, S.C., Reinhart, W.J. and Shtein, R.M. (2009) Descemet's Stripping Endothelial Keratoplasty: Safety and Outcomes: A Report by the American Academy of Ophthalmology. *Ophthalmology*, **116**, 1818-1830. http://dx.doi.org/10.1016/j.ophtha.2009.06.021

[2]   Suh, L., Yoo, S., Deobhakta, A., Donaldson, K., Alfonso, E., Culbertson, W., *et al.* (2008) Complications of Descemet's Stripping with Automated Endothelial Keratoplasty: Survey of 118 Eyes at One Institute. *Ophthalmology*, **115**,

1517-1524. http://dx.doi.org/10.1016/j.ophtha.2008.01.024

[3]   Busin, M. and Bhatt, M.R. (2008) Late Detachment of Donor Graft after Descemet Stripping Automated Endothelial Keratoplasty. *Journal of Cataract & Refractive Surgery*, **34**, 159-160. http://dx.doi.org/10.1016/j.jcrs.2007.08.027

[4]   Terry, M.A. and Ousley, P.J. (2006) Deep Lamellar Endothelial Keratoplasty: Early Complications and Their Management. *Cornea*, **25**, 37-43. http://dx.doi.org/10.1097/01.ico.0000164781.33538.b6

[5]   Price Jr., F.W. and Price, M.O. (2006) Descemet's Stripping with Endothelial Keratoplasty in 200 Eyes: Early Challenges and Techniques to Enhance Donor Adherence. *Journal of Cataract & Refractive Surgery*, **32**, 411-418. http://dx.doi.org/10.1016/j.jcrs.2005.12.078

[6]   Kim, P., Amiran, M.D., Lichtinger, A., Yeung, S.N., Slomovic, A.R. and Rootman, D.S. (2012) Outcomes of Descemet Stripping Automated Endothelial Keratoplasty in Patients with Previous Glaucoma Drainage Device Insertion. *Cornea*, **31**, 172-175. http://dx.doi.org/10.1097/ICO.0b013e318224820a

[7]   Suh, L.H., Kymionis, G., Culbertson, W.W., O'Brien, T.P. and Yoo, S.H. (2008) Descemet's Stripping with Endothelial Keratoplasty in Aphakic Eyes. *Archives of Ophthalmology*, **126**, 268-270. http://dx.doi.org/10.1001/archophthalmol.2007.32

[8]   Patel, A.K., Luccarelli, S., Ponzin, D. and Busin, M. (2011) Transcorneal Suture Fixation of Posterior Lamellar Grafts in Eyes With Minimal or Absent Iris-Lens Diaphragm. *American Journal of Ophthalmology*, **151**, 460-464. http://dx.doi.org/10.1016/j.ajo.2010.08.043

[9]   Price, M.O., Price Jr., F.W. and Trespalacios, R. (2007) Endothelial Keratoplasty Technique for Aniridicaphakic Eyes. *Journal of Cataract & Refractive Surgery*, **33**, 376-379. http://dx.doi.org/10.1016/j.jcrs.2006.10.052

[10]   Esquenazi, S., Schechter, B.A. and Esquenazi, K. (2011) Endothelial Survival after Descemet-Stripping Automated Endothelial Keratoplasty in Eyes with Retained Anterior Chamber Intraocular Lenses: Two-Year Follow-Up. *Journal of Cataract & Refractive Surgery*, **37**, 714-719. http://dx.doi.org/10.1016/j.jcrs.2010.10.054

[11]   Esquenazi, S. (2009) Safety of DSAEK in Pseudophakic Eyes with Anterior Chamber Lenses and Fuchs Endothelial Dystrophy. *British Journal of Ophthalmology*, **93**, 558-559. http://dx.doi.org/10.1136/bjo.2008.154914

[12]   Elderkin, S., Tu, E., Sugar, J., Reddy, S., Kadakia, A., Ramaswamy, R. and Djalilian, A. (2010) Outcome of Descemet Stripping Automated Endothelial Keratoplasty in Patients with an Anterior Chamber Intraocular Lens. *Cornea*, **29**, 1273-1277. http://dx.doi.org/10.1097/ICO.0b013e3181d00a5e

[13]   Groat, B., Ying, M.S., Vroman, D.T., Fernandez de Castro, L.E. (2007) Descemet-Stripping Automated Endothelial Keratoplasty Technique in Patients with Anterior Chamber Intraocular Lenses—Video Report. *British Journal of Ophthalmology*, **91**, 714. http://dx.doi.org/10.1136/bjo.2007.121343

[14]   Clements, J.L., Bouchard, C.S., Lee, W.B., Dunn, S.P., Mannis, M.J., Reidy, J., *et al.* (2011) Retrospective Review of Graft Dislocation Rate Associated with Descemet Stripping Automated Endothelia Keratoplasty after Primary Failed Penetrating Keratoplasty. *Cornea*, **30**, 414-418. http://dx.doi.org/10.1097/ICO.0b013e3181f7f163

[15]   Anshu, A., Price, M.O. and Price, F.W. (2011) Descemet's Stripping Endothelial Keratoplasty under Failed Keratoplasty: Visual Rehabilitation and Graft Survival Rate. *Ophthalmology*, **118**, 2155-2160. http://dx.doi.org/10.1016/j.ophtha.2011.04.032

[16]   Straiko, M.D., Terry, M.A. and Shamie, N. (2011) Descemet Stripping Endothelial Keratoplasty under Failed Penetrating Keratoplasty: A Surgical Strategy to Minimize Complications. *American Journal of Ophthalmology*, **151**, 233-237. http://dx.doi.org/10.1016/j.ajo.2010.08.017

[17]   Anandan, M. and Leyland, M. (2008) Suture Fixation of Dislocated Endothelial Grafts. *Eye*, **22**, 718-721. http://dx.doi.org/10.1038/sj.eye.6703000

[18]   Wu, W.K., Wong, V. and Chi, S. (2011) Graft Suturing for Lenticule Dislocation after Descemet Stripping Automated Endothelial Keratoplasty. *Journal of Ophthalmic & Vision Research*, **6**, 131-135

[19]   Macsai, M.S. and Kara-Jose, A.C. (2007) Suture Technique for Descemet Stripping and Endothelial Keratoplasty. *Cornea*, **26**, 1123-1126. http://dx.doi.org/10.1097/ICO.0b013e318124a443

[20]   Price, M.O. and Price, F.W. (2008) Endothelial Cell Loss after Descemet Stripping with Endothelial keratoplasty: Influencing Factors and 2-Year Trend. *Ophthalmology*, **115**, 857-865. http://dx.doi.org/10.1016/j.ophtha.2007.06.033

6

Optimization of the A Constant for the SRK/T Formula

John C. Merriam[1], Eva Nong[2], Lei Zheng[1], Malka Stohl[3]

[1]Edward S. Harkness Eye Institute, College of Physicians and Surgeons, Columbia University, New York, NY, USA
[2]Department of Ophthalmology, University of Maryland, Baltimore, MD, USA
[3]New York State Psychiatric Institute, New York, NY, USA
Email: jcm5@columbia.edu

Abstract

Purpose: To evaluate the effect of axial length (AL) and the average preoperative keratometry (K) on the A constant in the SRK/T formula. Methods: The retrospective, comparative case series includes 635 eyes from 407 cataract patients from Columbia University Medical Center from January 2006 to August 2010, operated by a single surgeon using a temporal incision and the Acrysof SN60WF IOL (Alcon Laboratories, TX). Using the postoperative manifest refraction and biometry data, we calculated the precise A constant (Ap) necessary to yield the postoperative spherical equivalent for each eye. To optimize the A constant, we developed three regression models (linear, quadratic, and categorical in 7 AL groups) to relate these precise A constants to AL and K. We verified our method with another series of 45 eyes for which we calculated mean errors (defined as the difference between the spherical equivalent of the postoperative refraction and the predicted postoperative refraction) using the optimized and manufacturer's suggested A constants. Results: There is a statistically significant relationship between AL (P < 0.001), K (P < 0.001) and the A constant. Ap increased as AL increased and as K decreased. In the validation data set, optimizing the A constant reduced mean errors from 0.50 D to 0.25 D and also reduced hyperopic refractive outcomes. Conclusions: The A constant for longer eyes with flatter corneas is larger than the A constant for shorter eyes with steeper corneas. Optimizing A constants using both AL and K improved the predictability of refractive outcomes without modification to the SRK/T formula.

Keywords

Cataract Surgery, SRK/T, A Constant

1. Introduction

In small incision cataract surgery, an accurate refractive outcome depends on a reliable intraocular lens (IOL) power formula, accurate biometry, and appropriate IOL constants. The SRK/T formula [1] is a third generation formula to determine the power of the implanted IOL. The IOL manufacturers suggest a lens-specific value for the A constant as a starting point for IOL calculation. Despite advances in surgical technique and biometry measurement, the post-operative refraction may deviate from the target refraction. Refinement of the constants of the IOL formulas may help to achieve the targeted refraction [2]-[4]. Olsen showed that incorporating the postoperative IOL position of the first eye improved the prediction accuracy for the second eye [5], and this method served as the basis for further studies [2] [6] [7]. Sheard and colleagues [8] reported that at the extremes of AL and K, the SRK/T was less accurate in calculating the corrected AL and corneal height, leading to inaccuracies in the IOL power prediction. Eom and colleagues showed that using A constants adjusted for corneal power improved refractive outcomes [9].

Authors of modern formulas have recommended many methods for optimizing IOL constants [10]-[12], but there is currently no standard method of optimization. Furthermore, patients with eyes at the extremes of axial length may be underrepresented [3]. This study examines the effect of AL and average preoperative keratometry (K) on the A constant using a large cohort of cataract surgery patients and the Acrysof SN60WF IOL. We developed regression models to optimize the A constant for each eye using its AL and K measurements. Our results suggest the use of these optimized A constants can improve the accuracy of the predicted postoperative refraction.

2. Methods

The Institutional Review Board of Columbia University approved this retrospective study of 635 cataract surgery cases (mean age 75 years, with 172 male eyes and 235 female eyes) with at least three consistent preoperative keratometry measurements and a consistent postoperative refraction. The study excludes patients unable to maintain fixation and those whose corneas were irregular due to conditions such as megalocornea or other congenital abnormalities, scars, dystrophies, or edema, or whose cataracts were too dense for accurate AL measurement with the IOLMaster (Carl Zeiss Meditec AG, Jena, Germany).

The surgeon selected the IOL power based on the preoperative biometry using the SRK/T formula. Keratometry measured with the IOLMaster was compared to manual keratometry, but in all cases the IOL calculation was based on the average keratometry values generated by the IOLMaster. A single surgeon (JCM) performed all procedures with local anesthesia and a temporal 2.2 or 2.6 mm clear corneal incision. The surgeon injected an Acrysof SN60WF (Alcon Laboratories, TX) into the capsule and dilated all patients postoperatively to be certain that both haptics of the IOL were within the capsule. The surgeon refracted all patients and entered the spherical equivalent of the stable postoperative manifest refraction into the IOLMaster's database.

The biometry data for each patient was extracted from the IOLMaster database by Zeiss in Jena, Germany. Using the biometry data and the spherical equivalent of the postoperative manifest refraction, we used the SRK/T formula to back calculate the precise A constant (Ap) for each eye.3 We ran multiple regression analyses to identify three possible models to optimize the A constant based on AL and Kavg 1) as linear variables, 2) AL as a quadratic variable, and 3) AL as a categorical variable with 7 subgroups in 1 mm increments ranging from less than 22 mm to greater than 27 mm. Optimized A constants from each model were used to predict the refractive outcome and the mean absolute error from the achieved refraction for each patient. The extracted data contained measurements from IOLMaster versions 3 and 5. Separate analysis of these two groups showed no significant difference between their Ap (P = 0.91), and the groups were merged for this paper.

Statistical Analysis

Mixed linear models were developed to describe the association between Ap and age, gender, AL, and Kavg. Variables with no significant effect on Ap were removed from the regression models, and SAS PROC MIXED (SAS software version 9.2, SAS Inc., Cary, NC) was used to account for the intra-class correlation between eyes of the same patient and to allow for a random intercept. Results were considered statistically significant if the P value was < 0.05.

3. Results

3.1. The Models to Optimize the A Constant

Table 1 shows Ap, AL, and K for both cohorts. The mean Ap of 119.3 mm is similar to the ULIB value of 119.0

Table 1. The mean, minimum, and maximum values of the data-adjusted precise A constant (Ap), AL, and Kavg.

Variable	Mean + StdDev	Min, Max Maximum	Mean + StdDev	Min, Max
Data Set for Developing Formulas (635 eyes)			Data Set for Validating Formulas (45 eyes)	
Ap (mm)	119.31 ± 0.51	117.44, 122.58	--	--
AL (mm)	24.1 ± 1.37	20.5, 30.0	23.9 ± 1.16	22.2, 27.5
Kavg (mm)	43.7 ± 1.42	39.4, 48.3	44.1 ± 1.48	40.2, 47.1

mm. The Ap almost always differed from the manufacturer's A constant of 118.7 mm. Linear regressions indicate that Ap has a significant correlation with both AL and K ($P < 0.0001$). No correlation is evident between Ap and age ($P = 0.92$). While a statistically significant relationship was also found between gender and the A-constant ($P = 0.005$), AL was highly correlated with gender, so gender provided no additional information to the model. Pearson correlation coefficients showed that AL (correlation coefficient 0.39) has a stronger effect than K (correlation coefficient −0.25) on Ap. AL and K are also inversely correlated with one another (correlation coefficient −0.23) ($P < 0.0001$). **Figure 1** shows the relationship between Ap and the corresponding AL for each eye, and a least squares polynomial regression of the plot suggests that the relationship between the A constant and AL is non-linear ($R^2 = 0.25$).

Regression analysis identified a linear model to describe the relationship between the A constant and both AL and K.

$$A = 119.94 + 0.11AL - 0.077K \tag{1}$$

In the linear model, an AL of 24 mm and K of 43.7 mm yield an optimized A constant of 119.22; and an AL of 27 mm and K of 43.7 m yield an A constant of 119.55.

In contrast, the quadratic model incorporates a quadratic AL term to allow for curvature to improve the fit.

$$A = 150.84 - 2.32AL + 0.049(AL)^2 - 0.096K \tag{2}$$

In the quadratic model, an AL of 24 mm and K of 43.7 mm yield an optimized A constant of 119.19; and an AL of 27 mm and K of 43.7 mm yield an A constant of 119.73.

Finally, the categorical model employs seven AL subgroups as categorical variables (in 1 mm increments from less than 22 mm to greater than 27 mm) with an AL correction factor X that adjusts the A constant for each AL subgroup (**Table 2**). The AL factor X variable is a significant predictor of the A constant ($p < 0.001$)

$$A = 123.93 + ALfactorX - 0.091K \tag{3}$$

In the categorical model, an AL of 24 mm and K of 43.7 mm and an AL factor of −0.64 result in an optimized A constant of 119.31 mm; and an AL of 27 mm and K of 43.7 mm and an AL factor of 0 result in an A constant of 119.95. For the same eye with AL 24 mm and K of 43.7 mm, all three regression models produce similar optimized A's that differ from the manufacturer's A. For eyes with the same AL, a steeper cornea would yield a smaller A value, and vice versa. For example, for eyes with AL of 24 mm and mean K of 42.0 and 47.0 mm, the categorical model yields an A of 119.47 and 119.01, respectively. In summary, both AL and K influence the A constant, which increases with increasing AL and decreasing K. In other words, a larger A is needed for longer eyes with flatter corneas.

3.2. Validating the Models

We used a data set of 45 eyes to evaluate the accuracy of the predicted postoperative refraction with the optimized A constants. With A constants derived from our three models, the ULIB website[1], and the manufacturer, the absolute value of the ME ranged from 0.00 to 1.25 D. The absolute value of the ME decreased from 0.50 D when using the manufacturer's A to 0.25 D when using optimized As from any of the three models. Furthermore, **Figure 2** shows that the optimized A constants decreased the percentage of eyes with positive mean errors, or hyperopia. Using the manufacturer's A constant, 22.2% of the eyes in the validation data set have hyperopic ME

---

[1]http://www.augenklinik.uni-wuerzburg.de/ulib/.

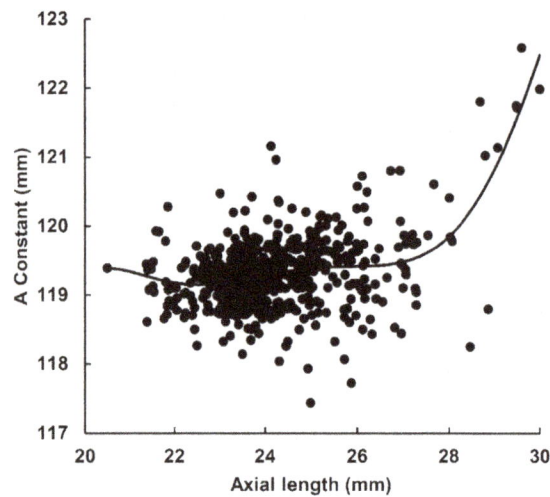

Figure 1. Axial lengths vs. precise A constants (A_p) for each eye. A_p increases with AL, especially with AL > 26 mm. A least squares polynomial regression of the plot illustrates that the relationship between the A_p and AL is non-linear ($R^2 = 0.25$).

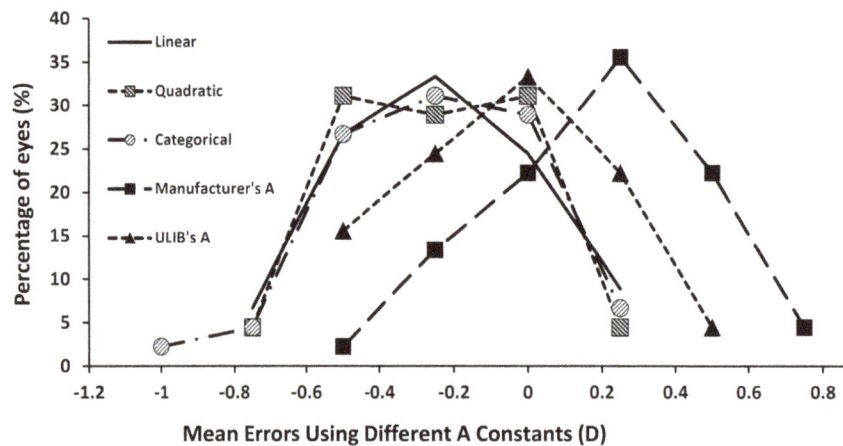

Figure 2. Histogram of mean errors (ME) calculated using A constants from the three models, the manufacturer (118.7), and the User Group for Laser Interference Biometry (ULIB) website (119.0). ME is the difference between the spherical equivalent of the achieved postoperative refraction and the predicted postoperative refraction using optimized and manufacturer's A constants. Optimized A constants from the models decreased the positive refractive or hyperopic errors, as predicted using the manufacturer's A.

Table 2. Correction factor X for the seven AL subgroups of the categorical model.

Axial Length (mm)	Number	X Frequency
<22.0	25	−0.59
22.0 to <23.0	80	−0.70
23.0 to <24.0	260	−0.76
24.0 to <25.0	142	−0.64
25.0 to <26.0	71	−0.57
26.0 and <27.0	32	−0.44
AL ≥ 27.0	25	0

greater than +0.5 D. Using optimized A constants, none of the eyes from the three optimization models had hyperopic MEs greater than +0.5 D.

3.3. Validating

Cataract surgery is a refractive procedure, and suboptimal refractive outcomes may temper patient satisfaction [13]. This study found a statistically significant correlation between AL, K, and the optimized A constant within the SRK/T formula. A single A constant is not optimal for all eyes with different AL and K values. We showed that a larger optimized A constant is needed for eyes with longer AL and flatter corneas. Optimized A in turn reduced the postoperative error and hyperopic outcomes compared to using the manufacturer's A. This is similar to the findings from previous studies that larger A constants may be needed to reduce hyperopic refractive errors [9].

Eom and colleagues examined the relationship between K, AL and predicted refractive error in 637 patients and found that the A constants decreased as K increased, consistent with our results. However, they concluded AL did not have a significant effect on postoperative error [9]. Our method differed, and we specifically evaluated the effect of AL on the optimized A constants, not on refractive errors. We showed that using optimized A constants in turn improved the postoperative refractive error. Our finding that both AL and K are important is consistent with the study by Wang and colleagues, who reported that inaccurate estimation of AL contributes to postoperative refractive error in long eyes >25 mm [14]. They found that optimized AL, sometimes smaller than the measured AL, reduced hyperopic outcomes in long eyes [14].

Clinicians may use the authors' A constants as a point of reference for each AL subgroup in the IOLMaster. A prior study found that optimizing IOL constants for the IOLMaster substantially improved refractive outcomes, far exceeding any additional benefit of personalizing IOL constants for individual surgeons [2]. Although all three regression models substantially improved the predicted refractive errors, the categorical model may be most easily programmed into the IOLMaster by creating AL groups. The optimized A constants in the categorical model were similar to As from the quadratic or linear models, and the A constant at high AL differs from the ULIB website's A constant of 119.0. While the standard interface of the IOLMaster assumes that one will use a single A constant for each IOL, the categorical model creates different As for groups of eyes with different AL, so longer eyes would warrant a larger A than shorter eyes. Once clinicians have amassed a critical number of eyes, they may use a set of A constants specific to their practices. Achieving targeted refractive outcomes is difficult in long eyes, which tend toward postoperative hyperopia [15]-[21]. When AL was measured with ultrasound, postoperative refractive errors were attributed to the inaccurate estimation of AL [14] [16] [18] [22]. After the introduction of more accurate laser interferometry measurements, however, the formula-dependent IOL power calculation is believed to contribute most to the error [22] [23]. All three regression models substantially improved the predicted refractive errors. It is not difficult to calculate an A constant for an individual eye with the quadratic model, but the categorical model may be most easily programmed into the IOLMaster by creating AL groups.

Low myopia after surgery may work as a substitute for accommodation and make patients more spectacle- independent [24] [25]. The manufacturer's A constant tends to produce more hyperopic errors than an optimized A constant [2], and hyperopia is a particularly undesirable outcome [2]. While other causes of postoperative hyperopia include posteriorly angulated IOLs from capsular fibrosis or late capsular bag distension syndrome [26]-[28], our study suggests that the optimized A constants may also reduce postoperative hyperopia.

The range of acceptable error depends on the clinical significance of the refractive error. With a large data base of 8108 eyes, Aristodemou *et al.* analyzed the benefits of IOL constant optimization based on refractive outcomes using manufacturers' and optimized IOL constants for the Hoffer Q, Holladay 1, and SRK/T formulas. They found that an A constant error exceeding 0.15 produced up to a 2.0% reduction in the percentage of eyes within ±0.50 D deviation from target refraction with the SRK/T formula [2]. Using the categorical model, an eye with an axial length of 24.08 mm and K of 43.68 mm has an optimized A constant of 119.32 mm, which is 0.62 greater than the manufacturer's recommended value of 118.7 mm and far exceeds this A constant error limit of 0.15. While the IOLMaster optimizes the A constant using data from 10 or more eyes, as many as 257 eyes may be required to optimize an IOL constant with an error margin of 0.10 [2]. Furthermore, the IOLMaster only generates one A constant for all eyes, while our regression models generate optimized A constants personalized for each eye.

It has been suggested that different IOL formulas may be used for different ALs. Aristodemou compared the

Hoffer Q, Holladay 1, and SRK/T formulas in 8108 eyes. They found that while all three tend to work equally well for medium length eyes, the Hoffer Q performed best in eyes with AL less than 22 mm and the SRK/T in eyes with AL > 27 mm [29]. In a separate study using the same database, Aristodemou also found that optimizing the IOL constant improved the predictability of refraction outcomes more than the choice of third-generation IOL formulas [2]. Nevertheless, for short eyes, the clinician may consider using or comparing the results with the Hoffer Q. This study suggests that surgeons may improve the refractive outcomes using SRK/T formula across AL ranges by considering each eye's AL and K measurements.

Acknowledgements

We would like to thank Stephen DeVience, PhD, for his support.

References

[1]   Retzlaff, J.A., Sanders, D.R. and Kraff, M.C. (1990) Development of the SRK/T Intraocular Lens Implant Power Calculation Formula. *Journal of Cataract & Refractive Surgery*, **16**, 333-340. http://dx.doi.org/10.1016/S0886-3350(13)80705-5

[2]   Aristodemou, P., Knox Cartwright, N.E., Sparrow, J.M. and Johnston, R.L. (2011b) Intraocular Lens Formula Constant Optimization and Partial Coherence Interferometry Biometry: Refractive Outcomes in 8108 Eyes after Cataract Surgery. *Journal of Cataract & Refractive Surgery*, **37**, 50-62. http://dx.doi.org/10.1016/j.jcrs.2010.07.037

[3]   Ladas, J.G. and Stark, W.J. (2011) Improving Cataract Surgery Refractive Outcomes. *Ophthalmology*, **118**, 1699-1700. http://dx.doi.org10.1016/j.ophtha.2011.05.038

[4]   Merriam, J.C., Zheng, L., Merriam, J.E., Zaider, M. and Lindström, B. (2003) The Effect of Incisions for Cataract on Corneal Curvature. *Ophthalmology*, **110**, 1807-1813. http://dx.doi.org10.1016/S0161-6420(03)00537-2

[5]   Olsen, T., Løgstrup, N., Olesen, H. and Corydon, L. (1993) Using the Surgical Result in the First Eye to Calculate Intraocular Lens Power for the Second Eye. *Journal of Cataract & Refractive Surgery*, **19**, 36-39.

[6]   Olsen, T. (2011) Use of Fellow Eye Data in the Calculation of Intraocular Lens Power for the Second Eye. *Ophthalmology*, **118**, 1710-1715. http://dx.doi.org/10.1016/j.ophtha.2011.04.030

[7]   Covert, D.J., Henry, C.R. and Koenig, S.B. (2010) Intraocular Lens Power Selection in the Second Eye of Patients Undergoing Bilateral, Sequential Cataract Extraction. *Ophthalmology*, **117**, 49-54. http://dx.doi.org/10.1016/j.ophtha.2009.06.020

[8]   Sheard, R.M., Smith, G.T. and Cooke, D.L. (2010) Improving the Prediction Accuracy of the SRK/T Formula: The T2 Formula. *Journal of Cataract & Refractive Surgery*, **36**, 1829-1834. http://dx.doi.org/10.1016/j.jcrs.2010.05.031

[9]   Eom, Y., Kang, S.Y., Song, J.S. and Kim, H.M. (2013) Use of Corneal Power-Specific Constants to Improve the Accuracy of the SRK/T Formula. *Ophthalmology*, **120**, 477-481. http://dx.doi.org/10.1016/j.ophtha.2012.09.008

[10] Hoffer, K.J. (1993) The Hoffer Q Formula: A Comparison of Theoretic and Regression Formulas. *Journal of Cataract & Refractive Surgery*, **19**, 700-712. http://dx.doi.org/10.1016/S0886-3350(13)80338-0

[11] Holladay, J.T. (1997) Standardizing Constants for Ultrasonic Biometry, Keratometry, and Intraocular Lens Power Calculations. *Journal of Cataract & Refractive Surgery*, **23**, 1356-1370. http://dx.doi.org/10.1016/S0886-3350(97)80115-0

[12] Petermeier, K., Gekeler, F., Messias, A., Spitzer, M.S., Haigis, W., and Szurman, P. (2009) Intraocular Lens Power Calculation and Optimized Constants for Highly Myopic Eyes. *Journal of Cataract and Refractive Surgery*, **35**, 1575-1581. http://dx.doi.org/10.1016/j.jcrs.2009.04.028

[13] MacLaren, R.E., Natkunarajah, M., Riaz, Y., Bourne, R.R., Restori, M. and Allan, B.D. (2007) Biometry and Formula Accuracy with Intraocular Lenses Used for Cataract Surgery in Extreme Hyperopia. *American Journal of Ophthalmology*, **143**, 920-931. http://dx.doi.org/10.1016/j.ajo.2007.02.043

[14] Wang, L., Shirayama, M., Ma, X.J., Kohnen, T. and Koch, D.D. (2011) Optimizing Intraocular Lens Power Calculations in Eyes with Axial Lengths above 25.0 mm. *Journal of Cataract & Refractive Surgery*, **37**, 2018-2027. http://dx.doi.org/10.1016/j.jcrs.2011.05.042

[15] Fechner, P.U., Kania, J. and Kienzle, S. (1988) The Value of a Zero Power Intraocular Lens. *Journal of Cataract & Refractive Surgery*, **14**, 436-440. http://dx.doi.org/10.1016/S0886-3350(88)80155-X

[16] Kora, Y., Koike, M., Suzuki, Y., Inatomi, M., Fukado, Y. and Ozawa, T. (1991) Errors in IOL Power Calculations for Axial High Myopia. *Ophthalmic Surgery*, **22**, 78-81.

[17] Kohnen, S. and Brauweiler, P. (1996) First Results of Cataract Surgery and Implantation of Negative Power Intraocular Lenses in Highly Myopic Eyes. *Journal of Cataract & Refractive Surgery*, **22**, 416-420.

http://dx.doi.org/10.1016/S0886-3350(96)80035-6

[18] Zaldivar, R., Shultz, M.C., Davidorf, J.M. and Holladay, J.T. (2000) Intraocular Lens Power Calculations in Patients with Extreme Myopia. *Journal of Cataract and Refractive Surgery*, **26**, 668-674. http://dx.doi.org/10.1016/S0886-3350(00)00367-9

[19] Tsang, C.S., Chong, G.S., Yiu, E.P. and Ho, C.K. (2003). Intraocular Lens Power Calculation Formulas in Chinese Eyes with High Axial Myopia. *Journal of Cataract & Refractive Surgery*, **29**, 1358-1364. http://dx.doi.org/10.1016/S0886-3350(02)01976-4

[20] MacLaren, R.E., Sagoo, M.S., Restori, M. and Allan, B.D. (2005) Biometry Accuracy Using Zero- and Negative-Powered Intraocular Lenses. *Journal of Cataract & Refractive Surgery*, **31**, 280-290. http://dx.doi.org/10.1016/j.jcrs.2004.04.054

[21] Pomberg, M.L. and Miller, K.M. (2005) Preliminary Efficacy and Safety of Zero Diopter Lens Implantation in Highly Myopic Eyes. *American Journal of Ophthalmology*, **139**, 914-915. http://dx.doi.org/10.1016/j.ajo.2004.11.031

[22] Olsen, T. (2012) Intraocular Lens Power Calculation Errors in Long Eyes. *Journal of Cataract & Refractive Surgery*, **38**, 733-734. http://dx.doi.org/10.1016/j.jcrs.2012.02.003

[23] Norrby, S. (2008) Sources of Error in Intraocular Lens Power Calculation. *Journal of Cataract & Refractive Surgery*, **34**, 368-376. http://dx.doi.org/10.1016/j.jcrs.2007.10.031

[24] Elder, M.J., Murphy, C. and Sanderson, G.F. (1996) Apparent Accommodation and Depth of Field in Pseudophakia. *Journal of Cataract & Refractive Surgery*, **22**, 615-619. http://dx.doi.org/10.1016/S0886-3350(96)80020-4

[25] Datiles, M.B. and Gancayco, T. (1990) Low Myopia with Low Astigmatic Correction Gives Cataract Surgery Patients Good Depth of Focus. *Ophthalmology*, **97**, 922-926. http://dx.doi.org/10.1016/S0161-6420(90)32480-6

[26] Nishi, O., Nishi, K. and Takahashi, E. (1998) Capsular Bag Distention Syndrome Noted 5 Years after Intraocular Lens Implantation. *American Journal of Ophthalmology*, **125**, 545-547. http://dx.doi.org/10.1016/S0002-9394(99)80195-0

[27] Wendrix, G. and Zeyen, T. (2006) Late-Onset Capsular Bag Distention Syndrome after Cataract Surgery: 2 Case-Reports. *Bulletin of the Belgian Society of Ophthalmology*, **30**, 67-69.

[28] Davison, J.A. (1993) Capsule Contraction Syndrome. *Journal of Cataract & Refractive Surgery*, **19**, 582-589. http://dx.doi.org/10.1016/S0886-3350(13)80004-1

[29] Aristodemou, P., Knox Cartwright, N.E., Sparrow, J.M. and Johnston, R.L. (2011) Formula Choice: Hoffer Q, Holladay 1, or SRK/T and Refractive Outcomes in 8108 Eyes after Cataract Surgery with Biometry by Partial Coherence Interferometry. *Journal of Cataract & Refractive Surgery*, **37**, 63-71. http://dx.doi.org/10.1016/j.jcrs.2010.07.032

7

The Corneal Endothelium in Children after Congenital Cataract Surgery—A Comparison of Pre- and Post-Operative Results

Ewa Porwik, Erita Filipek, Maria Formińska-Kapuścik

Ophthalmology Clinic and Department of Ophthalmology, School of Medicine in Katowice, Medical University of Silesia in Katowice, Katowice, Poland
Email: porwikewa@gmail.com

Abstract

Three months after surgery, the research group showed significantly statistical improvement in visual acuity, a statistically significant decrease in corneal endothelial cell density, a statistically significant increase in the percentage of 5 and 8 sided cells and a statistically significant decrease in the percentage of six sided cells. Central corneal thickness and the percentage of 4 and 7 and more than 8 sided did not change in a statistically significant way. Comparing the test group and control group, no statistically significant differences were detected in the examined parameters. The present study also shows that the cornea in the eyes with congenital cataract does not show statistically significant changes in the density and the morphology of the corneal endothelial cells and the thickness of the cornea and in terms of corneal thickness in comparison to the corneas of healthy eyes. Although in corneas undergoing cataract occurs statistically significant changes, the influence of the cornea does not affect the improvement in visual acuity which was also demonstrated in this study.

Keywords

Congenital Cataract Surgery, Corneal Endothelial Cells, Pleomorphism, Polimegatism

1. Introduction

The main function of the corneal endothelium is to maintain proper corneal hydration, thus ensuring transparency of the cornea through the activity of an ion pump which, in turn, is controlled by the endothelial cells' Na^+/K^+ ATP-asa. If there is a $500/mm^2$ loss in corneal endothelial density, the pump's endothelial cells are impaired, leading to corneal decompensation, haziness, and a resulting deterioration of the subject's vision. The cornea's endothelium has two primary functions: a barrier that permits a flow of dissolved nutrients and metabolites between the aqueous humor and the corneal stroma, and as a pump to maintain the correct tension of the cornea. The proper functioning of this pump ensures a translucent cornea. Changes in the quantitative and qualitative composition of the cornea's endothelium provide information about its operation. Many factors influence the corneal endothelium. These include systemic diseases such as diabetes, trauma, and the aging process. The corneal endothelium's fundamental characteristic is its endothelial cell density. This measurement can be supplemented by two additional evaluations: the endothelium's pleomorphism and its polimegatysm. Pleomorphism is an indicator of endothelial cell shape; polimegatysm is an indicator of the size of the endothelial cells. Using a microscope, endothelial abnormalities can be identified in a corneal endothelium's morphology. The corneal endothelium, consisting of hexagonal or hexagonal-like cells, is the cornea's single innermost mosaic. Doughty [1] observed that, these cells comprised around 60% of the cornea's cells; the remainder of them were exclusively four, five, seven or eight-sided cells [1]. Upon any loss of the normal hexagonal cells, the surrounding cells must then change their hexagonal shape, extending themselves to compensate for the endothelium's deficiencies caused by this cell loss. This results in an endothelium with a reduced number of properly hexagonal cells and an increased number of pleomorphic cells.

There are many factors that affect the corneal endothelium. Nucci *et al.*, Koraszewska-Matuszewska and Dong observed that the primary factor was the subject's age [2]-[4]. The current literature presents a fairly wide range for standard endothelial cell density, from 3000 to 7500 cells per mm^2. Following the first years of life, a sharp drop in the number of endothelial cells is observed, which is explained by the intensive growth of the eyeball during this time. It has been assumed by Nucci that, during the first year of life, the number of corneal endothelial cells reduces by 45% with the endothelial cell density falling to approximately 2700/mm^2 by the age of five years [2]. According to Koraszewska-Matuszewska from the age of 18 years onwards there is a corneal endothelial cell loss of 0.5% per year [3]. Bourne & McLaren observed that cell polimegatism increased with age, with the number of normal hexagonal cells decreasing [5]. While multiple publications have assessed age-related changes in corneal endothelial cell density, not one scientific report available has looked at changes in endothelial cell morphology such as the cells' size and their shape. It has been accepted that endothelial pump activity decreases with age, even though the process of endothelial cell loss has not yet been fully elucidated. Some authors, Cho, Rieck, and Wetson, have described the processes of induced apoptosis which could influence this aforementioned decrease [6]-[8]. The processes involved in release apoptosis in the human cornea were not fully understood, but Rieck considered that these may be a result of metabolic changes, mechanical stress, endotoxins, the loss of protective factors, or nutrient deprivations [7]. It has been described by Wetson how pro-inflammatory cytokines can cause corneal endothelial apoptosis [8]. In addition, many intracellular proteins are involved in either the induction, or the prevention, of apoptosis [8]. The corneal endothelium is affected by associated diseases such as glaucoma or inflammatory process in the anterior segment of the eye. It has been proven by Larsson that elevated intraocular pressure damages the corneal endothelium if it lasts for longer than three days [9]. The corneal endothelium is also affected by the wearing of contact lenses. Contact lenses worn for long periods of time alter the endothelium's morphology. Specular microscope studies have shown an increased polimegatism and polymorphism of endothelial cells, after the wearing of contact lenses. However, these changes were not observed by Cho to affect endothelial cell function or density [6]. Any trauma that disrupts the entire structure of the cornea is another factor that would influence the corneal endothelium. General diseases are another cause that affects the corneal endothelium, with the best-known general illness of this type being diabetes. While diabetes does not affect the density of the endothelial cells, it has been proven by Wetson and Larsson that it does cause an increase in corneal thickness and changes in endothelial cell morphologic characteristics [8] [9]. During surgery, any corneal rupture changes both the morphology and the density of endothelial cells. One example, cataract surgery, causes some endothelial cell loss, the extent of which is difficult to estimate prior to the surgery. Abnormalities in the density or morphology of endothelial cells prior to cataract surgery increase the risk of postoperative corneal decompensation. Such outcomes should be the subject of more extensive investigations.

Previous research has examined neither the distribution of corneal endothelial cells of different shapes in healthy corneas, nor if in some way this distribution differs from the endothelial cell distribution found in eyes with cataracts. The purpose of this paper is to present the distribution of different shapes of endothelial cells in the corneas of healthy eyes, in the corneas of those eyes with cataracts, and to compare the primary parameters of these two eye populations. In addition, this study seeks to compare preoperative with postoperative corneal parameters following surgery for congenital cataracts.

2. Patients and Methods

The research group consists of 31 eyes of 26 children (16 girls and 10 boys) aged 3 - 17 (mean age 8.46) with congenital cataracts. Unilateral cataract was observed in 21 children and bilateral cataract was observed in 5 children. Procedures were carried out in the years 2011-2013 in the Department of Pediatric Ophthalmology in Katowice. All children underwent cataract surgery by facoaspiration with simultaneous implanting an artificial intraocular lens foldable acrylic in the capsular bag. All patients were implanted with acrylic lens of the same model. Opacified lens was removed by irrigation and aspiration after a circular cut-out of the anterior capsule of the lens. The artificial lens was implanted into the capsular bag. In children under five years of age additional recess in the central portion of the posterior capsule of the lens was made and the cut out front of the vitreous body through this opening. Each patient enrolled in the study underwent, with their parents, a detailed interview. The following measurements were also collected: visual acuity at distance checked through the use of Snellen charts; the front section of each eye was examined using a slit lamp; and an endothelial microscope was used to collect the primary research parameters (polimegatism and pleomorphism). The studies used a microscope endothelial MOD SP-02 CSO (Costruzione Strumenti Oftalmici). These measurements were carried out one day before and three months after surgery undertaken to remove the lens and implant an artificial intraocular lens. The control group were children once tested before surgery—21 non-operated, healthy associated eyes in 21 children aged 3 to 17 years old children with unilateral cataracts (mean age 8.60).

The criteria for inclusion:
- congenital cataracts;
- aged younger than 18 years.

The criteria for exclusion:
- patients with a history of, or currently active, inflammatory process within the eyeball (with the exception of conjunctivitis);
- patients wearing contact lenses;
- patients with a history of surgery;
- patients with associated ocular diseases;
- patients with general diseases;
- patients with ocular trauma.

3. Results

Comparing the test group and the control group, no statistically significant differences were detected in the examined measurable properties. The pleomorphism seen in the test group and in the control group exhibited no statistically significant differences (**Table 1**, **Table 2**, **Figure 1**, **Table 3**).

Three months following the surgery, the research group showed a statistically significant improvement in visual acuity, a statistically significant increase in the percentage of five and eight-sided cells, a statistically significant decrease in the percentage of six sided cells and a statistically significant decrease in corneal endothelial

Table 1. Comparison of endothelial cells with specific number of sides in children in control group and in the analyzed group before operation.

Cell sides	Control group	Analyzed group before operation	p
4	1.428	1.937	0.340
5	17.5	17.656	0.979
6	61	59.750	0.685
7	18.142	18.656	0.667
8	1.523	2.000	0.465
8 + n	0.095	0.031	0.333

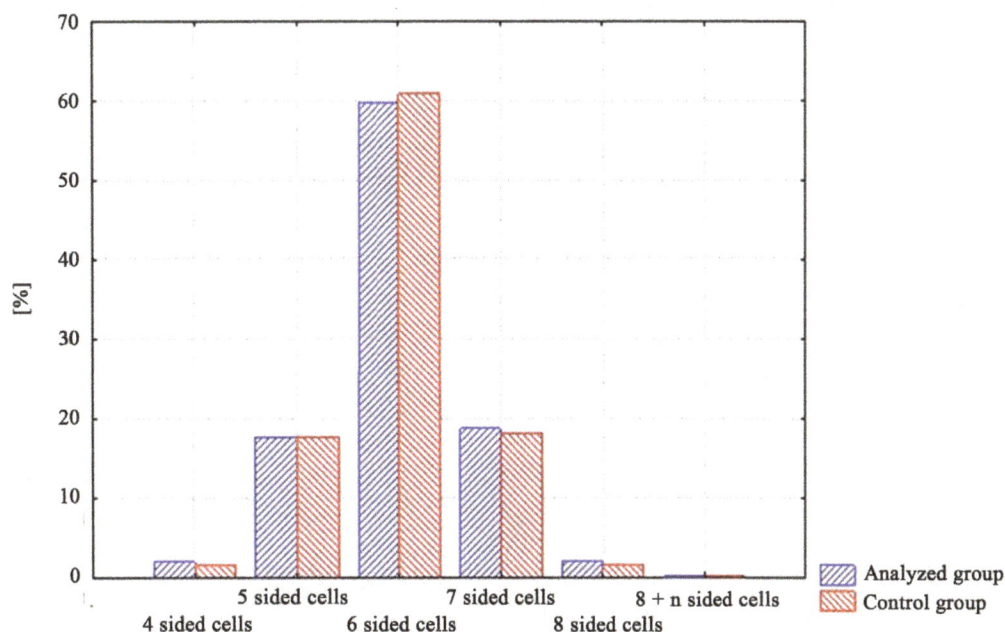

Figure 1. The proportion of endothelial cells with a specific number of sides in children in control and in the analyzed group.

Table 2. Standard deviation in evaluated parameters in control and analyzed group.

Parameter	Standard deviation (analyzed group)	Standard deviation (control group)
A4	2.16	1.86
A5	4.20	5.48
A6	7.43	11.30
A7	4.00	4.24
A8	2.80	2.58
A8 + n	0.18	0.18

Table 3. Comparison of endothelial cell density and central corneal thickness between control and analyzed group before operation.

Parameter	Analyzed group before operation	Control group	p	Significance
Endothelial cell density (cell/mm^2)	3,071,226	3200.571	0.379	NS
Central corneal thickness (μm^2)	590,096	605.714	0.176	NS

NS: statistically non significant, S: statistically significant.

cell density. Amongst the other measurable properties observed, the central corneal thickness and the percentage of four, seven, and more than eight-sided cells did not change in a statistically significant way (**Table 4**, **Figure 2**, **Table 5**, **Figure 3**, **Table 6**).

4. Discussion

The basic measurable property providing information about the outcome of cataract surgery is visual acuity. The results obtained from our investigation are in accordance with those found in the international literature; that is,

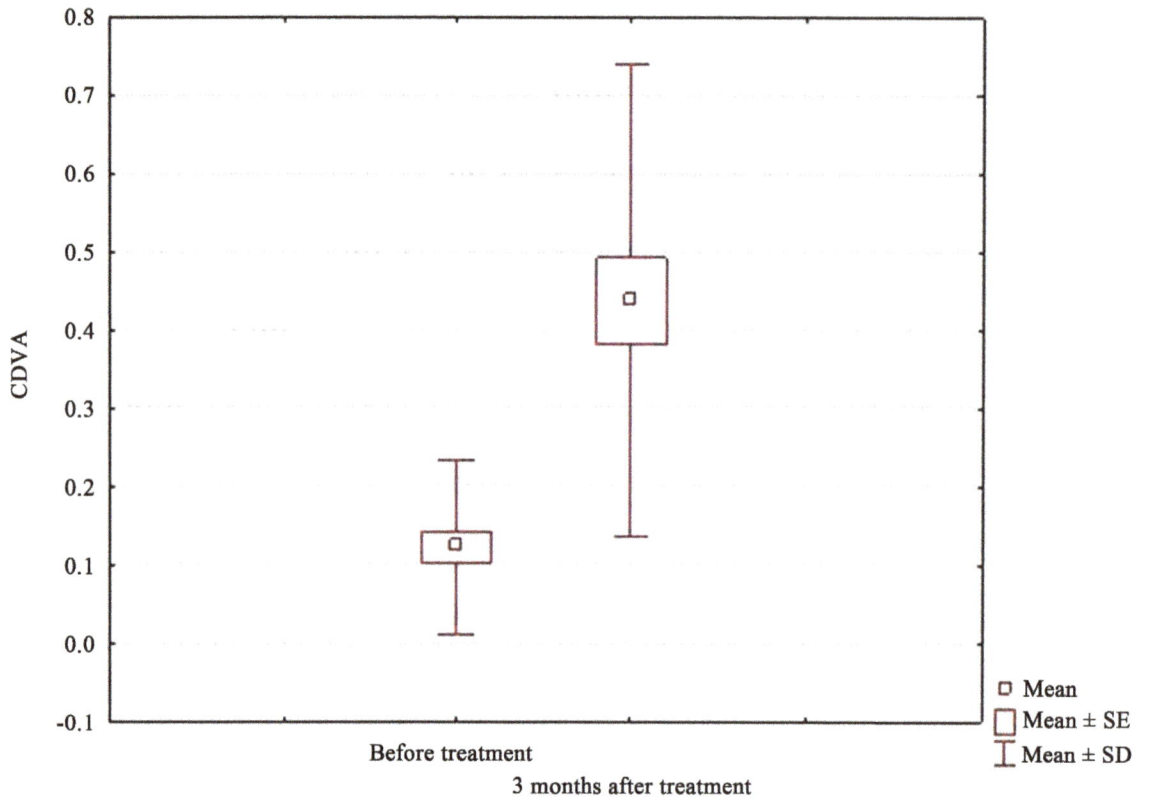

Figure 2. Comparison of corrected distance visual acuity before and 3 months after treatment in analyzed group.

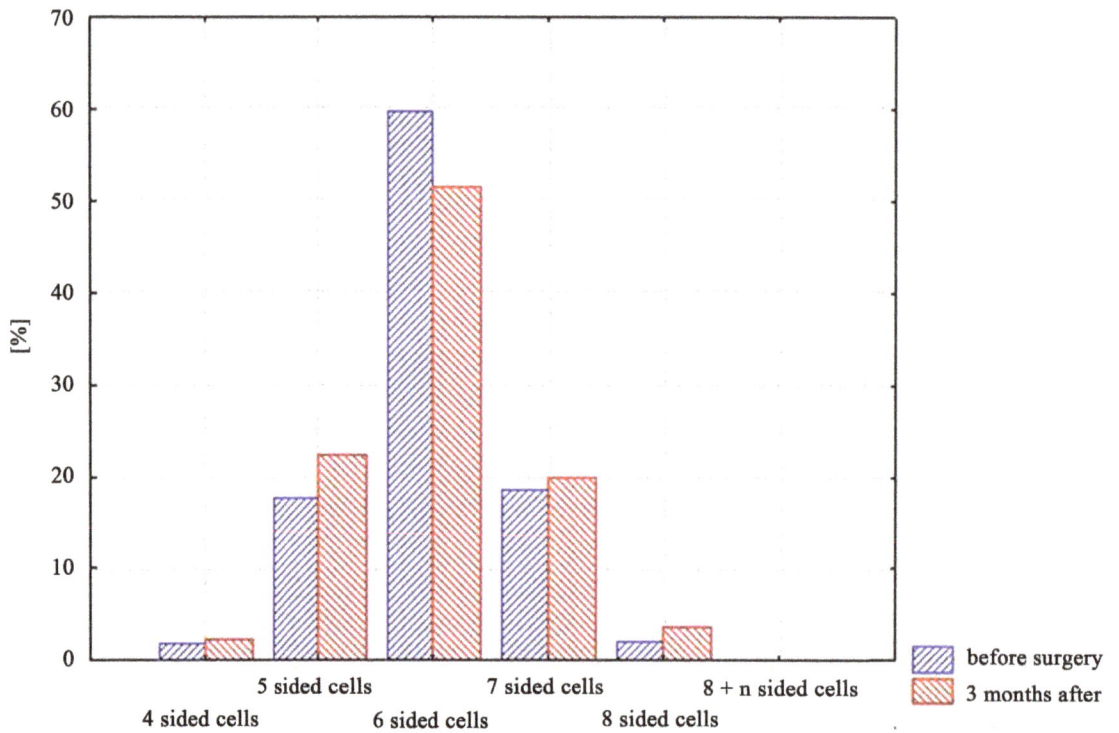

Figure 3. The proportion of endothelial cells with a specific number of sides in children before and 3 months after cataract surgery.

Table 4. Mean value of corrected distance visual acuity before and 3 months after treatment in analyzed group.

CDVA	Mean	p
Before treatment	0.1	p < 0.05
3 months after	0.4	

Table 5. Comparison of endothelial cells with a specific numbers of sides in children before and 3 months after treatment.

Cell sides	Analyzed group before treatment	Analyzed group 3 months after treatment	p
4	1.937	2.343	0.49
5	17.656	22.406	p < 0.05
6	59.750	51.531	p < 0.05
7	18.656	19.937	0.10
8	2.000	3.718	p < 0.05
8 + n	0.031	0.031	1.00

Table 6. Changes in three evaluated parameters before and 3 months after treatment in analyzed group.

Parameter	Analyzed group before treatment	Analyzed group 3 months after treatment	p	Significance
Endothelial cell density (cell/mm^2)	3071.226	2685.839	<0.05	S
Central corneal thickness (μm^2)	590.096	592.6129	0.834	NS

NS: statistically non significant, S: statistically significant.

in studies conducted by other researchers, the visual acuity was of a similar level as the visual acuity observed in our study. For example, for patients with traumatic and congenital cataracts, Bakunowicz-Łazarczyk gave a postoperative visual acuity in the range 0.1 - 0.4 in 65% of patients [10]. Brady studied children with bilateral cataract development and those with unilateral congenital or developmental cataracts [11]. All the children with bilateral cataracts had postoperative visual acuity of 0.5 or better. In children with unilateral cataracts, visual acuity was 0.1 - 0.5. Leurence reported that when examining children in whom an artificial posterior chamber lens had been implanted following a traumatic or congenital cataract, 90% of this sample achieved a visual acuity 0.3 [12]. Spierer studied 50 eyes of children with congenital cataract and found that postoperative visual acuity was 0.5 or better in one third of their patients [13]. Yao studied 27 eyes of children with congenital cataracts, finding that in all of these eyes the visual acuity after 10 months was 0.5 [14]. Filipek has noted that when 80 eyes of children were examined following developmental cataracts and the implantation of a posterior chamber foldable intraocular lens, the visual acuity achieved in all of these eyes was 0.6 [15]. Their observation period was, on average, 3.6 years. Filipek also present the results of tests on 105 eyes operated on due to developmental cataracts (the follow-up time here was 4.2 years), finding that the average visual acuity in children operated on due to unilateral cataracts was 0.3, while in children operated on due to bilateral cataracts it was 0.6 [16]. In the subsequent publication, Filipek wrote that 33 eyes operated on due to congenital cataracts (a mean follow-up time of 36.3 months), a visual acuity of 0.1 was achieved for those previously with unilateral cataracts cases, 0.2 for those formerly with bilateral cataracts [17]. The corneal endothelium is primarily responsible for the maintenance of normal turgor and transparency in the cornea. Thus, the endothelial condition should be evaluated *in vivo* both before and after surgery. Cell density is a good indicator of the endothelial state. It was proven by Szalai and Bourne that conducting research using an endothelial microscope allows for the detection of clinically normal corneas, the detection of small changes and of the pathological changes also seen in clinical examinations [18] [19]. To date there has been only a very small number of reports providing information on the loss of endothelial cells in children. All authors agree that the greatest loss of endothelial cells occurs in the early postoperative period (on a timescale of weeks); the existence of a corneal endothelium stabilization period remains controversial Liesang & Bourne and Galin & Lin hold that it is 3 months after surgery, Olsen 6 months after surgery and Mrzygłód hold the view that one year [20]-[23]. A large loss of endothelial cells has been associated with the material from which the lenses have been made. As medical science has developed, the material from which lens are constructed has improved, leading to better clinical results. According to the data provided by Urban, endothelial cell loss in children following cataract surgery with facoaspiration and artificial lens implantation was 10.94% after one month and 17.85% after six months [24]. According to a recent study by Vasavada three months after cataract surgery with simultaneous implantation of a lens, the corneal endothelial cell loss was 5.1% in children [25]. Basti have indicated that endothelial cell loss following extracapsular cataract surgery in children ranged from 5.28% to 7.50% during observation periods of 24 - 36 weeks [26]. According to Koraszewska-Matuszewska the average loss of endothelial cells in children six months after extracapsular congenital cataract surgery ranged from 8% to 27.8% (the mean loss was 11.2%) [3]. Most of the available research refers to changes in the corneal thickness seen in adults following cataract phacoemulsification surgery and intraocular lens implantation. The results obtained by this paper's authors: Hengerer and Lundberg are consistent with those observed elsewhere, in that they confirm that in the postoperative period there is an increase in the central corneal thickness (of around 6% to 15%) [27] [28]. There are, however, very few scientific reports that compare central corneal thickness before and after surgery for congenital cataracts accompanied by the implantation of an intraocular lens. Faramazi analyzed corneal thickness in 32 pseudophakic eyes and 15 aphakic eyes [29]. The tests were performed one month and six months after the operation. The average thickness of the cornea before surgery in the pseudophakic group of children was 540 ± 34; a month after surgery it was 587 ± 65. Six months after the procedure there was a return to pre-surgery levels, with central corneal thickness being found to be 540 ± 36. These changes were not statistically significant. Vasavada studied 100 eyes of children with congenital cataracts [25]. The central corneal thickness was measured before cataract surgery, after the implantation of an artificial lens, and three months following the surgery. Before surgery, the mean central corneal thickness was 529 ± 30; three months after surgery it was 527 ± 34. These changes were also not statistically significant. Pleomorphism is an indicator of the shape of the corneal endothelial cells. Polimegatism is an indicator of the size of the corneal endothelial cells. Polimegatism and pleomorphism are both measures that can be used to assess physiological imbalance or dysfunction in a cornea's endothelium. To date, the reported research has looked at changes in the hexagonal cells that are considered to form the physiological corneal endothelium. A high percentage of hexagonal cells has been used as an indicator of a healthy corneal endothelium. Vasavada have reported that the percentage of hexagonal cells dropped from 58.1 to 48.6 three months subsequent to congenital cataract surgery while, according to Basti this decrease is from 65.13% to 57.75% [25] [26]. The results obtained from our research are very similar to those presented here. However, no prior publication has described the changes seen in the shape of all of the cells that comprise the corneal endothelium. Also, none of the publications presented here has described changes in the size of the cells that comprise the corneal endothelium.

5. Conclusion

The above data indicate that the most sensitive evaluative parameters that can provide information about changes in the state of the cornea are the proportion of five-sided cells, the proportion of six-sided cells and changes in endothelial cell density. Eight-sided cells also serve as a sensitive indicator of the changes undergone by a cornea that has been subjected to surgery. Here, these indicators have neither been specifically studied nor described. The present study also demonstrates that in eyes with congenital cataracts, the cornea does not show any statistically significant change in the density or morphology of its corneal endothelial cells, nor in the cornea's thickness in comparison to healthy eyes' corneas. While, in corneas undergoing cataract surgery, there are statistically significant changes, the cornea does not appear to affect the improvement that is observed in visual acuity, an improvement that is also statistically significant as demonstrated in this study. This suggests that, in children, cataract surgery utilizing irrigation and aspiration is safe.

References

[1]   Douhty, M.J. (1998) Prevalence of "Non-Hexagonal" Cells in the Corneal Endothelium of Young Caucasian Adults, and Their Inter-Relationships. *Ophthalmic and Physiological Optics*, **18**, 415-422. http://dx.doi.org/10.1046/j.1475-1313.1998.00376.x

[2]   Nucci, P., Brancato, R., Mets, M.B. and Shevell, S.K. (1990) Normal Endothelial Cell Density Range in Childhood. *Archives of Ophthalmology*, **108**, 247-248. http://dx.doi.org/10.1001/archopht.1990.01070040099039

[3]   Koraszewska-Matuszewska, B., Samochowiec-Donocik, E., Papież, M., Filipek, E. and Bolek, S. (1992) Examination of Corneal Endothelium after Cataract Extraction in Children. *Klinika Oczna*, **94**, 338-340.

[4]   Dong, X.G. (1993) An Evaluation of Corneal Endothelial Damage Following Intraocular Lens Implantation. *Chinese Journal of Ophthalmology*, **29**, 346-348.

[5]   Bourne, W. and McLaren, J.W. (2004) Clinical Responses of the Corneal Endothelium. *Experimental Eye Research*, **78**, 561-572. http://dx.doi.org/10.1016/j.exer.2003.08.002

[6]   Cho, K.S., Lee, E.H., Choi, J.S. and Joo, C.K. (1999) Reactive Oxygen Species-Induced Apoptosis and Necrosis in Bovine Corneal Endothelial Cells. *Investigative Ophthalmology and Visual Science*, **40**, 911-919.

[7]   Rieck, P.W., Gigon, M., Jaroszewski, J., Pleyer, U. and Hartmann, C. (2003) Increased Endothelial Survival of Organ-Cultured Corneas Stored in FGF-2-Supplemented Serum-Free Medium. *Investigative Ophthalmology and Visual Science*, **44**, 3826-3832. http://dx.doi.org/10.1167/iovs.02-0601

[8]   Wetson, B.C., Bourne, W.M., Polse, K.A. and Hodge, D.O. (1995) Corneal Hydration Control in Diabetes Mellitus. *Investigative Ophthalmology and Visual Science*, **36**, 586-595.

[9]   Larsson, L.I., Bourne, W.M., Pach, J.M. and Brubaker, R.F. (1996) Structure and Function of the Corneal Endothelium in Diabetes Mellitus Type I and Type II. *Archives of Ophthalmology*, **114**, 9-14. http://dx.doi.org/10.1001/archopht.1996.01100130007001

[10] Bakunowicz-Łazarczyk, A., Stankiewicz, A., Urban, B. and Średzińska-Kita, D. (1996) Wyniki operacji zaćmy z wszczepieniem sztucznej soczewki u dzieci i młodzieży w latach 1990-1995 (materiał własny). *Klinika Oczna*, **98**, 295-297.

[11] Brady, K.M., Atkinskon, C.S., Kilty, L.A. and Hiles, D.A. (1995) Cataract Surgery and Intraocular Lens Implantation in Children. *American Journal of Ophthalmology*, **120**, 1-9.

[12] Leurence, C.L., Arne, J.L., Chapotot, E.C., Thouvenin, D. and Malecaze, F. (1998) Visual Outcome after Paediatric Cataract Surgery: Is Age a Major Factor? *British Journal of Ophthalmology*, **82**, 1022-1025. http://dx.doi.org/10.1136/bjo.82.9.1022

[13] Spierer, A., Desatnik, H., Rosner, M. and Blumenthal, M. (1998) Congenital Cataract Surgery in Children with Cataract as an Isolated Defect and in Children with Systemic Syndrome: A Comparative Study. *Journal of Pediatric Ophthalmology and Strabismus*, **35**, 281-285.

[14] Yao, Z., Xie, L., Huang, Y. and Wang, Z. (2002) Preliminary Results of Foldable Intraocular Lens Implantation in Children with Cataract. *Chinese Journal of Ophthalmology*, **38**, 488-490.

[15] Filipek, E., Formińska-Kapuścik, M., Nawrocka, L., Mrukwa-Kominek, E. and Pieczara, E. (2008) Ocena czynności oczu u dzieci i młodzieży po operacji zaćmy rozwojowej i pierwotnym wszczepieniu zwijalnej tylno komorowej soczewki wewnątrzgałkowej. *Okulistyka*, **4**, 29-32.

[16] Filipek, E., Formińska-Kapuścik, M., Nawrocka, L., Pieczara, E. and Domańska, O. (2006) Intraocular Lens Implantation after Congenital Cataract Extraction Infants and Small Children. *Polish Journal of Environmental Studies*, **15**, 73-77.

[17] Filipek, E., Formińska-Kapuścik, M., Nawrocka, L., Samochowiec-Donocik, E. and Pieczara, E. (2006) Visual Acuity and Amblyopia in Pseudophakic Children after Developmental Cataract Surgery. *Polish Journal of Environmental Studies*, **15**, 65-69.

[18] Szalai, E., Nemeth, G., Berta, A. and Modis Jr., L. (2011) Evaluation of the Corneal Endothelium Using Noncontact and Contact Specular Microscopy. *Cornea*, **30**, 567-570.

[19] Bourne, W.M. and Kaufman, H.E. (1976) Specular Microscopy of Human Corneal Endothelium *in Vivo*. *American Journal of Ophthalmology*, **81**, 319-323. http://dx.doi.org/10.1016/0002-9394(76)90247-6

[20] Liesegang, T.J., Bourne, W.M. and Ilstrup, D.M. (1984) Short- and Long-Term Endothelial Cell Loss Associated with Cataract Extraction and Intraocular Lens Implantation. *American Journal of Ophthalmology*, **97**, 32-39.

[21] Galin, M.A., Lin, L.L., Fetherolf, E., Obstbaum, S.A. and Sugar, A. (1979) Time Analysis of Corneal Endothelial Cell Density after Cataract Extraction. *American Journal of Ophthalmology*, **88**, 93-96.

[22] Olsen, T. (1980) Corneal Thickness and Endothelial Damage after Intracapsular Cataract Extraction. *Acta Ophthalmologica*, **58**, 424-433.

[23] Mrzygłód, S. and Warczyński, A. (1985) Examination of Corneal Endothelium by a Specular Microscope. I. The Types of Microscopes. *Klinika Oczna*, **87**, 23-24.

[24] Urban, B., Bakunowicz-Łazarczyk, A. and Krętowska, M. (2005) Ocena śródbłonka rogówki po operacjach usunięcia zaćmy u dzieci i młodzieży. *Klinika Oczna*, **107**, 43-45.

[25] Vasavada, A.R., Praveen, M.R., Vasavada, V.A., Shah, S.K., Vasavada, V. and Trivedi, R.H. (2012) Corneal Endothelial Morphologic Assessment in Pediatric Cataract Surgery with Intraocular Lens Implantation: A Comparison of Preoperative and Early Postoperative Specular Microscopy. *American Journal of Ophthalmology*, **154**, 259-265.

http://dx.doi.org/10.1016/j.ajo.2012.02.018

[26]   Basti, S., Aasuri, M.K., Reddy, S. and Raon, G.N. (1998) Prospective Evaluation of Corneal Endothelial Cell Loss af-
       ter Pediatric Cataract Surgery. *Journal of Cataract & Refractive Surgery*, **24**, 1496-1473.
       http://dx.doi.org/10.1016/S0886-3350(98)80168-5

[27]   Hengerer, F.H., Dick, H.B., Buchwald, S., Hutz, W.W. and Conrad-Hengerer, I. (2011) Evaluation of Corneal Cell
       Loss and Corneal Thickness after Cataract Removal with Light-Adjustable Intraocular Lens Implantation: 12 Month
       Follow-Up. *Journal of Cataract Refractive Surgery*, **37**, 2095-2100.

[28]   Lundberg, B., Jonsson, M. and Behndig, A. (2005) Postoperative Corneal Swelling Correlates Strongly to Corneal En-
       dothelial Cell Loss after Phacoemulsification Cataract Surgery. *American Journal of Ophthalmology*, **139**, 1035-1041.
       http://dx.doi.org/10.1016/j.ajo.2004.12.080

[29]   Faramazi, A., Javadi, M.A., Bonyadi, M.H.J. and Yaseri, M. (2010) Changes in Central Corneal Thickness after Con-
       genital Cataract Surgery. *Journal of Cataract & Refractive Surgery*, **36**, 2041-2047.
       http://dx.doi.org/10.1016/j.jcrs.2010.07.016

8

Toric Intraocular Lens Malposition Corrected by Lens Repositioning to Manifest Refractive Cylinder Axis in Patient with Irregular Astigmatism Due to Corneal Scar

Riley Sanders[1,2], Johnny Gayton[1,2]

[1]Mercer University School of Medicine, Macon, USA
[2]Eyesight Associates, Warner Robins, USA
Email: sanders_r@med.mercer.edu

Abstract

A case is presented of a patient with an unexpected poor visual result and subsequent correction following cataract removal surgery via phacoemulsification and intraocular lens implantation using a toric intraocular lens implant (IOL). The initial operation resulted in an uncorrected vision of 20/100 (0.70 logMAR). Retrospective analysis of the patient's corneal topography revealed irregular astigmatism secondary to remote trauma to the cornea. The cylinder axis on manifest refraction (MR) was significantly different from measured keratometry, so a second procedure was performed to align the cylinder axis of the IOL with the steep axis on MR. This repositioning procedure improved visual outcome to a final uncorrected vision of 20/25 (0.10 logMAR) and best corrected acuity of 20/20 (0.0 logMAR).

Keywords

Irregular Astigmatism, Toric IOL, IOL, Toric, Malposition, Reposition

1. Introduction

Toric intraocular lens implants (IOLs) used in cataract surgery are used to correct both sphere and cylinder refractive error, and are designed to neutralize preexisting corneal astigmatism. They have the potential to improve visual outcomes of astigmatic eyes in patients with regular or irregular astigmatism [1]. The Acrysof® Toricsingle-piece lens implant has demonstrated efficacy in refractive correction and minimal postoperative rotation [2].

Accurate biometry is crucial for calculating refractive power of the implant lens, and keratometry serves as the basis for determining placement of the toric lens's cylinder axis [3]. For reassurance of accurate and precise measurements, one may utilize several methods of keratometry including manual keratometers, optical low coherence reflectometry devices, and computerized corneal topography [4] [5].

Occasionally a patient may experience disturbing residual astigmatism following implantation of a toric IOL due to malposition on implantation, rotation of the IOL [6], surgically induced astigmatism [7], or ocular residual astigmatism not measurable preoperatively [8] [9]. Malposition can reduce the astigmatic correction, alter the astigmatic axis, and induce hyperopic spherical change [10].

In this case study, an astigmatic patient with misleading keratometry due to corneal irregularity from remote ocular trauma received a toric implant and was initially displeased with the result. Pre- and postoperative MR cylinder axis was found to differ from objective keratometry. Corneal topography revealed an unusual pattern of astigmatism created by the scarred area. Realignment of the toric IOL using the preoperative MR cylinder axis reduced astigmatism, improving vision and patient satisfaction.

2. Case History

The patient was a healthy 67-year-old Caucasian male with compound myopic astigmatism presenting with gradual decrease in best corrected visual acuity over a period of three years. His past history was significant for an injury to his eyes while grinding metal in the 1970s which required removal of metallic foreign bodies from both eyes and scarred the left cornea. His left eye's uncorrected vision was count-fingers at 5 feet (1.5 meters) with best corrected visual acuity of 20/40 (0.3 logMAR). His left eye manifest refraction was −8.50 + 1.50 × 032°. On exam he was found to have a well-healed stromal scar on the superior temporal left cornea, combined cataracts in both lenses, and no evidence of other ocular pathology. He was scheduled for phacoemulsification with IOL implantation, and a toric implant was chosen to correct astigmatism.

Ocular biometry for lensectomy and lens implantation was obtained with a manual keratometry (Topcon®), low coherence reflectometry (Zeiss IOL Master®) and computerized corneal topography (Zeiss Atlas®). The meridian of the flat and steep keratometry axis measured consistently between methods (steep axis range: 122° - 135°), although the cylinder power measured inconsistently and ranged from 0.75 to 2.25 diopters in the left eye depending on the method used (**Table 1**).

The Acrysof® Toric SN60T4 with 2.25 D cylinder power was selected to correct the patient's compound myopic astigmatism in the left eye. Measurements from manual keratometry and the IOL master were entered into The Acrysof Toric IOL Calculator™ online [11]. The software suggested the IOL be positioned with the steep axis at 120°.

The cataract was extracted via phacoemulsification through a temporal self-sealing incision and anterior capsulorhexis by forceps. An Acrysof Toric SN60T4 intraocular lens implant was inserted into the capsule and positioned at an axis of 120° without procedural complication.

Postoperatively, the patient's left eye uncorrected vision was 20/100 (0.70 logMAR) and best corrected acuity was 20/25 (0.10 logMAR) with a MR of −1.50 + 2.50 × 032. Examination and slit lamp photography confirmed the IOL to be in stable position with steep axis markings at 120°. Corneal topography was notable for a steep area surrounding his old corneal scar and separate from the bow-tie pattern of astigmatism across the central cornea (**Figure 1**). Due to the increase in manifest astigmatism at the same manifest axis, the surgeon decided to reopen the incision and reposition the lens to 30° based on his MR.

Following the repositioning, the patient's left eye saw 20/25 (logMAR 0.10) uncorrected with best corrected acuity of 20/20 (logMAR 0.0) with a MR of −0.75 + 0.75 × 005. The patient was pleased with this significant improvement from his prior vision. Informed consent was obtained prior to reporting the case.

Table 1. Preoperative keratometry measurements.

Keratometry	Flat K	Flat axis	Steep K	Steep axis	Avg. ΔD
Manual (Marco K1)	46.75 D	53°	47.25 D	127°	+0.75 D @127°
Zeiss IOL Master® (3 consecutive trials)	45.59 D ± 0.03	58° ± 1.63°	47.82 D ± 0.06	122° ± 1.63°	+2.24 D @122°
Zeiss Atlas® v. A12.2 (3 consecutive trials)	45.87 D ± 0.10	45° ± 12.7°	46.99 D ± 0.10	135° ± 12.7°	+1.12 D @134.7°

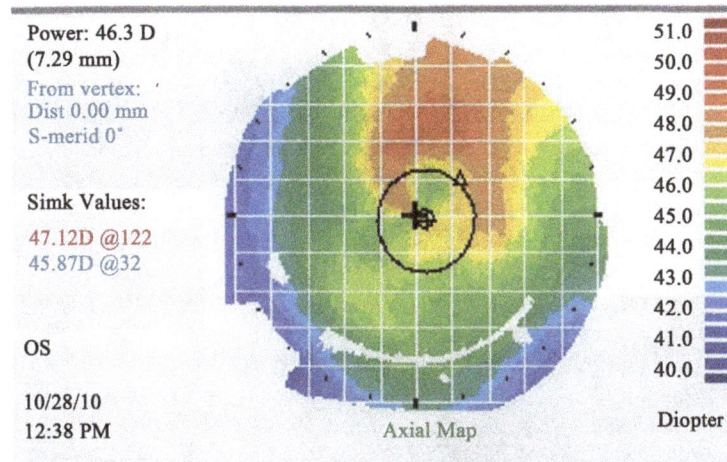

Figure 1. Corneal topography of OS showing superotemporal steepening outside of central bow-tie pattern astigmatism.

3. Discussion

Despite having high cylinder in his preoperative MR, this patient was a questionable candidate for a toric IOL implantation due to his unique corneal curvature secondary to scarring. It is imperative to obtain accurate and reproducible preoperative measurements when calculating IOL power; one must also consider patient preference and the effects of other ocular pathology.

This patient preferred a relatively high cylinder power in his corrective spectacles, so it seemed sensible to try a toric IOL. When keratometry consistently found a cylinder axis conflicting with the MR, the IOL implantation axis was planned for the keratometry axis rather than the MR axis. Positioning the steep meridian of a toric IOL along the keratometry axis is common practice because manifest astigmatism is understood to be the result of interaction between corneal curvature and internal factors including lenticular astigmatism [12]. Removing the crystalline lens removes its effect on manifest astigmatism, and thus corneal measurements are the primary concern when designating an axis for a toric lens implant.

This patient's measured keratometry was misleading and corneal topography provided a likely explanation. A small central bow-tie pattern was present and repeatedly measured while the scar position appeared to have been the true dominant astigmatic presence in the left cornea (**Figure 1**). As a result, the postoperative astigmatism after the first operation was worse by 1.00 diopter. Precisely calculating corneal refractive power is challenging since keratometry does not directly measure corneal power, and can be confounded by surgical or traumatic scars which change the relationship between the anterior and posterior cornea, altering the corneal refractive index [12]. Newer modalities such as rotating Scheimpflug imaging aim to improve measurement by scanning the anterior and posterior corneal surface [13].

The combined optical effects of the cornea and toric IOL can be considered as two obliquely crossed spherocylinders combined to form a new spherocylinder and more complex refractive status due to irregularities and optical aberrations. When there is an unsatisfactory refractive result following toric IOL implantation, options to correct the error include corrective lenses, laser vision correction, repositioning, or IOL exchange depending on the situation [10]. A repositioning procedure was appropriate in this case because of the high postoperative compound astigmatism. Repositioning to the MR axis resulted in improvement in this patient's vision. Cataract surgeons considering toric IOL implants should be cautious with patients having corneal scarring due to the risk of unexpected refractive changes postoperatively.

References

[1] Bauer, N.J.C., de Vries, N.E., Webers, C.A.B., Hendrikse, F. and Nuijts, R.M.M.A. (2008) Astigmatism Management in Cataract Surgery with the AcrySoftoric Intraocular Lens. *Journal of Cataract Refractive Surgery*, **34**, 1483-1488. http://dx.doi.org/10.1016/j.jcrs.2008.05.031

[2] Nuijts, R.M.M.A., Bauer, N.J.C. and Visser, N. (2009) Optimize Surgical Results with Toric IOLs. Cataract and Re-

fractive Surgery Today Europe, July/August, 17-25.

[3]   Koshy, J.J., Nishi, Y., Hirnschall, N., Crnej, A., Gangwani, V., Maurino, V. and Findl, O. (2010) Rotational Stability of a Single-Piece Toric Acrylic Intraocular lens. *Journal of Cataract Refractive Surgery*, **36**, 1665-1670. http://dx.doi.org/10.1016/j.jcrs.2010.05.018

[4]   Shirayama, M., Wang, L., Weikert, M.P. and Koch, D.D. (2009) Comparison of Corneal Powers Obtained from 4 Different Devices. *American Journal of Ophthalmology*, **148**, 528-535. http://dx.doi.org/10.1016/j.ajo.2009.04.028

[5]   Vogel, A., Dick, H.B. and Krummenauer, F. (2001) Reproducibility of Optical Biometry Using Partial Coherence Interferometry: Intraobserver and Interobserver Reliability. *Journal of Cataract Refractive Surgery*, **27**, 1961-1968. http://dx.doi.org/10.1016/S0886-3350(01)01214-7

[6]   Shah, G.D., Praveen, M.R., Vasavada, A.R., Vasavada, V.A., Rampal, G. and Shastry, L.R. (2012) Rotational Stability of a Toric Intraocular Lens: Influence of Axial Length and Alignment in the Capsular Bag. *Journal of Cataract Refractive Surgery*, **38**, 54-59. http://dx.doi.org/10.1016/j.jcrs.2011.08.028

[7]   Tejedor, J. and Perez-Rodriguez, J.A. (2009) Astigmatic Change Induced by 2.8-mm Corneal Incisions for Cataract Surgery. *Investigative Ophthalmology and Visual Science*, **50**, 989-994.
http://www.iovs.org/content/50/3/989.full.pdf
http://dx.doi.org/10.1167/iovs.08-2778

[8]   Alpins, N., Ong, J.K.Y. and Stamatelatos, G. (2014) Refractive Surprise after Toric Intraocular Lens Implantation: Graph Analysis. *Journal of Cataract Refractive Surgery*, **40**, 283-294. http://dx.doi.org/10.1016/j.jcrs.2013.06.029

[9]   Koch, D.D., Ali, S.F., Weikert, M.P., Shirayama, M., Jenkins, R. and Wang, L. (2012) Contribution of the Posterior Corneal Astigmatism to Total Corneal Astigmatism. *Journal of Cataract Refractive Surgery*, **38**, 2080-2087. http://dx.doi.org/10.1016/j.jcrs.2012.08.036

[10] Alcon, Inc. AcrySofToric IOL Web Based Calculator. www.acrysoftoriccalculator.com

[11] Jin, H., Limberger, I.J., Ehmer, A., Guo, H. and Auffarth, G.U. (2010) Impact of Axis Misalignment of Toric Intraocular Lenses on Refractive Outcomes after Cataract Surgery. *Journal of Cataract Refractive Surgery*, **36**, 2061-2072. http://dx.doi.org/10.1016/j.jcrs.2010.06.066

[12] Mohammadi, S., Tahvildari, M. and Z-Mehrjardi, H. (2012) Physiology of Astigmatism, Astigmatism—Optics, Physiology and Management. In: Goggin, M., Ed., InTech, 1-13.
http://www.intechopen.com/books/astigmatism-optics-physiology-and-management

[13] Lee, A.C., Qazi, M.A. and Pepose, J.S. (2008) Biometry and Intraocular Lens Power Calculation. *Current Opinion in Ophthalmology*, **19**, 13-17. http://dx.doi.org/10.1097/ICU.0b013e3282f1c5ad

9

Ocular Microsporidiosis—Our Experience in a Tertiary Care Centre in North India

Uma Sridhar[1], Amil Ausaf Ur Rahman[2], Jyoti Batra[1], Neelam Sapra[3]

[1]Cornea Department, ICARE Eye Hospital, Noida, India
[2]Training Centre, ICARE Eye Hospital, Noida, India
[3]Microbiology Depatment, Shroff Charity Eye Hospital, New Delhi, India
Email: u_sridhar@yahoo.com

Abstract

Microsporidia are obligate intracellular protozoal parasites. They are eukaryotic and spore forming. Increasing interest in this parasite as a pathogen in the ocular tissues in recent times is due to increasing awareness of microsporidia as an ocular pathogen and better methods of identification of the organism. It also can cause intestinal, sinus, pulmonary, muscular and renal diseases, in both immunocompetent and immunosuppressed patients. Ocular microsporidiosis can occur in isolation or as a part of systemic infections. In earlier published literature, ocular involvement in immunocompetent individuals was more in the form of stromal keratitis and immunocompromised individuals were seen to have keratoconjunctivitis. However, later studies show that this pattern has many variations. Occurrence in rainy season with exposure to muddy water and history of minor trauma is now a known factor. Identification by light microscopy from scrapings with KOH, Gram, Giemsa staining is possible. Growth of the organisms, however, is possible only by cell culture. Species identification is done by polymerase chain reaction and by electron microscopy. Immunofluorescent staining techniques are also available in advanced laboratories for species differentiation of microsporidia. Till date, treatment of ocular microsporidia has not been standardized and varies from simple debridement to use of various antibiotics, antiseptics antifungals and antiviral agents.

Keywords

Microsporidia, Keratoconjunctivitis, Stromal Keratitis

1. Introduction

Microsporidia are eukaryotic obligate intracellular parasitic organisms which are included as protozoans. The discovery of Microsporidia as pathogens in vertebrates and invertebrates was more than 100 years ago by Nageli who identified it as being causative organisms of a disease in silkworms [1]. Immunocompetent individuals can harbor microsporidia in their intestines as a part of normal flora [2]. Infection by microsporidia in humans was first reported by Matsubayashi *et al.* [3] in 1959. Ocular microsporidiosis was first reported by Ashton and Wirashinha in 1973 as encephalitozoan infection of cornea by *Nosema* sps. [4]. Earlier interest in these pathogens was due to their being opportunistic pathogens in immunocompromised patients and ocular involvement in the form of keratoconjunctivitis was also reported in these patients [5]. Recent reports in literature have been more often in immunocompetent individuals [6] [7]. The ocular manifestations include superficial punctate keratoconjunctivitis, and corneal stromal keratitis. The aim of this review is to focus on the epidemiology, pathogenesis, clinical manifestations, diagnosis and management of ocular microsporidiosis.

1.1. Epidemiology

Microsporidial infections occur in humans worldwide. It is identified now as a zoonotic disease as the genotypes that infect humans have been identified in animals [8]. It is also known have water borne transmission [9] and food borne transmission as a result of contaminated water used in irrigation [10]. Dairy cows' milk was also shown to be a mode of transmission of infection [11]. In areas with low socioeconomic conditions and poor sanitation, association with HIV infection is also common [12] [13]. Ocular infection occurs in immunocompetent and in immunocompromised individuals. Mode of transmission may be contact with contaminated water and soil after minor trauma. Occurrence in rainy season is common with minor epidemics being reported [14]. One of the earliest case reports of ocular involvement in humans was in a 11-year old boy who had stromal keratitis caused by microsporidia.[4]

1.2. Parasitology

Microsporidia are obligate, intracellular parasites. They have two developmental phases inside a host cell: schizogenic phase also called the feeding phase and the sporulation or sporogenic phase. The size of microsporidian spores varies from 1 µm to 20 µm. Spores can be spherical, oval or elongate. Each spore consists of sporoplasm and a tubular, polar filament with varying number of coils, depending on the species [15].

The infection is by direct inoculation where a polar filament is discharged into the host cell and a sporoplasm is introduced. The sporoplasm multiplies inside the host cell and develops into meronts (schizonts) and sporonts. Each sporont divides to form two sporoblasts, which, in turn, develop into spores at maturation [15]. Spores may disseminate from cell to cell inside the host or can be excreted via the skin or urine. Urine to finger to eye transmission may be responsible for horizontal spread in humans [16] [17].

The only stage of microsporidia outside the host cell is that of infective spores. There are two distinct phases in the development of microsporidia: a proliferative phase (merogony) responsible for a massive increase in number inside the host cell and a sporogonic phase (sporogony), in which sporonts produce sporoblasts which mature into spores

Taxonomically, the microsporidia were grouped and classified on the basis of their natural hosts and ultrastructural features such as size of the developing and mature organisms, nucleus arrangement (monokaryon or diplokaryon), number of polar filament coils, interface with the host cell during development (e.g., direct contact with host cell cytoplasm, replication within a host-cell derived parasitophorous vacuole, replication of organisms surrounded by endoplasmic reticulum, sporogony within a parasite-generated sporophorous vesicle), and mode of cell and nuclear division (binary division, karyokinesis with delayed cytokinesis) [15].

1.3. Genus and Species Specific Characteristics

There are seven genera that infect humans. These parasites can be distinguished by their developmental cycle and host-parasite relationships in infected cells.

1.3.1. *Encephalitozoon*

Encephalitozoon cuniculi are unikaryotic. They develop within host cells in vacuoles bounded by a membrane that is thought to be of host cell origin. The spores are ellipsoid and measure approximately 2.5 × 1.5 mm They have a corrugated exospore surface, a thick endospore, four to seven (usually five or six) coils of the polar tubules, and often a polar vacuole [1] [18].

1.3.2. Nosema

Some of the structures lie in cysts bounded by membranes, but most of the parasites are in direct contact with the cytoplasm. There is no vacuole present. Spores are oval, measuring approximately 2.5 - 5 mm × 2 mm. Nuclei in the diplokaryon arrangement are seen in all forms. There is diplosporoblastic sporogony. The polar tube has about 11 coils [1] [18].

1.3.3. *Pleistophora*

Organisms resembling microsporidia of the genus *Pleistophora* have been recognized in one human patient. The spores were oval, approximately 2.8 × 3.2 - 3.4 mm. Not all developmental stages were seen. Unkaryotic with sporophorous vesicle. The spore wall is typical for many microsporidia, having a thin electron-dense exospore layer, a thick electron-lucent endospore, and a thin internal plasmalemma. Approximately 11 cross sections of the polar tubule were recognized in spores [1] [18].

1.3.4. Vittaform Cornea

Spores measure 3.05 - 4.55 × 0.77 - 1.27 mm. It is diplokaryotic. There is no vacuole in direct contact with host cell cytoplasm. Band like sporonts are seen. All stages are surrounded by a cistern of host endoplasmic reticulum [1] [18].

1.3.5. *Enterocytozoon*

Enterocytozoon bienusi is the microsporidian parasite most commonly recognized in humans and, so far, has been detected only in enterocytes. All stages are seen in direct contact with the host cell cytoplasm. Early developmental stages may have diplokaryotic nuclei but later stages display isolated nuclei. The parasites are small, approximately 2 to 4 mm in diameter, and have a simple plasma membrane during the early stages of division. Spores are approximately 1.1 - 1.6 × 0.7 - 1.0 mm in tissue section and differ from other microsporidia by having a very thin endospore layer [1] [18].

The other two genera are Trachipleistophora and Anncaliia (Brachiola) [18]. Classification of microsporidia in humans has depended on transmission electron microscopy (TEM) [19]. The presence of a polar tubule classifies an organism as a member of the phylum Microspora. Species differentiation using ultrastructural examinations is usually possible.

The fine structure of the spores with the unique coiled polar tube, the nature of host-parasite interface, and the method of division are criteria for diagnosis and species differentiation of microsporidia [18].

1.4. Non Ocular Presentation

Microsporidia can cause a variety of human diseases, involving multiple organ systems which include intestinal, ocular, sinus, pulmonary, muscular and renal diseases, in both immunocompetent as well as immunocompromised patients [20]. A case report of a Japanese boy with severe headache, vomiting and seizures in whom microsporidia was isolated by inoculation of mouse with his cerebrospinal fluid and urine was published in 1959 [21]. After this case report, many years ellapsed before a similar case was reported [18].

E. bieneusi and E. intestinalis are common pathogens in HIV infected patients with severe immunodeficiency and low CD 4 counts [22]. Enterocytozoon bieneusi and Encephalitozoon intestinalis have also been associated with cholangitis including sclerosing cholangitis [23]. Hepatitis and peritonitis may also be caused by microsporidia [18].

1.5. Ocular Manifestations

Keratitis in a Sri Lankan boy was reported in 1973 [4] by Ashton and Wirashinha in the British Journal of Ophthalmology which was histopathologically proven as microsporidiosis. Initial reports of microsporidiosis were in HIV positive patients. Cases of related cases of keratoconjunctivitis typically described the lesions as coarse, punctate epithelial lesions which may stain positive with fluorescein dye. Organism found in conjunctiva and cornea was Encephalitozoon hellem [24] [25]. In a case series from New York, keratoconjunctivitis in HIV positive individuals revealed Encephalitozoon cuniculi spores on conjunctival biopsy [26], In HIV positive patients, chronic keratoconjunctivitis has been more commonly found, whereas both deep stromal keratitis and keratoconjunctivitis have been described in immunocompetent individuals [27]-[29]. Contact lenses may harbor the organisms and cause corneal infections. In a case series, of microsporidial keratitis reported from Singapore, 20.1% (25 out of 124) had a history of contact lens wear [30].

Domestic animals such as cats may harbor the organism and close contact with them may cause ocular infection [24]. Use of topical corticosteroids can also predispose to superadded infection with microsporidia. Infection after corneal grafting has been reported due to local immunosuppression with corticosteroids [31].

Exposure to muddy water, especially in rainy season has been reported as a predisposing factor in causing an outbreak in Singapore [32].

1.6. Spectrum of Ocular Microsporidiosis

Deep stromal keratitis and superficial punctate keratopathy are the main manifestations in the cornea. Conjunctival involvement may occur along with the keratitis. Keratoconjunctivits mimicking adenoviral keratoconjunctivitis may occur especially in the rainy season. A mixed follicular and papillary reaction may occur in the conjunctiva. Sclera and uvea may also be involved.

In cases of keratoconjunctivitis, the presenting symptoms are photophobia, blurred vision, and foreign body sensation. Conjunctiva usually is chemosed, with decreased luster. The corneal involvement is in the form of superficial punctate keratopathy with coarse fluorescein staining and non-staining epithelial opacities. The lesions are limited to the level of the epithelium and can be debrided.

Several case series describing keratoconjunctivits in immunosuppressed and in later publications, immunocompetent patients have been published in the last two decades [26]-[32].

1.7. Our Experience of Keratoconjunctivitis

Between August 2013 to March 2014 25 cases of microsporidiosis were seen in our opd. All patients had history of exposure to rain water or to muddy water. A family of seven patients had exposure to water from their overhead tank and presented with a similar picture of conjunctival congestion, chemosis raised epithelial lesions and some target shaped epithelial lesions (**Figure 1** and **Figure 2**). Corneal scraping in all the patients was done and stained with Gram stain.

Spores of microsporidia were detected in all the specimens.

Most of the patients who were clinically suspected to have microsporidial keratitis in our opd were subjected to corneal scraping. All the specimens were either stained with Gram stain or with Geimsa stain (**Figure 3**). All the specimens were showed spores of microsporidia.

Patient responded to topical fluoroquinolones and oral albendazole 400 mg once daily for seven days.

Three patients also showed signs of anterior uveitis on follow up with nummular corneal opacities and had to

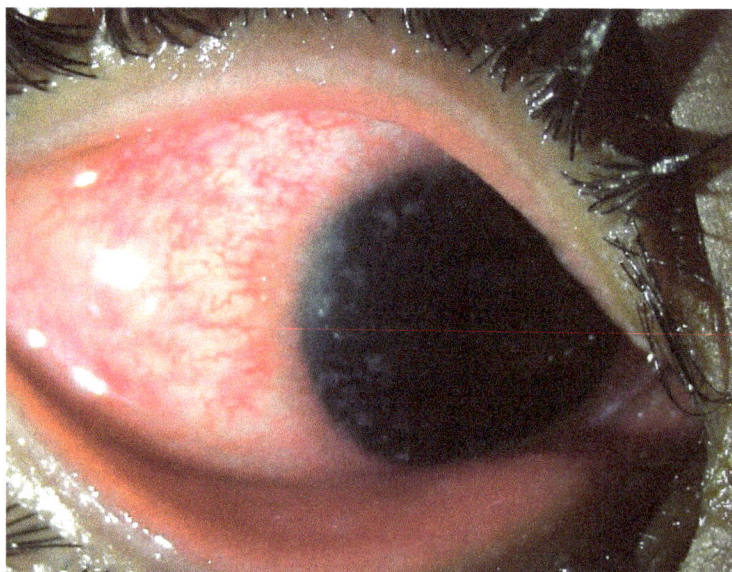

Figure 1. Raised coarse epithelial lesions on cornea in a case of microsporidia keratoconjunctivitis.

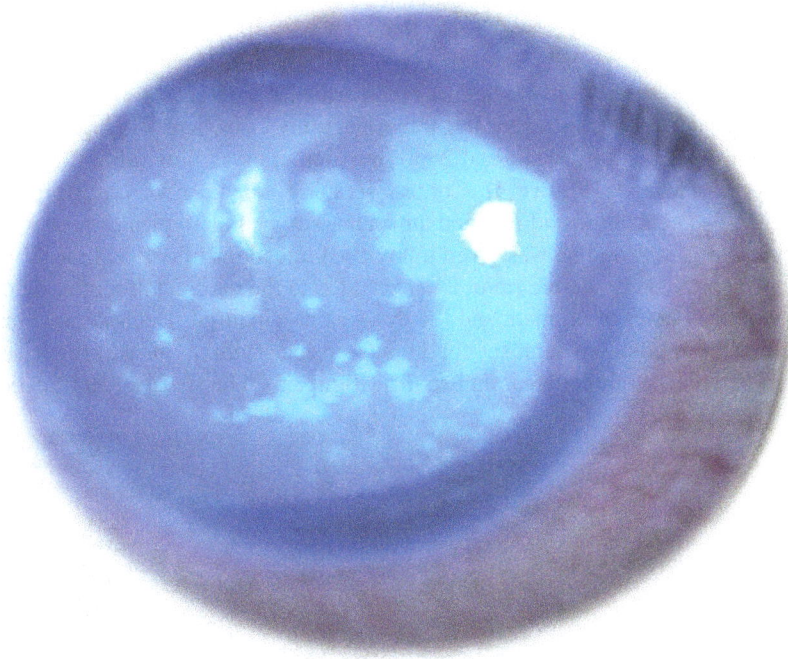

Figure 2. Fluorescein staining of punctate raised epithelial lesions in acase of microsporidia keratoconjunctivitis.

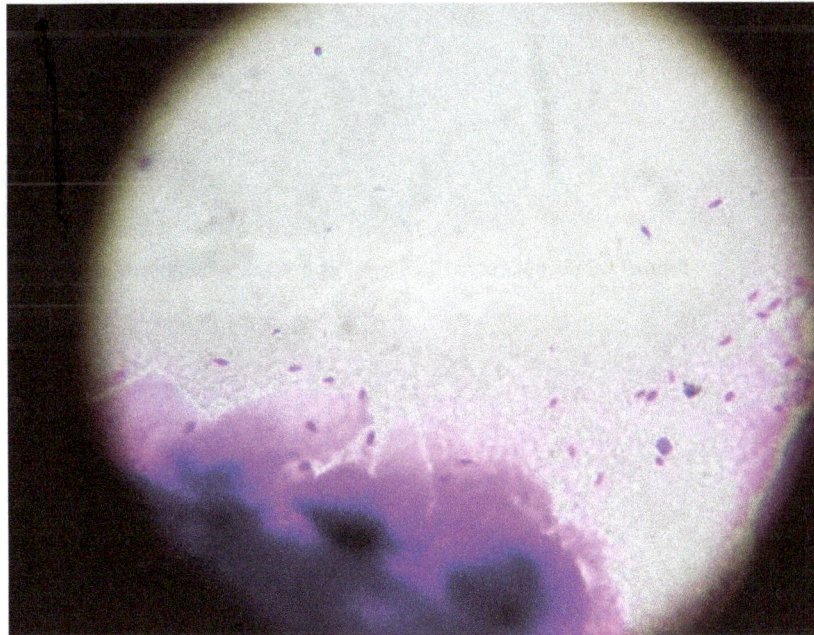

Figure 3. Giemsa staining showing microsporidia spores.

be given a short course of topical steroids.

Stromal Keratitis

Stromal keratitis due to microsporidia is rarer than superficial keratoconjunctivitis. It occurs mainly in immuno-competent patients. Stromal keratitis due to microsporidia can be mistaken for Herpes Simplex virus keratitis. A case report of a patient who had dense greyish white stromal infiltrates in the cornea which had a crystalline keratopathy-like pattern and was treated initially as Herpes simplex virus stromal keratitis was reported by Font *et al.* [33]. Corneal biopsy showed microsporidial keratitis. Since there was no improvement with oral albendazole and topical fumagillin even after 6 weeks, lamellar keratoplasty and later penetrating keratoplasty (PK) was done. The organism was identified as Nosema corneum (renamed Vittaforma corneae).

In our experience, a 70 year old gentleman presented with a diagnosis of chronic endophthalmitis in his right eye, having undergone cataract surgery and trabeculectomy elsewhere. He had perception of light with inaccurate projection in that eye. Cornea showed 2 × 3 mm area of crystalline infiltrates in the stroma near the temporal cataract surgery wound, (**Figure 4**). Corneal scraping did not reveal any organisms. He was empirically treated with fortified cefazoline and fortified amikacin, suspecting atypical mycobacterial infection. Vitritis was seen on ultrasound B scan and he was given intravitreal injections of ceftazidime. Vitreous biopsy did not show any organism. Topical and systemic steroids were added to the treatment regimen as the patient developed more inflammation in the posterior segment and the eye was now painful. Decision was made to eviscerate the right eye as the corneal and posterior segment condition worsened with no visual prognosis. Corneal button on histopathology showed plenty of microsporidial spores (**Figure 5**). The species identification was not done. This was

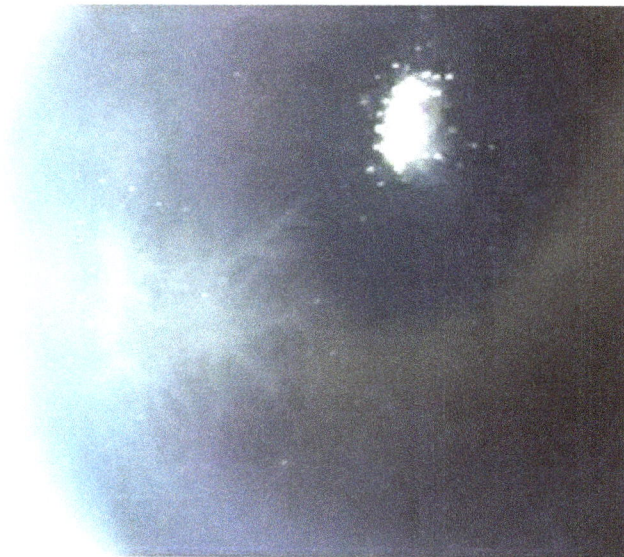

Figure 4. Infectious crystalline keratopathy due to microsporidia.

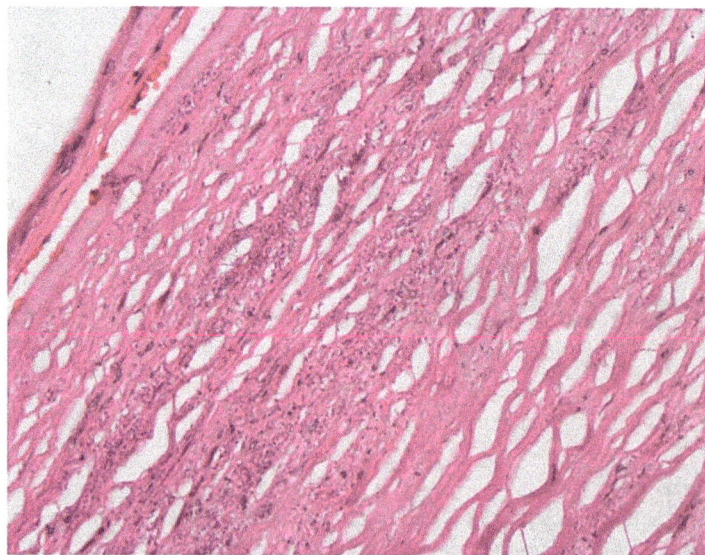

Figure 5. Histopathology of corneal button of the case of infectious crytalline keratopathy due to microsporidia.

a case of crystalline keratopathy due to microsporidia which was not clinically diagnosed and was negative on scraping. Associated posterior segment inflammation was also a feature.

Another case report of stromal keratitis mistakenly diagnosed as viral keratitis in an 82-year-old patient was reported by Fogla et al. [34]. Initially the peripheral mid stromal infiltrates seemingly resolved with acyclovir and topical prednisolone acetate. The lesion recurred a month later as a full thickness stromal infiltrate. therapeutic penetrating keratoplasty was performed and the histopathology of the corneal button showed microsporidia spores.

Cellular reaction in the anterior chamber is common but posterior segment involvement from microsporidial infection rare. Meitz et al. [35] have reported a case of sclerouveitis with retinal detachment. There was no corneal infiltrate in the sixty six year old woman who had progressive loss of vision. There were keratic precipitates in the cornea. Diagnostic vitrectomy revealed infection with microsporidia; she was treated with oral albendazole 400 mg twice daily. Endophthalmitis due to microsporidia was also reported in a patient with acute myelogenous leukemia [36].

2. Diagnostic Methods

2.1. Non Invasive Techniques

Clinically diagnosis of microsporidia has been done in cases of keratoconjunctivitis based on history of exposure to muddy water especially in the rainy season and the presence of coarse epithelial lesions along with conjunctival chemosis and follicular and papillary reaction. Stromal keratitis however may be more difficult to distinguish from Herpes simplex stromal keratitis clinically. When the infiltrate does not respond to topical antivirals and steroids, then resort has to be made to other means like confocal microscopy and corneal biopsy. Sometimes therapeutic penetrating or lamellar keratoplasty and histopathology may be the only means of diagnosis.

2.2. Confocal Microscopy

Hyperreflective spots seen on confocal microscopy in keratoconjunctivitis due to microsporidia have been reported and the diagnosis later confirmed by corneal scraping [37]. In stromal keratitis also confocal microscopy has been useful to detect microsporidia and the diagnosis has been later confirmed by biopsy [38]. Confocal microscopy, thus may be a simple and non-invasive technique to detect the organism in deep seated infections and to monitor the effectiveness of treatment.

2.3. Microbiological Diagnosis

Corneal and conjunctival scraping can be effective in diagnosis. Various staining methods have been used. 10% KOH mount (potassium hydroxide) plain or with calcofluor white.

3. Laboratory Diagnosis

Identification by light microscopy from scrapings with KOH, KOH+CFW (potassium hydroxide plus calcofluor white), Gram, Giemsa and modified Ziehl-Neelsen (1% H_2SO_4 cold) staining is possible. KOH + CFW staining is observed under a fluorescence microscope with cube U having filter combinations for the excitation spectrum region near 365 nm for a DAPI (4', 6'-diamidino-2-phenylindole) stain. In various studies, the KOH + CFW stain along with the modified Ziehl-Neelsen stain most frequently detected microsporidia, followed by the Gram stain, while Giemsa staining had the least detection efficacy among the four. KOH + CFW and acid-fast stains were to be most efficient (29/30 [96.7%] and 28/30 [93.3%], respectively) in the diagnosis of microsporidial keratitis.

Microsporidal spores as observed under various stains on corneal scrapings. a) KOH + CFW stain (magnification, ×1000). Organisms were seen as bright turquoise to white oval bodies, often clustered in groups, against a relatively dark background. The spores displayed variable fluorescence intensities. Depending on the orientation of the microsporidia, the anterior end appeared concave. b) Gram stain (magnification, ×1000). Spores appeared ovoid and refractile and bright purple, resembling gram-positive organisms. The spores were scattered or highly clustered within the cytoplasm of occasional epithelial cells. Microsporidial spores show a dark staining belt girding them either diagonally or equatorially. c) Giemsa stain (magnification, ×1000). This stain is not taken up by the cell wall, and only the cytoplasm gets stained. The spores appear smaller than those in the other stains.

There was also poor differentiation from other bacteria and debris. The darkly stained belt could be identified in 18/30 cases, aiding preliminary diagnosis. d) Modified Ziehl-Neelsen stain (magnification, ×1000). Except for two, all cases of microsporidial spores were acid fast (1% H_2SO_4). The acid-fast spores appeared bright red on a blue background, and a posterior vacuole and central diagonal strip within the spores were often visible. Bacteria and other cell debris appeared blue, owing to methylene blue counterstain.

Growth of the organisms, however, is possible only by cell culture. Species identification is done by polymerase chain reaction and by electron microscopy. Immunofluorescent staining techniques are also available in advanced laboratories for species differentiation of microsporidia.

References

[1] Nageli, K.W. (1857) Uber die neue Krankheit der Seidenraupe und verwandte Organismen. *Bot Z*, **15**, 760-761.

[2] Nkinin, S.W., Asonganyi, T., Didier, E.S., *et al.* (2007) Microsporidian Infection is Prevalent in Healthy People in Cameroon. *Journal Clinical Microbiology*, **45**, 2841-2846. http://dx.doi.org/10.1128/JCM.00328-07

[3] Matsubayashi, H., Koike, T., Mikata, T. and Hagiwara, S. (1959) A Case of Encephatitozoon like Body Infection in Man. *Archives of Pathology*, **67**, 181-187.

[4] Ashton, N. and Wirashinha, P.A. (1973) Encephalitozoonosis (Nosematosis) of the Cornea. *British Journal of Ophthalmology*, **57**, 669-674. http://dx.doi.org/10.1136/bjo.57.9.669

[5] Cali, A., Meisler, D.M., Lowder, C.Y., *et al.* (1991) Corneal Microsporidiosis: Characterization and Identification. The *Journal of Protozoology*, **38**, S215-S217.

[6] Chan, C.M., Theng, J.T., Li, L., *et al.* (2003) Microsporidial Keratoconjunctivitis in Healthy Individuals: A Case Series. *Ophthalmology*, **110**, 1420-1425. http://dx.doi.org/10.1016/S0161-6420(03)00448-2

[7] Quek, D.T., Pan, J.C., Unny Krishnan, P. and Zhao, P.S. (2011) Teoh SCB Microsporidial Keratoconjunctivitis in the Tropics: A Case Series. *The Open Ophthalmology Journal*, **5**, 42-47. http://dx.doi.org/10.2174/1874364101105010042

[8] Mathis, A., Weber, R. and Deplazes, P. (2005) Zoonotic Potential of the Microsporidia. *Clinical Microbiology Reviews*, **18**, 423-445. http://dx.doi.org/10.1128/CMR.18.3.423-445.2005

[9] Didier, E.S., Stovall, M.E., Green, L.C., *et al.* (2004) Epidemiology of Microsporidiosis: Sources and Modes of Transmission. *Veterinary Parasitology*, **126**, 145-166.

[10] Calvo, M., Carazo, M., Arias, M.L., *et al.* (2004) Prevalence of *Cyclospora* sp., *Cryptosporidium* sp., Microsporidia and *Fecal coliform* Determination in Fresh Fruit and Vegetables Consumed in Costa Rica. *Archivos Latinoamericanos de Nutrición*, **54**, 428-432.

[11] Lee, J.H. (2008) Molecular Detection of *Enterocytozoon bieneusi* and Identification of a Potentially Human-Pathogenic Genotype in Milk. *Applied and Environmental Microbiology*, **74**, 1664-1666. http://dx.doi.org/10.1128/AEM.02110-07

[12] Sarfati, C., Bourgeois, A., Menotti, J., Liegeois, F., Moyou-Somo, R., Delaporte, E., *et al.* (2006) Prevalence of Intestinal Parasites Including Microsporidia in Human Immunodeficiency Virus-Infected Adults in Cameroon: A Cross-Sectional Study. *The American Journal of Tropical Medicine and Hygiene*, **74**, 162-164.

[13] Chacin-Bonilla, L., Panunzio, A.P., Monsalve-Castillo, F.M., Parra-Cepeda, I.E. and Martinez, R. (2006) Microsporidiosis in Venezuela: Prevalence of Intestinal Microsporidiosis and Its Contribution to Diarrhea in a Group of Human Immunodeficiency Virus-Infected Patients from Zulia State. *The American Journal of Tropical Medicine and Hygiene*, **74**, 482-486.

[14] Tan, J., Lee, P., Lai, Y., Hishamuddin, P., Tay, J., Tan, A.L., Chan, K.S., Lin, R., Tan, D., Cutter, J. and Goh, K.T. (2013) Microsporidial Keratoconjunctivitis after Rugby Tournament, Singapore. *Emerging Infectious Diseases*, **19**, 1484-1486. www.cdc.gov/eid

[15] Current, W.L. and Owen, R.L. (1989) Cryptosporidiosis and Microsporidiosis. In: Farthing, M.J.G. and Keusch, G.T., Eds., *Enteric Infection. Mechanisms, Manifestations and Management*, 11th Edition, Chapman and Hall, London, 203-207.

[16] Bryan, R.T., Cali, A., Owen, R.L. and Spencer, H.C. (1991) Microsporidia: Opportunistic Pathogens in Patients with AIDS. In: Sun, T., Ed., *Progress in Clinical Parasitology*, Vol. 2, Field and Wood Medical Publishers, New York, 1-26.

[17] Lowder, C.Y. (1993) Ocular Microsporidiosis. *International Ophthalmology Clinics*, **33**, 145-151. http://dx.doi.org/10.1097/00004397-199303310-00012

[18] Sharma, S., Das, S., Joseph, J., Vemuganti, G.K. and Murthy, S. (2011) Microsporidial Keratitis: Need for Increased Awareness. *Survey of Ophthalmology*, **56**, 1-22.

[19] Sprague, V. and Vaˊvra, J. (1977) Systematics of the Microsporidia. In: Bulla Jr., L.A. and Cheng, T.C., Eds., *Com-*

parative Pathobiology, Vol. 2. Plenum Press, New York, 1-510.

[20] Weber, R., Bryan, R.T., Schwartz, D.A. and Owen, R.L. (1994) Human Microsporidial Infections. *Clinical Microbiology Reviews*, **7**, 426-461.

[21] Franzen, C. (2008) Microsporidia: A Review of 150 Years of Research. *The Open Parasitology Journal*, **2**, 1-34. http://dx.doi.org/10.2174/1874421400802010001

[22] Kotler, D.P. and Orenstein, J.M. (1998) Clinical Syndromes Associated with Microsporidiosis. *Advances in Parasitology*, **40**, 321-349. http://dx.doi.org/10.1016/S0065-308X(08)60126-8

[23] Costa, S.F. and Weiss, L.M. (2000) Drug Treatment of Microsporidiosis. *Drug Resistance Updates*, **3**, 384-399. http://dx.doi.org/10.1054/drup.2000.0174

[24] Didier, E.S., Didier, P.J., Friedberg, S.M., Stenson, D.N., Orenstein, J.M., Vee, R.W., *et al.* (1991) Isolation and Characterization of a New Human Microsporidian, *Encephalitozoon hellem* (n. sp.), from Three AIDS Patients with Keratoconjunctivitis. *The Journal of Infectious Diseases*, **163**, 617-621. http://dx.doi.org/10.1093/infdis/163.3.617

[25] Grossnikiaus, H.E., Diesenhouse, M.C., Wilson, L.A., Corrent, G.F., Visvesvara, G.S. and Bryan, R.T. (1993) Treatment of Microsporidial Keratoconjunctivitis with Topical Fumagillin. *American Journal of Ophthalmology*, **115**, 293-298. http://dx.doi.org/10.1016/S0002-9394(14)73578-0

[26] Friedberg, D.N., Stenson, S.M., Orenstein, J.M., Tierno, P.M. and Charles, N.C. (1990) Microsporidial Keratoconjunctivitis in Acquired Immunodeficiency Syndrome. *Archives of Ophthalmology*, **108**, 504-508. http://dx.doi.org/10.1001/archopht.1990.01070060052047

[27] Joseph, J., Sridhar, M.S., Murthy, S. and Sharma, S. (2006) Clinical and Microbiological Profile of Microsporidial Keratoconjunctivitis in Southern India. *Ophthalmology*, **113**, 531-537. http://dx.doi.org/10.1016/j.ophtha.2005.10.062

[28] Moon, S.J., Mann, P.M. and Matoba, A.Y. (2003) Microsporidial Keratoconjunctivitis in a Healthy Patient with a History of LASIK Surgery. *Cornea*, **22**, 271-272. http://dx.doi.org/10.1097/00003226-200304000-00020

[29] Sridhar, M.S. and Sharma, S. (2003) Microsporidial Keratoconjunctivitis in a HIV-Seronegative Patient Treated with Debridement and Oral Itraconazole. *American Journal of Ophthalmology*, **136**, 745-746. http://dx.doi.org/10.1016/S0002-9394(03)00391-X

[30] Loh, R.S., Chan, C.M., Ti, S.E., Lim, L., Chan, K.S. and Tan, D.T.H. (2009) Emerging Prevalence of Microsporidial Keratitis in Singapore: Epidemiology, Clinical Features, and Management. *Ophthalmology*, **116**, 2348-2353. http://dx.doi.org/10.1016/j.ophtha.2009.05.004

[31] Kakrania, R., Joseph, J., Vaddavalli, P.K., Gangopadhyay, N. and Sharma, S. (2005) Microsporidia Keratoconjunctivitis in a Corneal Graft. *Eye*, **20**, 1314-1315. http://dx.doi.org/10.1038/sj.eye.6702178

[32] Das, S., Sharma, S., Sahu, S.K., Nayak, S.S. and Kar, S. (2008) New Antimicrobial Spectrum of Epidemic Keratoconjunctivitis: Clinical and Laboratory Aspects of an Outbreak. *British Journal of Ophthalmology*, **92**, 861-862.

[33] Font, R.L., Samaha, A.N., Keener, M.J., Chevez-Barrios, P. and Goosey, J.D. (2000) Corneal Microsporidiosis. Report of Case, Including Electron Microscopic Observations. *Ophthalmology*, **107**, 1769-1775. http://dx.doi.org/10.1016/S0161-6420(00)00285-2

[34] Fogla, R., Padmanabhan, P., Therese, K.L., Biswas, J. and Madhavan, H.N. (2005) Chronic Microsporidial Stromal Keratitis in an Immunocompetent, Noncontact Lens Wearer. *Indian Journal of Ophthalmology*, **53**, 123-125. http://dx.doi.org/10.4103/0301-4738.16177

[35] Mietz, H., Franzen, C., Hoppe, T. and Bartz-Schmidt, K.U. (2002) Microsporidia-Induced Sclerouveitis with Retinal Detachment. *Archives of Ophthalmology*, **120**, 864-865.

[36] Yoken, J., Forbes, B., Maguire, A.M., Prenner, J.L. and Carpentieri, D. (2002) Microsporidial Endophthalmitis in a Patient with Acute Myelogenous Leukemia. *Retina*, **22**, 123-125. http://dx.doi.org/10.1097/00006982-200202000-00028

[37] Shah, G.K., Pfister, D., Probst, L.E., Ferrieri, P. and Holland, E. (1996) Diagnosis of Microsporidial Keratitis by Confocal Microscopy and the Chromatrope Stain. *American Journal of Ophthalmology*, **121**, 89-91. http://dx.doi.org/10.1016/S0002-9394(14)70538-0

[38] Sagoo, M.S., Mehta, J.S., Hau, S., Irion, L.D., Curry, A. and Bonshek, R.E. (2007) Microsporidium Stromal Keratitis: *In Vivo* Confocal Findings. *Cornea*, **26**, 870-873. http://dx.doi.org/10.1097/ICO.0b013e31806c7a3c

10

Diagnostics and Prediction of Glaucoma in Patients with Familial Congenital Iris Hypoplasia

Tatiana Iureva[1,2], Andrey Shchuko[1], Yulia Pyatova[1]

[1]Irkutsk Branch, S. Fyodorov Eye Microsurgery Federal State Institution, Irkutsk, Russia
[2]Irkutsk State Medical Academy for Postgraduate Education, Irkutsk, Russia
Email: tnyurieva@mail.ru

Abstract

Purpose: To identify the clinical features of the syndrome Frank-Kamenetsky and determine the criteria of early formation of glaucoma. Materials and Methods: We observed 52 patients. Follow up period was from 5 to 22 years. The first group (juvenile) consisted of males who had the first signs of glaucoma diagnosed before the age of 12 (n = 22). The average age of the group was 10.1 ± 2.4 years. The control group included healthy males (n = 30) in the same age range (average age 7.2 ± 1.6 years). The second group (adults) consisted of patients who had the first signs of glaucoma diagnosed after the age of 18 and elder. The average age of the group was 32.44 ± 6.28 years. The control group had males (n = 30) in the same age range (average age 26.59 ± 4.12 years). The inclusion criterion was: the presence of congenital bilateral mesodermal iris leaf hypoplasia, trabecular dysgenesis signs, the presence of blood relatives on the maternal line (grandfather, uncle) male with similar changes iridociliary zone and glaucoma. Criteria of glaucoma formation were: increased IOP more than 21 mmHg with accompanying it expansion of the cup/disc ratio, reducing the thickness of the nerve fiber layer (RNFL) according to OCT. Results: It was found that Frank-Kamenetsky Syndrome had an X-linked with sex, recessive inheritance and was characterized by bilateral congenital irisdysgenesis and goniodysgenesis with the accession glaucoma. Predictors of glaucoma formation in early childhood are a combination of: 1) congenital subtotal atrophy of iris mesodermal layer (from 0 to 30 mkm) with signs of progressive dystrophy; 2) nonprogressive congenital megalocornea (cornea diameter 12 - 14 mm); 3) iridotrabecular dysgenesis of II-III degree; 4) hyperopic refraction in axial myopia.

Keywords

Glaucoma, Megalocornea, Congenital Mesodermal Iris Atrophy, Goniodysgenesis

1. Introduction

To our knowledge, this syndrome was first described in Russia in 1925, was characterized by congenital atrophy of the mesodermal layer of the iris and goniodysgenesis and led to the development of glaucoma [1]-[3]. It was later named as Frank-Kamenetsky Syndrome in honor of the discoverer. This syndrome is different from "congenital hypoplasia of the iris stroma" because it is an X-linked recessive as opposed to autosomal dominant in its inheritance. In addition, the long-term (over 20 years) patient follow up period allowed revealing of features for the syndrome and glaucoma [4]-[6].

In a retrospective study of medical records, it is found that the formation of glaucoma in these patients occurs either in a child aged from 0 to 12 years or in an adult in their second or third decade of life. The cause of congenital glaucoma formation changes in iridocorneal angle, "cog" fixing of the iris and the gray veil mesodermal tissue inclusions in the trabecular zone. In contrast to other forms of congenital glaucoma, forming of buphthalmos and acute IOP decompensation never occurs. Glaucoma occurs as open angle form, which makes it difficult to diagnose in the early stages of development. It is suggested that the mechanisms of glaucoma development in different ages can have fundamental differences. These differences are dependent on the combination of several characteristics of mesenchymal dysgenesis inherited in this syndrome.

2. Purpose

To identify the clinical features of the Frank-Kamenetsky syndrome and determine the criteria of early formation of glaucoma

3. Materials and Methods

The study was conducted in accordance with the Declaration of Helsinki and approved by the Ethics Committee of the institution. All patients signed an Informed Consent form prior to participation in the study.

4. Subjects

52 patients (males) with Frank-Kamenetsky syndrome. The control group included 60 patients (males).

Therefore, in the future, all patients were divided into two groups according to their glaucoma development time to identify specific symptoms and patterns of disease formation:

1) The first group (juvenile), consisted of males who had the first signs of glaucoma diagnosed before the age of 12 (n = 22). The average age of the group was 10.1 ± 2.4 years. The control group included healthy males (n = 30) in the same age range (average age 7.2 ± 1.6 years).

2) The second group (adults), consisted of patients who had the first signs of glaucoma diagnosed after the age of 18 and elder. The average age of the group was 32.44 ± 6.28 years. The control group were males (n = 30) in the same age range (average age 26.59 ± 4.12 years).

The inclusion criterion were: the presence of congenital bilateral mesodermal iris leaf hypoplasia, trabecular dysgenesis signs, the presence of blood relatives on the maternal line (grandfather, uncle) male with similar changes iridociliary zone and glaucoma. Criteria of glaucoma formation were: increased IOP more than 21 mmHg with accompanying it expansion of the cup\disc ratio, reducing the thickness of the nerve fiber layer (RNFL) according to OCT.

5. Ophthalmological Examination

Ophthalmological examination included standard methods of diagnosis (visual acuity measurement, biometry, refractometry, ophthalmoscopy, gonioscopy) as well as examinations of morphology iris and optic nerve-optical coherence tomography (Cirrus HD-OCT, Carl Zeiss Meditec Inc., USA), ultrasound biomicroscopy imaging (UBM-840, Hamphrey).

6. Statistical Analysis

The statistical data on all the studied parameters was represented as the mean value ± standard deviation. The difference between the treatment groups and control group was defined using Mann-Whitney U-test. The critical level of significance P upon the examination of statistical hypotheses was 0.05. All the calculations were made using the program STATISTICA 8.0, Stat Soft. Inc., USA.

7. Results

7.1. The Study of the Iris.

In the process of examination and long-term follow up of the patients with the syndrome, it was found that the symptomatic feature is a peculiar congenital hypoplasia of the iris stroma with exposure of its pigment epithelium. In addition this is always a bilateral process (*i.e.* both eyes are affected). While the defect of the front mesodermal iris layer is congenital, the destruction of the backsheet is acquired, appearing later in life and progressing throughout. External changes in the iris are so consistent and typical that after the examination of the patients it seems that they are close relatives or brothers (**Figure 1**).

While the normal pupillary zone [7] of an iris is darker than a ciliary zone, all patients with the syndrome have thicker, light gray or yellow, lackluster pupillary zone, devoid of the normal luster. The periphery of the iris looks like a wide ring of contrasting brown or blue-purple. The reason for the color contrast is the hypoplasia of the iris stroma, through which the pigment epithelium is seen.

In 44.4% of the cases of the patients in the juvenile group, and in 6.8% of the cases of the patients in the adult group in addition to the two-color staining there was also rough damage of the iris:

1) Iridoschizis and radial zones of the transillumination around the iris periphery.
2) Slotted through-defects of the iris in the ciliary zone (**Figure 2**).
3) Polycoria (**Figure 3**).
4) Ectopia and pupillary ring deformation (**Figure 4**).

Long-term iris monitoring in patients of this group has revealed that the iris abnormalities are the successive stages of the progressive atrophy of the stroma and the destruction of the pigment epithelium.

The study of the iris by the OCT method [8] confirmed the presence of rough congenital bilateral hypoplasia of the stroma in patients of the juvenile group (**Figure 5**). In the control group, the thickness of the iris stroma was from 460 to 283 microns. The iris stroma of the juvenile group was severely thinner, up to its complete absence in the ciliary zone (from 126.0 mkm to 0 mkm) and was 3 - 5 times thinner than that of healthy children. In the adult group, the thickness of the iris stroma was also thinner and it was on average 209.27 ± 44.27 mkm ($P = 0.001$). The pigment layer in all patients with the syndrome was dramatically thickened, up to 70 microns at the limbus and up to 90 microns in the pupil area, which is almost 1.5 times higher than normal (**Figure 6**).

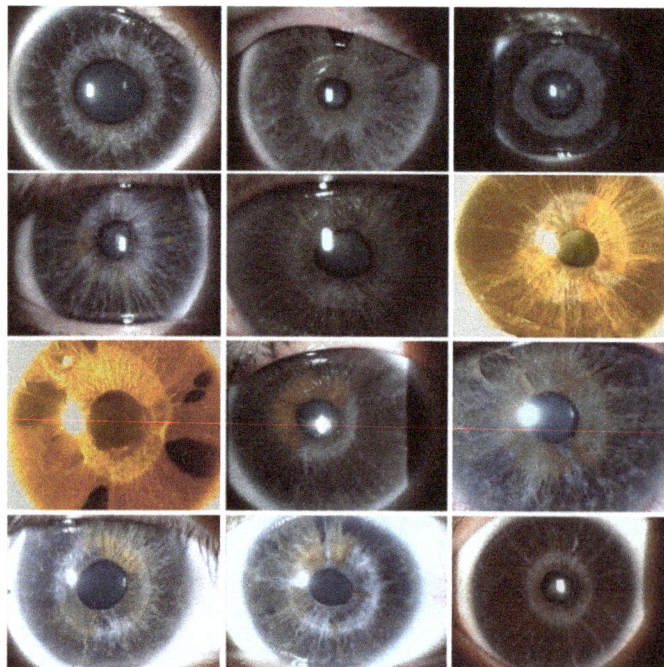

Figure 1. Photos of iris of 12 patients of the juvenile group.

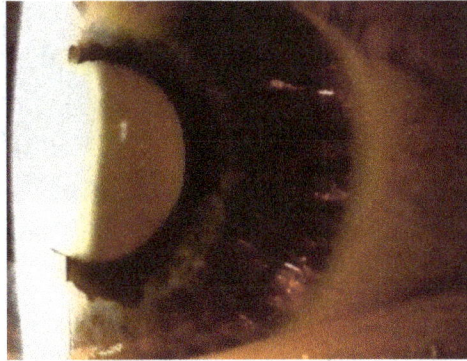

Figure 2. Radial zones of transillumination around the periphery of iris.

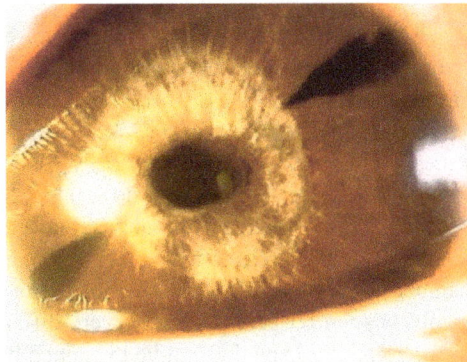

Figure 3. Large triangular breaks of the iris.

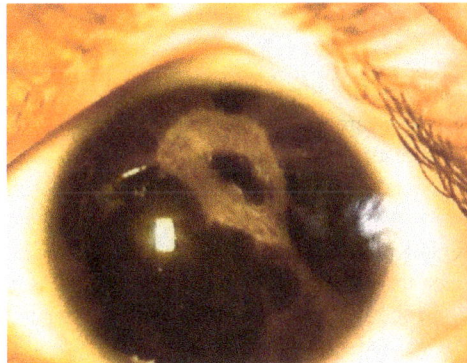

Figure 4. Ectopia of the pupil, large iris breaks.

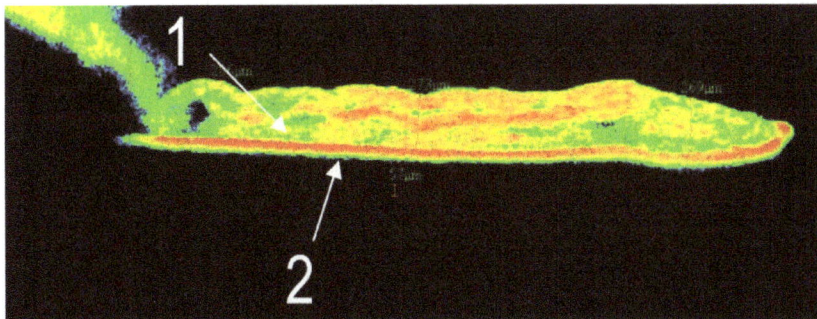

Figure 5. OCT imaging of the iris in healthy eyes: 1—stroma 236 - 405 microns, 2—pigment epithelium 57 - 60 microns.

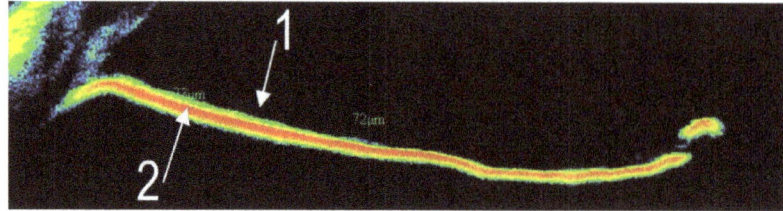

Figure 6. OCT imaging of the iris of a 6 year-old patient with glaucoma: 1—iris stroma—0 micron, 2—pigment epithelium—72 - 78 microns.

The smallest thickness of the pigment layer was registered next to the iris through-defects. That is, with the progression of the process there is rupture and wrinkling of the tissues, rather than atrophy of the tissue.

7.2. Features of the Iridocorneal Angle

Goniodysgenesis is characterized by the front fastening of the iris above the trabecular meshwork or fastening of the iris to the modified anterior border of the Schwalbe's ring, which was protruding into the anterior chamber in the form of the crest and was characterized as a posterior embryotoxon. Posterior embryotoxon was detected in patients of the juvenile group in 100% of the cases (**Figure 7**).

The degree of goniodysgenesis (classification Hoskins HD Jr., Shaffer RN: 1—Trabeculodysgenesis, 2—partial iridotrabekulodysgenesis, 3—full iridotrabekulodysgenesis)), evaluated by a point system, in this group of patients juvenile group was 2.1 ± 0.71, in individuals of adult group 1.19 ± 0.04, which significantly exceeds the control group -0.05 ± 0.22 and 0.07 ± 0.26 respectively ($P = 0.004$ and $P = 0.05$). Despite the fact that such a condition of the anterior chamber angle should lead to a complete pre-trabecular meshwork retention, acute decompensation of IOP in patients was not observed, which is very different for this form of glaucoma in comparison with simple congenital glaucoma. Perhaps this can be explained by the hypoplasia of iris stroma in patients with the syndrome when the partial drainage of aqueous humor is preserved. It was found that the through-defects of an iris are formed at the initial stromal thickness of up to 30 microns.

7.3. Cornea

It was found that the clinically significant corneal pathology [9] [10] was diagnosed in the majority of the juvenile group patients. There was an increase in congenital corneal diameter of more than 12 mm (**Figure 8**) with normal values of intraocular pressure in 20 of the researched cases, which determined a significant difference (F-criterion—4.33 with a significance level of $P = 0.05$) on the basis of the control group. This condition was diagnosed as megalocornea.

Corneal thickness of patients with megalocornea averaged 591.57 ± 52.67 mkm, resulting in an increase in the average thickness of the cornea in juvenile group patients of 50 microns, compared with healthy children.

In addition, it was found that the increase of the cornea diameter in patients born with the Frank-Kamenetsky Syndrome is detected at birth, is independent of the IOP level, is not progressive and, as opposed to simple congenital glaucoma, is accompanied by thickening (not thinning) of the cornea. Therefore, such cornea condition is one of the manifestations of congenital malformations of the eye's mesenchymal tissue.

Due to the fact that mesenchymal dysgenesis involves changing of all structures of the anterior segment of an eye, the following was studied in great detail: parameters of the cornea, lens and anterior chamber angle values, changes in the ways of the outflow of aqueous humor, the state of the iris at all stages of the disease (**Table 1**).

7.4. Discriminant Analysis of the Study's Results of the "Juvenile" and "Adult" Groups of Patients

Informative attributes, calculated from the F-Fisher criterion, are distributed as follows (**Table 2**). The most informative attributes were the thickness of the iris stroma (F-score 22.1) and the degree of goniodysgenesis (F-score 22.16), with a significance level of $P < 0.00001$. It was observed that such features as the thickness of the cornea (the F-score 6.16) and the diameter of the cornea (F-criterion 1.9) appeared to have the same degree of canonical value construction with $P < 0.05$. In addition, the discriminant analysis revealed the possible impact indicators such as the degree of refraction (F-score 3.2 for $P = 0.07$), the length of an eyeball (F-score 5.64), the

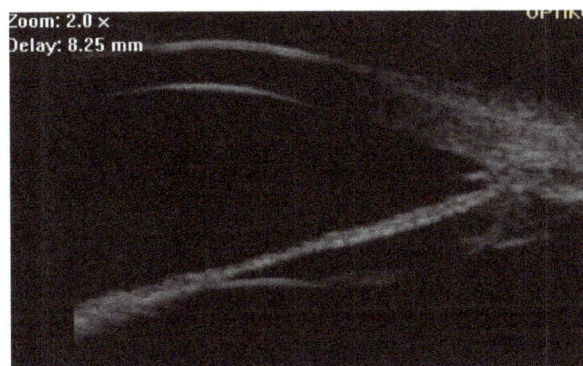

Figure 7. UBM of the anterior segment of the eye of Patient K. In the top of the anterior chamber angle-protrusion of an anterior border of the Schwalbe's ring-posterior embryotoxon.

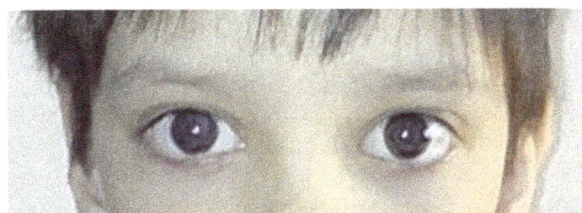

Figure 8. Photo of the patient with a corneal diameter of 14 mm.

Table 1. Results of a comparative analysis of the parameters of the visual system of patients with the syndrome and the control group (M ± s).

Data	1-control group, n = 30, males, average age 7.2 ± 1.6	2-"juvenile" group, n = 22, males, average age 10.1 ± 2.4	3-control group, n = 30, males, average age 26.59 ± 4.12	4-"adult" group, n = 28, males, average age 32.44 ± 6.28	P, Mann-Whitney
Refraction of an eye	+0.4 ± 0.28	+0.41 ± 1.75	−0.16 ± 0.67	−0.72 ± 1.58	3 - 4 = 0.008
Diameter of the cornea, mm	10.32 ± 0.40	12.48 ± 0.96	10.18 ± 0.39	10.83 ± 0.67	1 - 2 = 0.045
CCT, microns	546.28 ± 37.94	591.57 ± 52.67	558.94 ± 33.22	548.63 ± 38.09	1 - 2 = 0.007
Thickness of the iris stroma, microns (OCT)	334.57 ± 30.12	100.57 ± 27.25	328.94 ± 30.20	209.27 ± 44.27	1 - 2 = 0.001 3 - 4 = 0.001
Thickness of the iris pigment epithelium, microns (OCT)	62.75 ± 5.54	72.61 ± 7.58	62.11 ± 5.54	79.52 ± 6.75	1 - 2 = 0.006 3 - 4 = 0.004
Availability through-defects of the iris, %	-	44.4	-	6.8	1 - 2 = 0.002 3 - 4 = 0.002
Degree of a goniodisgenesis	0.05 ± 0.22	2.10 ± 0.71	0.07 ± 0.26	1.19 ± 0.40	1 - 2 = 0.004 3 - 4 = 0.05

magnitude of the anterior chamber (F-criterion 3, 3 for $P = 0.07$).

Therefore, the most important signs determining the formation of glaucoma in children are congenital subtotal dysplasia of the iris stroma, goniodysgenesis and corneal changes by type of megalocornea characterized by increase of the diameter and CCT of the cornea. Other signs altogether characterize the discrepancy between the length of the eyeball and the degree of refraction, because myopic component in these patients is compensated by a weak refractive power of the cornea with its congenital dysgenesis.

7.5. The Types of Inheritance of the Gene

The conducted Genealogical Analysis showed that all of the patients were Caucasian and did not have any other somatic or eye diseases [11] [12]. During the cytogenetic examination of the probands in families A, B, and C (pedigrees #1, 2, 3) no chromosomal abnormalities were found, which may indicate the monogenetic nature of the disease. The most common ways of inheritance of the Frank-Kamenetsky Syndrome are seen in the P. family (**Chart 1**).

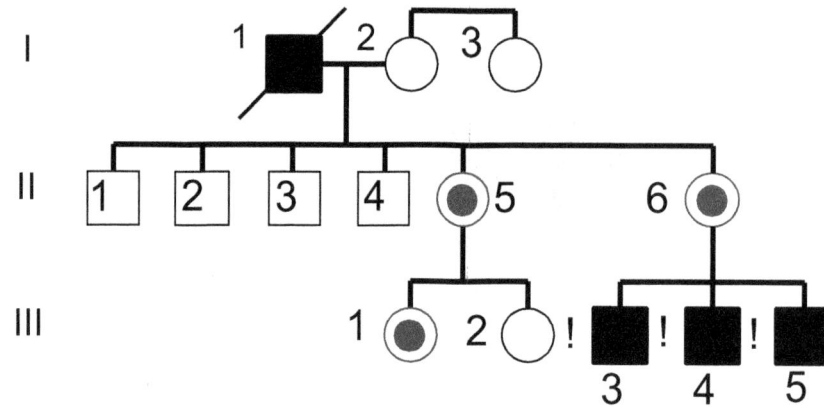

Chart 1.
I (1)—proband, died blind at 58 years old.
II (5)—no eye pathology, 37 years old.
II (6)—no eye pathology, 43 years old.
III (3)—proband-1, glaucoma since age 5.
III (4)—sibs, glaucoma since age 21.
III (5)—sibs, no glaucoma, 28 years old.

Female, carrier of pathological gene (carrier)—

Healthy Female—
Individual with Frank-Kamenetsky Syndrome—

Healthy Male—

According to the provided genealogical **Chart 1**, 3 boys with congenital hypoplasia of the iris are observed within the P. family. The oldest brother's glaucoma was diagnosed at the age of 5, the middle brother's IOP began to increase at the age of 21, and the younger brother had a phenotypic syndrome only at the age of 28. Their maternal grandfather was blind from glaucoma, and died at the age of 58. Proband's and sibling's mother does not have any vision problems but has micro signs of the disease.

Thus, the mechanism of inheritance of pathological signs in this syndrome corresponds to x-linked recessive manner on the following criteria:

1) Common in men.

2) All female children of an affected father will be carriers. (Daughters possess their father's X-chromosome in 100% cases). The sons of the daughter will have a 50% probability to be affected.

3) No male children of the sick father will be affected. (Sons do not inherit their father's X-chromosome).

4) Heterozygous females are considered carriers and generally will not manifest clinical symptoms of the disease, but some of them may have varying degrees of severity of the disease.

The presence of such micro phenotypic symptoms of the syndrome can be taken into consideration in a prenatal genetic diagnosis.

8. Discussion

According to the study results, the initial mesodermal layer thickness of the iris at birth is a sign of dysgenesis, which is directly correlated with the degree of goniodysgenesis, abnormalities of the cornea, and the presence of partial or complete posterior embryotoxon. In general, alteration of the iris may determine the degree of anterior segment dysgenesis [13]-[15]. Formation of glaucoma in children is caused by a combination of congenital abnormalities of the cornea, iris, and the iridocorneal angle, as well as the presence of coarse dysgenesis of the anterior segment of the eye. These are, namely, the association of subtotal hypoplasia of the iris's mesodermal sheet (thickness from 0 to 30 mkm) with symptoms of progressive dystrophy, congenital megalocornea, posterior embryotoxon, and dysgenesis of iridocorneal angle of II-III degree.

Identification of the criteria and mechanisms of glaucoma is important as it allows not only to diagnose the disease at early preclinical stages of development but also to assign pathogenetically-based treatment soon

Table 2. Classification features of the syndrome of the juvenile group.

	Data	% contribution	F-criterion	P-level
X7	Thickness of the iris stroma	25.25%	66.61	0.00001
X6	Degree of goniodysgenesis	19.85%	22.16	0.00001
X4	Thickness of the cornea	11.76%	5.64	0.034
X5	Diameter of the cornea	6.50%	6.16	0.03
X1	Magnitude of the anterior chamber	8.16%	3.2	0.07
X3	Refraction of the eye	8.66%	3.3	0.071
X2	Length of an eyeball	11.11%	3.2	0.07

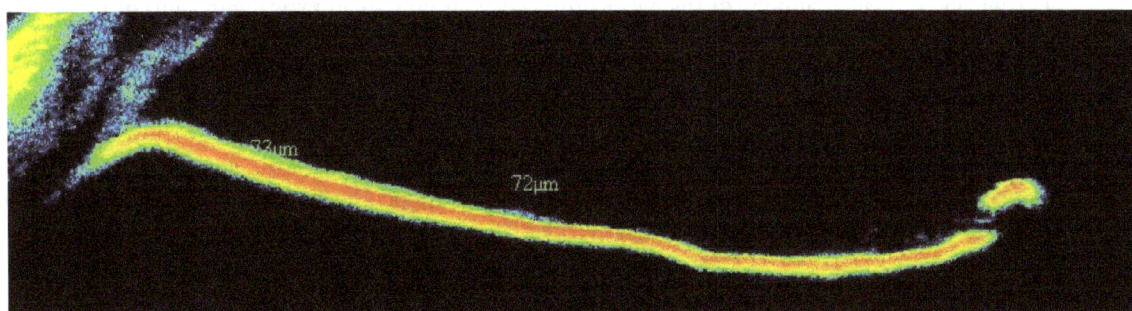

(a)

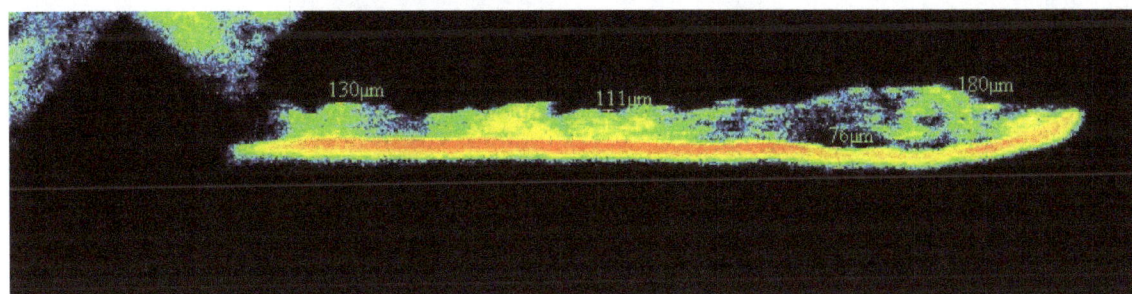

(b)

Figure 9. (a) OCT of the iris of Patient D., 11 years old. Stroma 0. Pigment layer (1) 72 - 78 mkm, (b) OCT of the iris of D.'s brother, 14 years old, Stroma 111 - 180 mkm (2). Pigment layer (1) 76 mkm, compacted, transparency reduced.

enough. The special importance in juvenile patients with glaucoma is the diminished visual function for several reasons. First, the development of glaucoma is an asymptomatic process, therefore an ophthalmologist is not involved until a later stage of the disease progression. Second, antihypertensive drug therapy has a weak hypotensive effect on this type of glaucoma. Third, is the progressive destruction of the iris, leading to impairment of accommodation and diaphragm function, which causes light scattering and further reduces a patient's visual acuity. Pathological process usually ends in late detection of glaucoma with blindness or poor vision at 40 - 50 years of age.

The combination of moderate iris hypoplasia with gonidysgenesis of I degree causes formation of glaucoma after the age of 20 - 30, sometimes after reaching 40 years of age. At the same time the structure of the trabecular meshwork becomes differentiated and hydrodynamic blocks can be associated with the anatomical features of the trabecular meshwork structure. Glaucoma in these cases has a relatively benign course that is observed in adult patients.

Case History

Patient D., 11 years old, has complex pathological changes of the anterior eye segment: megalocornea, corneal diameter of 13 mm, posterior embryotoxon, front fixing of the iris, and the thickness of the iris stroma is 10 - 0 mkm (**Figure 9a**). Glaucoma developed at the age of 5.

D.'s brother was first examined 5 years ago at the age of 14. At that time the typical two-tone coloring of the iris was identified, the anterior chamber angle was open, the trabecula was partially covered with gray fibrous tissue, and the thickness of the iris stroma was 180 mkm (**Figure 9b**). Data for glaucoma for the period of examination and in the present time are not found.

9. Conclusions

Thus, the study of patients with inherited congenital mesenchymal dysgenesis and pathogenetic mechanisms of both the Frank-Kamenetsky Syndrome and glaucoma is allowed to determine the differences in the two clinical groups and to identify the criteria for early glaucoma development in patients with such syndrome.

Such criteria are a combination of:

1) Congenital subtotal atrophy of iris mesodermal layer (from 0 to 30 mkm) with signs of progressive dystrophy;

2) Nonprogressive congenital megalocornea (cornea diameter 12 - 14 mm);

3) Iridotrabecular dysgenesis of II-III degree;

4) Hyperopic refraction in axial myopia.

Thus, the formation of glaucoma in children is caused by dysgenesis of the anterior segment of the eye—a combination of congenital anomalies of the iris, cornea, and iridocorneal angle, which implies the inherited defects in the embryonic development of all germ layers of mesenchymal tissue.

References

[1]   Becker, B. and Shaffer, R. (2004) Diagnosis and Therapy of the Glaucomas. Mosby, St. Louis.

[2]   Frank-Kamenetskiy, Z.G. (1951) To the Question of Congenital Histoplasia of the Iris with Secondary Glaucoma. *Proceedings of the Irkutsk Medical Institute*, Dedicated to the 30th Anniversary of Its Existence, IGMI, Irkutsk, 281-288.

[3]   Frank-Kamenetskiy, Z.G (1925) The Peculiar Form of Hereditary Glaucoma. *Russian Ophthalmological Journal*, No. 3, 203-219.

[4]   Brémond-Gignac, D. (2007) Glaucoma in Aniridia. *Journal Français d'Ophtalmologie*, **2**, 196-199. http://dx.doi.org/10.1016/S0181-5512(07)89576-3

[5]   Iureva, T.N. (2012) Mechanisms of Formation of Glaucoma Associated with Alteration of the Iris. Ph.D. Dissertation, Siberian Branch of the Russian Academy of Medical Sciences, Irkutsk.

[6]   Levin, A.V. (2003) Congenital Eye Anomalies. *Pediatric Clinics of North America*, **1**, 55-76. http://dx.doi.org/10.1016/S0031-3955(02)00113-X

[7]   Apple, D.J. and Naumann, G.O.H. (1997) General Anatomy and Development of the Eye. *Pathology of the Eye*, 1-19.

[8]   Radhakrishan, S., Rollins, A. and Roth, J. (2001) Real-Time Optical Coherence Tomography of the Anterior Segment at 1310 nm. *Archives of Ophthalmology*, **119**, 1179-1185. http://dx.doi.org/10.1001/archopht.119.8.1179

[9]   Shchuko, A.G. and Iureva, T.N. (2009) Glaucoma and Pathology of the Iris. Borges, Moscow.

[10]   Smelser, G.K. and Duke-Elder, S. (1990) Morphological and Functional Development of the Cornea. Symposium Abstract Book: The Transparency of the Cornea, Springfield, 23-39.

[11]   Clemente, C.D. (2007) Anatomy: A Regional Atlas of the Human Body. Lippincott Williams & Wilkins, Philadelphia.

[12]   MacDonald, I.M., Tran, M. and Musarella, M.A. (2004) Ocular Genetics: Current Understanding. *Survey of Ophthalmology*, **2**, 159-196. http://dx.doi.org/10.1016/j.survophthal.2003.12.003

[13]   Deepak, P.E. and Kaufman, L.M. (2003) Anatomy, Development, and Physiology of the Visual System. *Pediatric Clinics of North America*, **1**, 1-23.

[14]   Idrees, F., Vaideanu, D. and Fraser, S.G. (2006) A Review of Anterior Segment Dysgeneses. *Survey of Ophthalmology*, **3**, 213-231. http://dx.doi.org/10.1016/j.survophthal.2006.02.006

[15]   Rodrigues, M.M., Jester, J.V. and Richards, R. (1985) Essential Iris Atrophy. A Clinical, Immunohistologic, and Electron Microscopic Study in an Enucleated Eye. *Ophthalmology*, **95**, 69-73. http://dx.doi.org/10.1016/S0161-6420(88)33234-3

11

Surgically Induced Corneal Astigmatism Following Cataract Surgery

Derya Buran Kağnici¹, Tolga Kocatürk²*, Harun Çakmak², Sema Oruç Dündar²

¹Department of Ophthalmology, Aydın State Hospital, Aydın, Turkey
²Department of Ophthalmology, Adnan Menderes University Medical Faculty, Aydın, Turkey
Email: *tolgakocaturk@gmail.com

Abstract

Aim: To study the surgically induced astigmatism (SIA) caused by two different type main incisions in phacoemulsification. **Methods:** Sixty-eight eyes of 65 patients who underwent phacoemulsification were randomly divided into two groups according to main incision type: 2.8 mm superior limbal incision (in Group 1) and 2.8 mm upper clear corneal incision (in Group 2). Surgical techniques did not differ between the groups except for the main incisions. All patients received detailed ophthalmological examination in addition to keratometry at the pre- and post-operatively. The preoperative and postoperative astigmatisms were calculated by the vector analysis method and the SIA was compared between the groups. **Results:** The mean SIA values were 1.3 ± 0.67 D, 0.89 ± 0.47 D, 0.77 ± 37 D in Group 1 and 1.42 ± 0.62 D, 1.15 ± 0.54 D, 0.94 ± 0.47 D in Group 2 on the first day, first week and first month postoperatively, respectively. According to the vector analysis, SIA was less in Group 1 than Group 2; although the difference was not statistically significant (p > 0.05). **Conclusion:** Although less astigmatism was detected in the superior limbal incision group, this difference was not statistically significant.

Keywords

Cataract, Phacoemulsification, Surgically Induced Astigmatism

1. Introduction

Cataract is the leading treatable cause of blindness in the world and it is treated by surgery only. Due to fast visual improvement and lower complication rate, cataract extraction by phacoemulsification and the insertion of a foldable intraocular lens (IOL) through a small incision is the preferred surgical method [1].

---

*Corresponding author.

Currently, cataract surgery is considered as a type of refractive surgery and reduction of refractive defects to the lowest level is possible, leading to increased expectations of patients. Astigmatism due to surgery may affect vision quality and varies related to the type and size of the incision and suture utilization [2].

In this study, surgically induced astigmatism (SIA) following phacoemulsification by 2.8 mm superior limbal incision and superior clear corneal incision were compared.

2. Materials and Method

Patients with the diagnosis of cataracts over the age of 50 subjected to phacoemulsification and IOL implantation were enrolled in this study. Ethical approval was obtained from the local institutional ethics committees and informed consent was obtained from all patients. The study adhered to the tenets of the Declaration of Helsinki. Patients with previous ocular surgery, diabetes, systemic connective tissue disorder, severe dry eye, pytergium, corneal scar, degeneration and ectasia, pseudoexfoliation, uveitis, glaucoma, high myopia and retinal diseases were excluded. In addition, patients with complications such as non-completed capsulorhexis during the operation, zonule dialysis, posterior capsule opening, patients with sutured incisions and patients without regular post-op follow up were excluded.

Ophthalmologic evaluation included best corrected visual acuity (BCVA) by Snellen chart, refraction, keratometry, biomicroscopy, detailed fundus examination, and intraocular pressure (IOP) measurement and corneal topography (Orbscan 2z, B & L, USA). IOL diopter was calculated by Lensstar (Haag Streit Eyesuite™, USA) biometry instrument according to SRK-T formula. Pre- and post-operative astigmatism was calculated by vector analysis and the effect of the incision site on astigmatism due to surgery was compared.

All operations were performed by two surgeons (TK, HC) under topical anesthesia by proparacaine HCl 0.5% (Alcaine; Alcon, Puurs, Belgium). Patients were assigned randomly into two groups. Main incision was made with two sided 2.8-mm blade. One-step superior limbal incision was done in Group 1 and superior clear corneal incision in Group 2. There was no difference between the groups, except location of incision, in any aspects of surgery. Nucleus was broken by "horizontal chop" method and was emulsified using a Sovereign Compact (AMO Laboratories, USA) phacoemulsification instrument. Hydrophobic acrylic IOL (Acriva UD 613.VSY, Istanbul, Turkey) was placed by injector-cartridge system.

In this study, surgical SIA Calculator Version 2.1 vector analysis program developed by Sawhney and Aggarwal, was used. SPSS (Statistical Package for Social Sciences) 17.0 program was used for statistical analysis. Mann Whitney U, Friedman and t tests were used for data comparison. Any p value less than 0.05 ($p < 0.05$) was accepted as significant. Power analysis recommended a minimum of 33 eyes per group in order to obtain an efficacy size of 0.8, alpha value 0.05 and statistical power of 0.8.

3. Results

Sixty-eight eyes of 65 patients (31 females, 34 males) were included. Superior limbal incision was used in 35 patients (13 female, 22 male) (Group 1) and superior clear corneal incision in 33 patients (18 female, 15 male) (Group 2). Mean age was 64.00 ± 8.83 and 64.12 ± 10.30 years in Group 1 and 2, respectively. No statistical differences were present between the two groups in terms of mean age (p = 0.959) and gender distribution (p = 0.150).

Mean BCVAs in Group 1 were 0.19 ± 0.11, 0.36 ± 0.23, 0.70 ± 0.23 and 0.92 ± 0.08 pre-operatively, and postoperatively first day, first week and first month, respectively; same parameters were 0.17 ± 0.11, 0.38 ± 0.24, 0.72 ± 0.20 and 0.94 ± 0.08 in Group 2. No statistical difference was found between the groups in terms of these values (p = 0.512, p = 0.808, p = 0.686 and p = 0.150).

Mean IOP measured by non-contact tonometry in Group 1 were 12.71 ± 3.81 mmHg, 15.06 ± 3.39 mmHg, 12.85 ± 3.54 mmHg, and 12.66 ± 3.71 mmHg pre-operatively, postoperatively first day, first week and first month, respectively; same parameters were 13.09 ± 2.98 mmHg, 15.27 ± 4.93 mmHg, 13.00 ± 3.93 mmHg, 12.97 ± 2.70 mmHg in Group 2. No statistical difference was found between the two groups in terms of these values (p = 0.643, p = 0.567, p = 0.875 and p = 0.715).

Mean SIA calculated by vector analysis method was smaller in Group 1 than those in Group 2 however; the difference was not statistically significant between the groups (**Table 1** and **Figure 1**). In-group comparison, significant decrease was seen in astigmatism during postoperative wound healing period when analyzed by Friedman test (p values for Group 1 and 2 respectively, 0.045 and <0.001).

Mean SIA centroid values calculated by vector analysis method in Group 1 and 2 were seen in **Table 2** and **Figure 2**. Mean SIA centroid axial values revealed that patients in Group 1 had irregular astigmatism whereas oblique astigmatism were seen in Group 2 postoperatively.

Correlation between mean SIA calculated by vector analysis and mean IOP was evaluated and no significant correlation was detected by assessing the effect of mean IOP on SIA (r < 0.50) (**Table 3**).

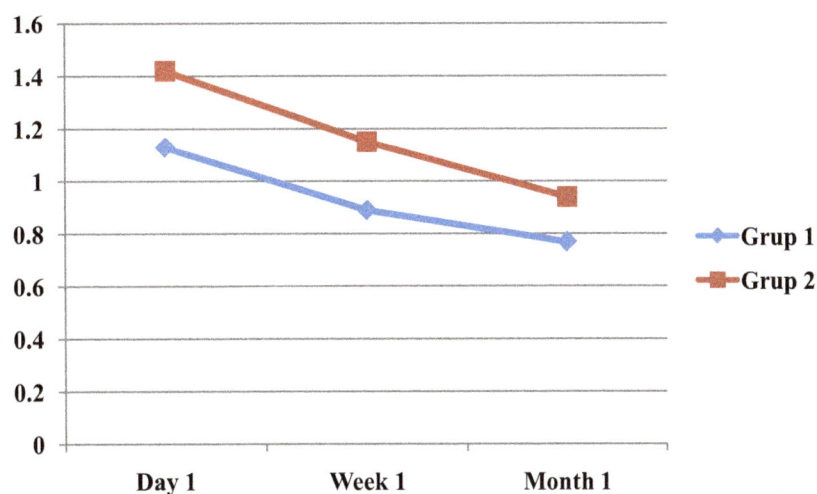

Figure 1. Mean SIA in both groups (diopter) calculated by vector analysis method in both groups on postoperative 1st day, 1st week and 1st month.

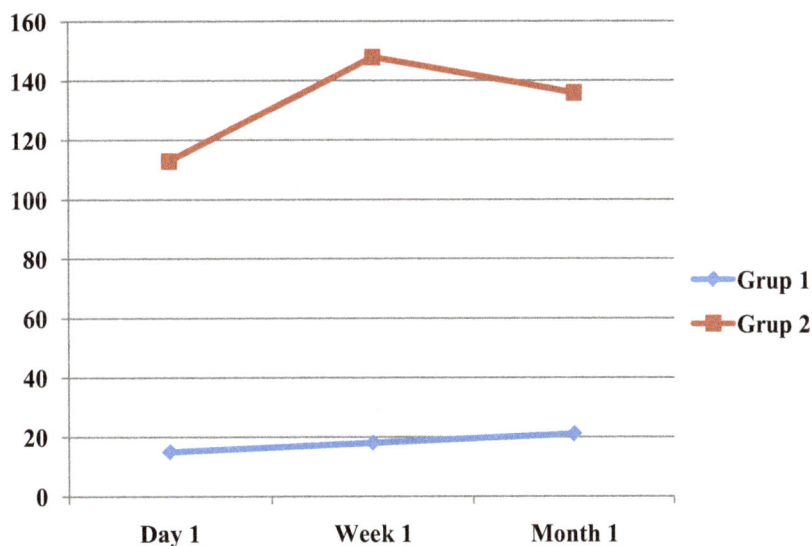

Figure 2. Mean SIA centroid axial values (degree) in both groups calculated by vector analysis method in both groups at postoperative 1st day, 1st week and 1st month.

Table 1. Surgery-related astigmatism ± SD (diopter) calculated by vector analysis method in both groups on postoperative 1st day, 1st week and 1st month.

Postoperative	Group 1	Group 2	t/u value	p value
1st day	1.13 ± 0.67	1.42 ± 0.62	−1.721 (t)	0.090
1st week	0.89 ± 0.47	1.15 ± 0.54	392 (u)	0.054
1st month	0.77 ± 0.37	0.94 ± 0.47	519 (u)	0.473

Table 2. Mean surgery-related astigmatism centroid (c) in both groups calculated by vector analysis method in both groups on postoperative 1st day, 1st week and 1st month.

Postoperative	Group 1		Group 2	
	Centroid	Axis	Centroid	Axis
1st day	0.81	15	0.31	113
1st week	0.60	18	0.26	148
1st month	0.43	21	0.46	136

Table 3. Correlation between mean surgery-related astigmatism calculated by vector analysis and mean IOP postoperative 1st day, 1st week, 1st month in both groups.

Postoperative	Group 1		Group 2	
	r value	p value	r value	p value
1st day	−0.21	0.219	−0.08	0.634
1st week	−0.27	0.116	−0.02	0.878
1st month	−0.14	0.421	0.18	0.300

4. Discussion

Phacoemulsification and IOL implantation technique is currently the most widely used ocular surgery. Corneal interventions affect corneal curve and refraction power. Post-surgical high astigmatism is one of the reasons behind unsatisfying visual outcomes of cataract procedure. Phacoemulsification provides faster visual improvement, smaller surgical incision and less irregular astigmatism than other techniques. Foldable IOL usage leads to small incision site and minimal SIA. Post operative astigmatism after cataract surgery is related to two factors: preoperative astigmatism of patient and SIA [3] [4].

Surgically induced astigmatism is a frequent complication of cataract surgery and plays an important role in postoperative visual acuity. Astigmatic variation is mostly due to corneal contour changes in SIA. Surgically induced astigmatism varies related to type, length and site of the incision, suture utilization, distance of incision to the optic center of cornea. Even lower astigmatism is important, since this would affect distance sight of patients [3] [5].

Incision site is an important factor affecting SIA. While superior corneal or limbal incision leads to irregular astigmatism, temporal corneal incision leads to regular astigmatism. One or two sided temporal incisions lead to minimal astigmatism; however three sided and deep groove incisions lead to increased astigmatism [6]. Kohnen et al. [7] showed more SIA in nasal incisions in their study. They suggested that this could be due to more stress and corneal stretch in the wound site related to more perpendicular entrance to cornea in nasal incision and also to the closer location of nasal incision to corneal center.

Wirbelauer et al. [8] compared superior, temporal and oblique vertical axial scleral tunnel incisions of 7.0 mm and detected flattening of vertical axis and steepening in horizontal axis. In addition, increased degrees of astigmatism were seen in superior incisions than all other incisions. Şimşek et al. [9] compared temporal clear corneal incision and superior clear corneal incision; they showed statistically significantly more and irregular astigmatism in superior corneal incisions.

In another study, Pakravan et al. [10] compared biplanar temporal and nasal clear corneal incisions of 3.2 mm and they determined statistically significantly less astigmatism for temporal incision (0.26 D) compared to nasal incision (0.92 D) at 6th month. Özkurt et al. [11] compared the effects of superior-nasal and superior-temporal clear corneal incisions on total astigmatism and they showed statistically significantly less total and SIA in temporal incision at 6th week. Long et al. [12] compared corneal tunnel incisions from vertical axis of 3.0 - 3.2 and 3.5 mm. Incisions on vertical meridian were reported to lead to more astigmatic change than ones at horizontal meridian. Kılıç et al. [13] compared superior temporal and superior nasal clear corneal incisions of 3.2 mm in their study. Surgically induced astigmatism was statistically significantly more frequent with nasal incision. Yaycıoğlu et al. [14] compared nasal, temporal, superior temporal or superior clear corneal incisions to vertical axis and they showed less SIA with temporal and superior temporal incisions. Rainer *et al.* [15] compared temporal and superior-lateral clear corneal incisions of 3.0 mm and they observed corneal flattening at incision site of all types, being more frequent with superior-lateral incisions. In these studies comparing temporal, nasal and superior corneal incisions, astigmatism was less frequent with temporal incisions. This was related to the existence of more distance of temporal incision to central cornea than superior incision due to ellipsoid figure of cornea. The other cause was reported to be fluctuation of wound site due to pressure of superior lid. This was related with both scleral tunnel incisions and clear corneal incisions [8]-[15]. Ermiş *et al.* [16] compared superior temporal and superior nasal clear corneal incisions of 3.3 - 3.5 mm in their study and they found no statistically significant difference in terms of SIA. Tejedor *et al.* [17] found out less corneal alterations by temporal incision in patients without preoperative corneal astigmatism. Furthermore, when surgery was performed by temporal clear corneal incisions in eyes with preoperative irregular astigmatism, it was observed that astigmatism decreased in the postoperative period [18] [19]. Temporal incision was recommended in patients with preoperative regular lower astigmatism and preoperative neutral patients [10] [11] [13].

In our study, superior limbal incision of 2.8 mm was used in Group 1 and superior clear corneal incision of 2.8 mm in Group 2. Post-operative surgery related centroid axis values were detected as irregular astigmatism in Group 1 on first day, first week and first month. In Group 2, post-operative surgery related axis were oblique at all measurements on first day, first week and first month.

Type of incision site is an important factor affecting astigmatism. He *et al.* [20] compared astigmatism parameters measured by keratometry for clear temporal corneal incision and superior scleral tunnel incision in terms of astigmatic effect following phacoemulsification.

Postoperatively, more astigmatism was present with corneal incision at first month. However, no statistically significant difference was present between two groups on postoperative third month.

Barequet *et al.* [21] reported that no conjunctival scar developed with clear corneal incisions, thus conjunctiva were preserved for possible future glaucoma surgery. They also reported that conjunctival hemorrhage, hyphema risk and post-operative blood-aqueous changes were low, and also that shorter tunnel incision provided better vision and more comfortable surgery. Therefore, clear corneal incisions were found to be more advantageous than cornea-scleral incisions. Stabilization of corneal tunnel incision lasts postoperative two to six weeks [21]. Astigmatism increased as incision approached the corneal center. Ernest *et al.* [22] compared phacoemulsification with 2.2 mm posterior limbal incision by one surgeon and surgery of 2.2 mm clear corneal incision by five different surgeons and they reported that SIA with posterior limbal incision was statistically significantly less (0.25 D) than all other lowest SIA (0.38). Limbus and cornea are structurally different. Thus, their patterns of wound healing would be different. Cornea is an avascular and starched tissue with dense fibroblasts. Limbus has vascular structures constituting the source of fibroblasts, resulting in a faster wound healing. Wound healing occurs within seven days at limbus however this period may be extended to 60 days for cornea [23]. Since limbus is more resistant than cornea against the pressure, clear corneal incision has 5.8 times more risk of endophthalmitis than limbal and scleral tunnel incisions [24]. In our study, superior limbal incision was used in Group 1 and superior clear corneal incision was used in Group 2. Mean SIA was less in the group with limbal incision than in the group with corneal incision on postoperative first day, first week and first month. However, this difference was not statistically significant. In-group comparison, during wound healing process, decrease in astigmatism is more prominent in Group 2 in the first month postoperatively.

Suture is also an important factor for astigmatism. Suture and tissue adhesive reduce tissue elasticity. Suture at appropriate stretch and localization may reduce SIA. However, stretched and misplaced sutures may flatten the incision site and increase astigmatism in that meridian by steepening in the central optic zone [25]. In our study, we have no patients with suture.

Corneal burn due to phacoemulsification also leads to serious SIA especially in clear corneal incision. Same amount of corneal burn results in more SIA in clear corneal incision than in limbal incision.

Reducing SIA is an important issue in modern cataract surgery. Currently, cataract surgery is considered as a kind of refractive surgery. Development of modified techniques may reduce post-operative astigmatism. Examples of these methods are incision at vertical axis of cornea, corneal-limbal relaxing incisions, toric IOL implantation and excimer laser. Preoperative astigmatism of 1.5 D may be corrected by incision at vertical corneal axis. Astigmatism of >1.5 D may require additional relaxing incisions or other methods. In patients with preoperative irregular astigmatism, temporal incision may reduce astigmatism [3] [4]. Tejedor *et al.* [17] reported that clear corneal incisions reduce preoperative astigmatism by performing incision at vertical axis. In patients without preoperative astigmatism, superior corneal incision may lead to more astigmatism than temporal incision, especially incision at vertical axis should be recommended in preoperative astigmatism of 1.50 D and more at vertical axis of 90° and preoperative astigmatism of 0.75 D and more at vertical axis of 180°. He *et al.* [20] reported that refractive stabilization of cornea may take three months. Therefore, in cases of additional corneal limbal relaxing suture or incision on wound site, they would be done within postoperative three months. SIA may be reduced by toric-multifocal IOL [26]. In patients with preoperative astigmatism of >1 D multifocal IOL may be used [27].

5. Conclusion

In conclusion, no differences were present in our study in terms of incision site and size between groups. Mean SIA was lower in limbal incision group than clear corneal incision group on postoperative first day, first week and first month. However, no statistically significant difference was present.

Declaration of Interest

None.

Conflicts

The authors report no conflicts of interest.

Fund

No financial support was received for this submission.

References

[1]   Jackson, T.L. (2008) Moorfields Manual of Ophthalmology. Mosby Elsevier, Philadelphia, 6.

[2]   Henderson, B., Pineda, R., Ament, C., Chen, S. and Kim, J. (2007) Essentials of Cataract Surgery. Slack Incorporated, Online Library, Chapter 2.

[3]   Albert, D.M., Miller, J.W., Azar, D.T. and Blodi, B.A. (2008) Principles and Practice of Ophthalmology. 3rd Edition, Saunders Company, Philadelphia, Chapter 120.

[4]   Henderson, B., Pineda, R., Ament, C., Chen, S. and Kim, J. (2007) Essentials of Cataract Surgery. Slack Incorporated, Online Library, Chapter 7.

[5]   Kohnen, T. (1997) Corneal Shape Changes and Astigmatic Aspects of Scleral and Corneal Tunnel Incisions. *Journal of Cataract Refractive Surgery*, **23**, 301-302. http://dx.doi.org/10.1016/S0886-3350(97)80168-X

[6]   Henderson, B., Pineda, R., Ament, C., Chen, S. and Kim, J. (2007) Essentials of cataract surgery. Slack Incorporated, R2 Online Library, Chapter 6.

[7]   Kohnen, S., Neuber, R. and Kohnen, T. (2002) Effect of Temporal and Nasal Unsutured Limbal Tunnel Incisions on Induced Astigmatism after Phacoemusification. *Journal of Cataract Refractive Surgery*, **28**, 821-825. http://dx.doi.org/10.1016/S0886-3350(01)01215-9

[8]   Wirbelauer, C., Anders, N., Pham, D.T. and Wollensak, J. (1997) Effect of Incision Location on Preoperative Oblique Astigmatism after Scleral Tunnel Incision. *Journal of Cataract Refractive Surgery*, **23**, 365-371. http://dx.doi.org/10.1016/S0886-3350(97)80181-2

[9]   Simsek, S., Yasar, T., Demirok, A., Cinal, A. and Yılmaz, O.F. (1998) Effect of Superior and Temporal Clear Corneal Incisions on Astigmatism after Sutureless Phacoemulsification. *Journal of Cataract Refractive Surgery*, **24**, 515-518. http://dx.doi.org/10.1016/S0886-3350(98)80294-0

[10]   Pakravan, M., Nikkhah, H., Yazdani, S., Shahabi, C. and Rahimabadi, M.S.M. (2009) Astigmatic Outcomes of Temporal versus Nasal Clear Corneal Phacoemulsification. *Journal of Ophthalmic Vision Research*, **4**, 79-83.

[11]   Ozkurt, Y., Erdogan, G., Guveli, A.K., *et al.* (2008) Astigmatism after Superonasal and Superotemporal Clear Corneal Incisions in Phacoemulsification. *International Ophthalmology*, **28**, 329-332. http://dx.doi.org/10.1007/s10792-007-9141-y

[12]   Long, D.A. and Monica, M.L. (1996) A Prospective Evaluation of Corneal Curvature Changes with 3.0 to 3.5 mm Corneal Tunnel Phacoemulsification. *Ophthalmology*, **103**, 226-232. http://dx.doi.org/10.1016/S0161-6420(96)30712-4

[13] Kılıc, A., Gul, A., Yener, H.I., Cınal, A. and Demirok, A. (2010) Surgically Induced Astigmatism after Superotemporal or Superonasal Clear Corneal Incision in Phacoemulsification Surgery. *Van Medical Journal*, **17**, 84-88.

[14] Yaycioglu, A., Akova, Y.A., Akca, S., Gur, S. and Oktem, C. (2007) Effect on Astigmatism of the Location of Clear Corneal Incision in Phacoemulsification of Cataract. *Journal of Refractive Surgery*, **23**, 515-518.

[15] Rainer, G., Menapace, R., Vass, C., Annen, D., Findl, O. and Schmetterer, K. (1999) Corneal Shape Changes after Temporal and Superolateral 3,0 mm Clear Corneal Incisions. *Journal of Cataract Refractive Surgery*, **25**, 1121-1126. http://dx.doi.org/10.1016/S0886-3350(99)00132-7

[16] Ermis, S.S., Inan, U.U. and Ozturk, F. (2004) Surgically Induced Astigmatism after Superotemporal and Superonasal Clear Corneal Incisions in Phacoemulsification. *Journal of Cataract Refractive Surgery*, **30**, 1316-1319. http://dx.doi.org/10.1016/j.jcrs.2003.11.034

[17] Tejedor, J. and Murube, J. (2005) Choosing the Location of Corneal Incision Based on Preexisting Astigmatism in Phacoemulsification. *American Journal of Ophthalmology*, **139**, 767-776. http://dx.doi.org/10.1016/j.ajo.2004.12.057

[18] Kohnen, T., Dick, B. and Jacobi, K.W. (1995) Comparison of the Induced Astigmatism after Temporal Clear Corneal Tunnel Incisions of Different Sizes. *Journal of Cataract Refractive Surgery*, **21**, 417-424. http://dx.doi.org/10.1016/S0886-3350(13)80532-9

[19] Huang, F.C. and Tseng, S.H. (1998) Comparison of Surgically Induced Astigmatism after Sutureless Temporal Clear Corneal and Scleral Frown Incisions. *Journal of Cataract Refractive Surgery*, **24**, 477-481. http://dx.doi.org/10.1016/S0886-3350(98)80287-3

[20] He, Y., Zhu, S., Chen, M. and Li, D. (2009) Comparison of the Keratometric Corneal Astigmatic Power after Phacoemulsification: Clear Temporal Corneal Incision versus Superior Scleral Tunnel Incision. *Journal of Ophthalmology*, **2009**, Article ID: 210621.

[21] Barequet, I., Yu, E., Vitale, S., Cassard, S., Azar, D.T. and Stark, W.J. (2004) Astigmatism Outcomes of Horizontal Temporal versus Nasal Clear Corneal Incision Cataract Surgery. *Journal of Cataract Refractive Surgery*, **30**, 418-423. http://dx.doi.org/10.1016/S0886-3350(03)00492-9

[22] Ernest, P., Hill, W. and Potvin, R. (2011) Minimizing Surgically Induced Astigmatism at the Time of Cataract Surgery Using a Square Posterior Limbal Incision. *Journal of Ophthalmology*, **2011**, Article ID: 243170.

[23] Ernest, P., Tipperman, R., Eagle, R., *et al.* (1998) Is There a Difference in Incision Healing Based on Location? *Journal of Cataract Refractive Surgery*, **24**, 482-486. http://dx.doi.org/10.1016/S0886-3350(98)80288-5

[24] ESCRS Endophthalmitis Study Group (2007) Prophylaxis of Postoperative Endophthalmitis Following Cataract Surgery: Results of the ESCRS Multicenter Study and Identification of Risk Factors. *Journal of Cataract Refractive Surgery*, **33**, 978-988. http://dx.doi.org/10.1016/j.jcrs.2007.02.032

[25] Henderson, B., Pineda, R., Ament, C., Chen, S. and Kim, J. (2007) Essentials of Cataract Surgery. Slack Incorporated, On Line Library.

[26] Hill, W. and Potvin, R. (2008) Monte Carlo Simulation of Expected Outcomes with the AcrySof® Toric Intraocular Lens. *BMC Ophthalmology*, **8**, 1-9. http://dx.doi.org/10.1186/1471-2415-8-22

[27] Hayashi, K., Manabe, S., Yoshida, M. and Hayashi, H. (2010) Effect of Astigmatism on Visual Acuity in Eyes with a Diffractive Multifocal Intraocular Lens. *Journal of Cataract Refractive Surgery*, **36**, 1323-1329. http://dx.doi.org/10.1016/j.jcrs.2010.02.016

12

The Prevalence and Risk Factors for Dry Eye Disease among Older Adults in the City of Lodz, Poland

Michal S. Nowak[1], Janusz Smigielski[2]

[1]Department of Ophthalmology and Visual Rehabilitation, Medical University of Lodz, Lodz, Poland
[2]Department of Geriatrics, Medical University of Lodz, Lodz, Poland
Email: michaelnovak@interia.pl, janusz.smigielski@umed.lodz.pl

Abstract

Purpose: To estimate the prevalence and risk factors for dry eye disease (DED) in a sample population of Polish older adults. Material and methods: Cross-sectional and observational study of 1107 men and women of European Caucasian origin aged 35 - 97 years, who were interviewed and underwent detailed ophthalmic examinations. DED was defined as presence of a previous clinical diagnosis of dry eye with concomitant dry eye treatment. Results: The overall prevalence of DED in the researched population was 6.7% (95% CI 5.2 - 8.2). The prevalence of DED increased with age from 4.8% in age group 35 - 59 years to 8.3% in group aged ≥60 years. The prevalence of DED was also higher in women 8.1% than in men 4.7%. In multiple logistic regression modelling with age, gender, presence of cataract surgery and glaucoma or ocular hypertension (OHT) treatment, DED was significantly associated with older age (OR 1.99, 95% CI 1.21 - 3.30) and with female gender (OR 1.76, 95% CI 1.05 - 2.96). Conclusions: The prevalence of DED in our study population was comparable with the findings of other studies from Europe and the United States, with significantly higher rates among women and elderly subjects.

Keywords

Dry Eye Disease, Older Adults

1. Introduction

"Dry eye disease (DED) is a multifactorial disease of the tears and the ocular surface that results in symptoms of discomfort, visual disturbance, and tears film instability with potential damage to the ocular surface. It is accompanied by increased osmolarity of the tear film and the inflammation of the ocular surface [1]". Dry eye is a serious health problem, with limited treatment options. DED has also a substantial economic burden on the society estimated to be 55.4 billion dollars in the United States [2] [3]. On the basis of available reports, the prevalence of DED among older adults varies from 5% to 34% [4] [5]. Although it is a common ocular problem, the number of studies concerning the prevalence of DED in Eastern European nations (post-soviet countries) is still very few. The aim of this study was the assessment of the prevalence and risk factors for dry eye disease in a sample population of Polish older adults.

2. Materials and Methods

The study design was an observational and cross-sectional. The methodology of the recruitment and subjects sampling for the current study has been described earlier. In brief: "sample size for the study was calculated with 99% confidence, within an error bound of 5%. The sample size requirement was 661, as calculated by

$$n = Z^2 / 4d^2 ,$$

where $Z = 2.57$ for 99% confidence interval and $d = 0.05$ for 5% error bound. After allowing for an arbitrary 50% increase in sample size to accommodate possible inefficiencies associated with the sample design, the sample size requirement increased to 991 subjects [6] [7]". We defined an older adult as a person aged ≥35 years because in our previous reports conducted on young males in the military population we considered young adult as person aged 18 - 34 years [8] [9]. "We used simple systematic sampling to select our study population. In total 14,110 outpatients were examined in the Department of Ophthalmology and Visual Rehabilitation of the Medical University of Lodz in year 2012 and we included into the study every tenth subject aged 35 years and older [7]". Basing on age, our study participants were divided into two groups; group I aged 35 - 59 years, and group II aged 60 years and older. All selected subjects were interviewed and underwent detailed ophthalmic examinations. Dry eye disease (DED) was defined as presence of a previous clinical diagnosis of DED with concomitant dry eye treatment (artificial tear drops or gel) like in other studies [2] [5]. This was assessed by two questions: 1) have you ever been diagnosed (by an ophthalmologist) as having dry eye disease? and 2) do you currently use any artificial tear drops or gel? Only if answer was "Yes" to both questions DED was diagnosed. For this report we used the data concerning the prevalence of cataract surgery, glaucoma and ocular hypertension (OHT) in the researched population from our recent paper [7]. All statistical analyses were performed using STATISTICA v. 10.1 PL (StatSoft Polska, Krakow, Poland) software. Prevalence rates of dry eye disease (DED) in whole population and according to the subjects' age and gender were calculated. Multiple logistic regression statistics were used to investigate the association of DED with age, gender as well as with the presence of cataract surgery and glaucoma or OHT treatment. Odds ratios (ORs) were computed, the differences were significant at $p < 0.05$. All confidence intervals (CIs) were 95% CI. The study was approved by the institutional review board of the Medical University of Lodz and was conducted in accordance with the provisions of Declaration of Helsinki for research involving human subjects.

3. Results

The demographic characteristics of all participants in the study and statistical analyses are presented in **Table 1**. A total of 1107 subjects aged ≥35 years were successfully enumerated and included into the study. All of them were of European Caucasian origin. According to 2011 national census, they were a fair representation of the population of the city of Lodz in terms of sex distribution (statistical analysis-chi square test: $\chi^2 = 3.64$, $p > 0.05$) and socioeconomic status [10]. The city of Lodz is the second largest city in Poland and consists of seven hundred forty thousand inhabitants (2011 national census), mostly of middle socioeconomic level [10]. The mean age of our study participants was 60.4 ± 7.1 years (range, 35 to 97 years). There were 642 women (58.0%) and 465 men (42.0%) and they were divided into two age groups: 520 (47.0%) subjects were aged 35 - 59 years, and 587 (53.0%) subjects were aged ≥60 years. The overall prevalence of dry eye disease in the researched population (diagnosed by clinician with concomitant dry eye treatment) was 6.7% (95% confidence interval [CI] 5.2 - 8.2). The prevalence of DED increased with age from 4.8% (95% CI 3.0 - 6.6) in age group 35 - 59 years to 8.3% (95% CI 6.1 - 10.6) in group aged ≥60 years (**Figure 1**). The prevalence of dry eye was also higher in women 8.1% (95% CI 6.0 - 10.2) than in men 4.7% (95% CI 2.8 - 6.7) (**Figure 2**). Statistical analysis revealed that the differences between prevalence rates of dry eye disease (DED) among genders and particular age groups were

Table 1. The demographic characteristics of examined group.

Examined group	Number of subjects: n (%)	Min	Max	Mean	Med	Std. dev.	Men	Women
All	1107 (100%)	35.0	97.0	60.4	61.0	12.8	465 (100%)	642 (100%)
35 - 59 years	520 (47.0%)	35.0	59.0	49.3	50.0	7.1	230 (49.5%)	290 (45.2%)
≥60 years	587 (53.0%)	60.0	97.0	70.1	69.0	7.8	235 (50.5%)	352 (54.8%)

Examined group	Number of subjects: n (%)	Min	Max	Mean	Med	Std. dev.	35 - 59 years	≥60 years
All	1107 (100%)	35.0	97.0	60.4	61.0	12.8	520 (100%)	587 (100%)
Men	465 (42.0%)	35.0	97.0	59.8	60.0	14.1	230 (44.2%)	235 (40.0%)
Women	642 (58.0%)	35.0	93.0	60.7	61.0	11.7	290 (55.8%)	352 (60.0%)

χ^2 test p = 0.158.

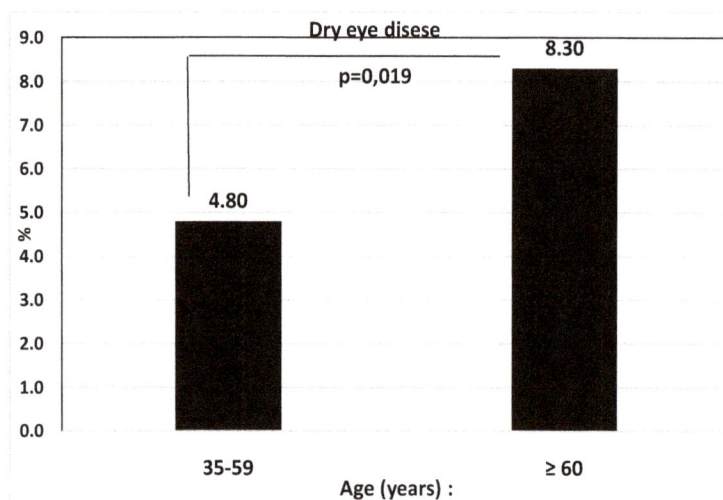

Figure 1. The prevalence of dry eye disease as a function of age.

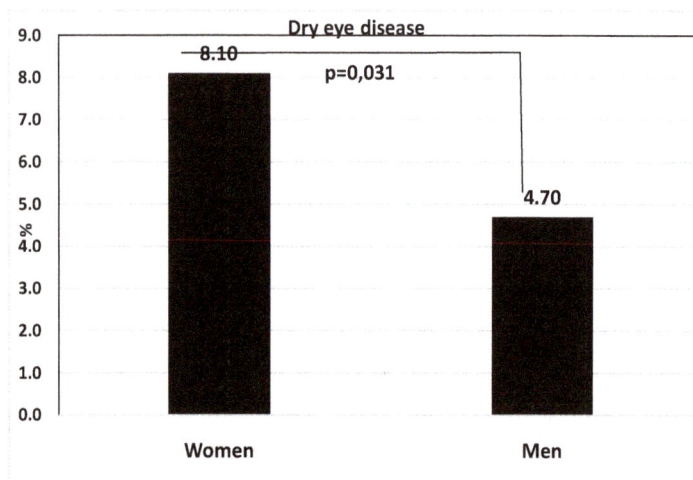

Figure 2. The prevalence of dry eye disease among genders.

statistically significant (χ^2 test p = 0.031 and p = 0.019 respectively). As reported earlier 8.04% (95% CI 6.44 - 9.64) of all participants in the study had cataract surgery in either eye. Various types of glaucoma were diagnosed in 5.51% (95% CI 4.17 - 6.85) of subjects and 2.62% (95% CI 1.68 - 3.56) had ocular hypertension (OHT). Multivariate logistic regression model was constructed to analyze the risk factors for dry eye in this population. In multiple logistic regression modelling with age, gender, presence of cataract surgery and glaucoma or ocular hypertension (OHT) treatment, dry eye disease (DED) was significantly associated with older age (OR 1.99, 95% CI 1.21 - 3.30) and with female gender (OR 1.76, 95% CI 1.05 - 2.96). However no association was found between DED and the presence of cataract surgery and glaucoma or OHT treatment.

4. Discussion

The current study provides for the first time reliable data concerning the prevalence and risk factors for dry eye disease (DED) in a large unselected population of Polish citizens aged 35 years and older. Overall the prevalence of DED in the examined population was rather low (6.7%) and was higher in women (8.1%) than in men (4.7%). The prevalence of DED was also significantly higher in the age group ≥60 years. Direct comparison of our results to the results of other studies on DED is limited due to differences in study design and population sampling. The major limitation is the fact that the presence of DED was determined by subject self-reported history of dry eye. We did not perform any diagnostic tests *i.e.* Schirmer test, tear break-up time measurement (TBUT), rose bengal staining or fluoresceine staining to confirm the clinical diagnosis of DED. However our prevalence rate of dry eye was closer to the results obtained in a British female cohort study, in which they used the same definition of DED and found that 9.6% of women had a DED diagnosis with concomitant dry eye treatment [2]. In addition our results were similar to those reported in large epidemiological studies from the United States (Women's Health Study and Physician's Health Study), which indicated that the prevalence of symptomatic dry eye disease is about 7% in women and 4% of men over the age of 50 years [4] [11] [12]. Although previous studies identified several risk factors for the development of DED like aging, gender, hormonal changes, contact lens wear, certain medications and surgical procedures [4], in the present study multiple regression analysis showed that DED was only associated with older age and with female gender.

5. Conclusion

In conclusion, the prevalence of DED in our study population was comparable with the findings of other studies from Europe and the United States, with significantly higher rates among women and elderly subjects. Further studies are needed to confirm some of the previously identified risk factors.

Conflict of Interests

The authors declare that there is no conflict of interests regarding the publication of this paper.

References

[1]   (2007) The Definition and Classification of Dry Eye Disease: Report of the Definition and Classification Subcommittee of the International Dry Eye Workshop (2007). *The Ocular Surface*, **5**, 75-92.
       http://dx.doi.org/10.1016/S1542-0124(12)70081-2

[2]   Vehof, J., Kozareva, D., Hysi, P.G. and Hammond, C.J. (2014) Prevalence and Risk Factors of Dry Eye Disease in a British Female Cohort. *British Journal of Ophthalmology*, **98**, 1712-1717.
       http://dx.doi.org/10.1136/bjophthalmol-2014-305201

[3]   Yu, J., Asche, C.V. and Fairchild, C.J. (2011) The Economic Burden of Dry Eye Disease in the United States: A Decision Tree Analysis. *Cornea*, **30**, 379-387. http://dx.doi.org/10.1097/ICO.0b013e3181f7f363

[4]   Gayton, J.L. (2009) Etiology, Prevalence, and Treatment of Dry Eye Disease. *Clinical Ophthalmology*, **3**, 405-412.
       http://dx.doi.org/10.2147/OPTH.S5555

[5]   Galor, A., Feuer, W., Lee, D.J., Florez, H., Carter, D., Pouyeh, B., Prunty, W.J. and Perez, V.L. (2011) Prevalence and Risk Factors of Dry Syndrome in a United States Veterans Affairs Population. *American Journal of Ophthalmology*, **152**, 377-384. http://dx.doi.org/10.1016/j.ajo.2011.02.026

[6]   Nowak, M.S. and Smigielski, J. (2015) The Prevalence and Causes of Visual Impairment and Blindness among Older Adults in the City of Lodz, Poland. *Medicine* (*Baltimore*), **94**, e505. http://dx.doi.org/10.1097/MD.0000000000000505

[7]   Nowak, M.S. and Smigielski, J. (2015) The Prevalence of Age-Related Eye Diseases and Cataract Surgery among
      Older Adults in the City Lodz, Poland. *Journal of Ophthalmology*, Article ID: 605814.
      http://dx.doi.org/10.1155/2015/605814

[8]   Nowak, M.S., Goś, R., Jurowski, P. and Śmigielski, J. (2009) Correctable and Non-Correctable Visual Impairment
      among Young Males: A 12-Year Prevalence Study of the Military Service in Poland. *Ophthalmic and Physiological
      Optics*, **29**, 443-448. http://dx.doi.org/10.1111/j.1475-1313.2008.00628.x

[9]   Nowak, M.S., Jurowski, P., Goś, R. and Śmigielski, J. (2010) Ocular Findings among Young Men: A 12 Year Preva-
      lence Study of Military Service in Poland. *Acta Ophthalmologica*, **88**, 535-540.
      http://dx.doi.org/10.1111/j.1755-3768.2008.01476.x

[10] The National Census of Population and Housing 1 April - 30 June 2011. Zakład Wydawnictw Statystycznych. Wars-
      zawa 2013. http://www.stat.gov.pl/gus/nsp

[11] Schaumberg, D.A., Sullivan, D.A., Buring, J.E. and Dana, M.R. (2003) Prevalence of Dry Eye Syndrome among US
      Women. *American Journal of Ophthalmology*, **136**, 318-326. http://dx.doi.org/10.1016/S0002-9394(03)00218-6

[12] Schaumberg, D.A., Dana, R., Buring, J.E. and Sullivan, D.A. (2009) Prevalence of Dry Eye Disease among US Men:
      Estimates from the Physicians' Health Studies. *Archives of Ophthalmology*, **127**, 763-768.
      http://dx.doi.org/10.1001/archophthalmol.2009.103

13

Repair of Spontaneous Corneal Perforation in Pellucid Marginal Degeneration Using Amniotic Membrane

Martin Heur[1], Samuel Yiu[2]*

[1]Department of Ophthalmology, Keck School of Medicine of the University of Southern California, Los Angeles, CA, USA
[2]Department of Ophthalmology, The Wilmer Eye Institute, The John Hopkins University, Baltimore, Maryland, USA
Email: *syiu2@jhmi.edu

Abstract

A 47-year-old woman with a history of pellucid marginal degeneration was referred for management of hydrops and peripheral perforation of the right cornea. The initial management with cyanoacrylate tissue adhesive and bandage contact lens did not preclude aqueous leakage the next day. Amniotic membrane grafting using both a surgical graft and a bandage patch was thus performed in the operating room the following day. There was no aqueous leakage on the first postoperative day. The corneal integrity was restored with resolution of the corneal edema; and the visual acuity improved from 20/400 before surgery to 20/40 three months later. This case illustrates the clinical efficacy of amniotic membrane grafting as an effective alternative in the management of spontaneous corneal perforation resulted from pellucid marginal degeneration.

Keywords

Pellucid Marginal Degeneration, Corneal Perforation, Cyanoacrylate Tissue Adhesive, Amniotic Membrane

1. Introduction

Pellucid marginal degeneration is a non-inflammatory corneal ecstatic disorder characterized by inferior peri-

---

*Corresponding author.

pheral thinning with rare spontaneous perforation [1]-[6]. Surgical management in the acute phase can be challenging. Here, we presented a case in which we used cryopreserved amniotic membrane as a patch graft and a Prokera device as a biologic bandage to achieve surgical repair of the perforation.

2. Case Presentation

A 47-year-old female with bilateral pellucid marginal degeneration was referred to the Cornea Service at the Doheny Eye Institute for management of acute hydrops and spontaneous perforation of the right cornea. The patient presented with pain and photophobia of the right eye (OD) that began the morning of the day of presentation. She denied trauma and was evaluated by an ophthalmologist, who subsequently referred her for the management of a peripheral perforation of the right cornea. The patient suffered from pellucid marginal degeneration and wore rigid gas permeable contact lenses (RGPCL). She reported difficulty tolerating the RGPCL in the same eye for two days prior to presentation. She was not on any medication, and past medical history, family history and review of systems were unremarkable.

On examination, the uncorrected visual acuity was 20/400, right eye, and RGPCL-corrected visual acuity OS was 20/40, left eye. Pupils were reactive both eyes and no afferent pupillary defect was noted. Confrontational visual fields were full and the external examination was unremarkable. Slit lamp evaluation revealed right corneal hydrops with 8 mm by 2 mm inferior peripheral epithelial defect. Aqueous leakage was noted in the area of the epithelial defect, and the anterior chamber was flat. The right lens was clear. The slit lamp examination showed inferior peripheral thinning of the left corneal stroma. The right inferior corneal perforation was initially managed with cyanoacrylate tissue adhesive and a bandage contact lens. The anterior chamber deepened slightly after the tissue adhesive application. The patient was started on moxifloxacin four times a day in the right eye.

The next day, the patient's symptoms persisted. Slit lamp examination confirmed aqueous leakage around the tissue adhesive and a shallow anterior chamber. The patient consented with surgical repair of the perforation in the operating room the following day.

Under the operating microscope, we noted an edematous cornea and shallow anterior chamber (**Figure 1(a)**). The cyanoacrylate tissue adhesive was debrided and the cornea denuded with 4% cocaine solution. One layer of cryopreserved amniotic membrane (Bio-Tissue, Miami, FL) was secured onto the cornea using fibrin tissue adhesive, and its corners were transfixated to the conjunctiva using interrupted 8-0 polyglactin sutures. A Prokera

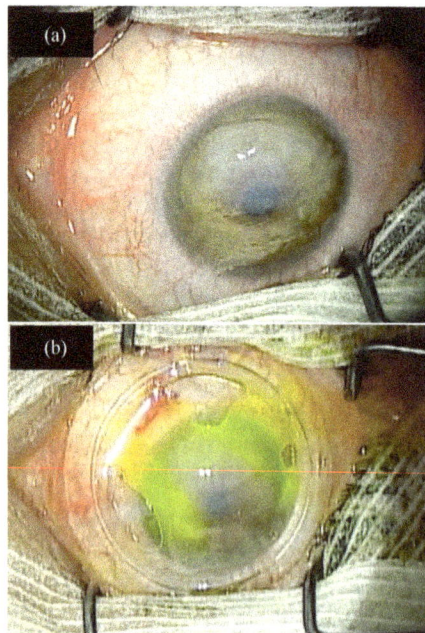

Figure 1. (a) The surgeon's view of the cornea OD shows the presence of hydrops and inferior corneal perforation prior to the surgical repair. (b) The surgeon's view of the cornea OD shows how amniotic membrane was used as a surgical graft and a bandage patch via the insertion of Prokera (Bio-Tissue, Miami, FL).

device (Bio-Tissue, Miami, FL), amniotic membrane on a polycarbonate symblepharon ring, was then mounted on top of the amniotic membrane (**Figure 1(b)**). On the first post-operative day, the patient reported improvement in her symptoms. The slit lamp examination showed persistent corneal edema but a formed anterior chamber. The amniotic membrane dissolved over time. The polycarbonate ring was removed two weeks postoperatively. The patient improved gradually and she noted resolution of pain and photophobia (**Figure 2(a)**) on postoperative month 3. The uncorrected visual acuity OD had improved to 20/40, and slit lamp examination revealed marked improvement in the corneal edema (**Figure 2(b)**).

3. Discussion

Pellucid marginal degeneration is a non-inflammatory corneal ecstatic disorder characterized by inferior peripheral thinning producing high against the rule astigmatism. Acute hydrops due to rupture of Descemet's membrane is a recognized sequelae in pellucid marginal degeneration. Spontaneous perforation of the cornea in pellucid marginal degeneration is exceedingly rare but had been reported [1]-[6]. Hydrops and peripheral perforation present a unique challenge for surgical management with traditional penetrating keratoplasty in the acute setting. Cyanoacrylate tissue adhesive is an alternative temporizing measure to seal the perforation and facilitate deturgescence prior to surgical repair [7]. However, as demonstrated by this present case, it is not always possible to seal a large defect. A peripheral crescentic lamellar graft combined with concurrent central penetrating keratoplasty has been proposed as a surgical technique to repair advanced cases of pellucid marginal degeneration. Technical challenge would ensue in the setting of an acute perforation with hydrops [6] [8]. Herein, we present a case in which we used cryopreserved amniotic membrane as a patch graft and a Prokera device as a temporary bandage to achieve surgical repair of the perforation. Amniotic membrane is a unique tool in the armamentarium for ocular surface reconstruction [9]-[13], as it offers several advantages in situations as illustrated in the present case. Firstly, commercial availability of amniotic membranes reduces the concern of donor cornea shortage. Secondly, amniotic membrane transplantation is technically facile, compared to a penetrating or lamellar keratoplasty. Thirdly, less surgically induced astigmatism by amniotic membrane transplantation improves visual rehabilitation. Finally, amniotic membrane grafting obviates the risk of allograft rejection that is common when corneal transplantation is performed in acute, inflamed and perforated status. Collectively, these advantages of amniotic membrane offer a viable surgical management option for cases presenting with large corneal perforation that is not amenable to initial management with cyanoacrylate tissue adhesive.

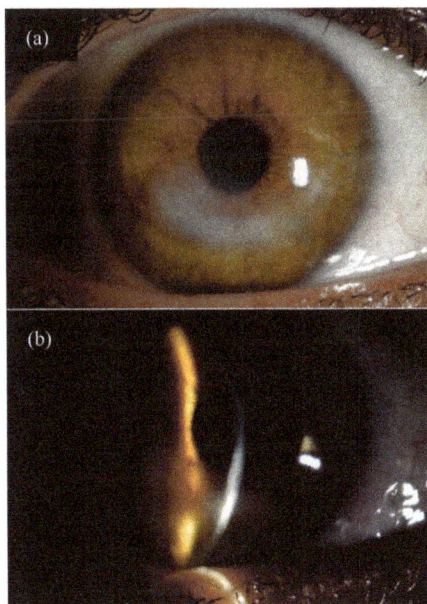

Figure 2. (a) The photograph of the cornea OD shows the restoration of corneal integrity and a marked improvement in hydrops. (b) The slit beam photograph of the cornea OD shows the marked resolution of stromal edema in the affected area.

4. Discussion

Although the amniotic membrane grafting has successfully been used for treating corneal perforation caused by diverse underlying etiologies, the present case report is the first demonstration for pellucid marginal degeneration.

Disclosure

a. Financial Support: An unrestricted grant from Research to Prevent Blindness

b. Financial Disclosure(s): The authors have no financial interests in the topic of this manuscript. No conflicting relationship exists for any author.

References

[1] Akpek, E.K., Altan-Yaycioglu, R., Gottsch, J.D. and Stark, W.J. (2001) Spontaneous Corneal Perforation in a Patient with Unusual Unilateral Pellucid Marginal Degeneration. *Journal of Cataract & Refractive Surgery*, **27**, 1698-1700. http://dx.doi.org/10.1016/S0886-3350(01)00792-1

[2] Aldave, A.J., Mabon, M., Hollander, D.A., *et al.* (2003) Spontaneous Corneal Hydrops and Perforation in Keratoconus and Pellucid Marginal Degeneration. *Cornea*, **22**, 169-174. http://dx.doi.org/10.1097/00003226-200303000-00019

[3] Lee, W.B., O'Halloran, H.S. and Grossniklaus, H.E. (2008) Pellucid Marginal Degeneration and Bilateral Corneal Perforation: Case Report and Review of the Literature. *Eye & Contact Lens*, **34**, 229-233. http://dx.doi.org/10.1097/ICL.0b013e318164771b

[4] Lucarelli, M.J., Gendelman, D.S. and Talamo, J.H. (1997) Hydrops and Spontaneous Perforation in Pellucid Marginal Corneal Degeneration. *Cornea*, **16**, 232-234. http://dx.doi.org/10.1097/00003226-199703000-00018

[5] Orlin, S.E. and Sulewski, M.E. (1998) Spontaneous Corneal Perforation in Pellucid Marginal Degeneration. *The CLAO Journal*, **24**, 186-187.

[6] Symes, R.J., Catt, C.J., Sa-ngiampornpanit, T. and Males, J.J. (2007) Corneal Perforation Associated with Pellucid Marginal Degeneration and Treatment with Crescentic Lamellar Keratoplasty: Two Case Reports. *Cornea*, **26**, 625-628.

[7] Yiu, S.C., Thomas, P. and Nguyen, P. (2007) Review: Corneal Surface Reconstruction: Recent Advancements and Future Outlooks. *Current Opinion in Ophthalmology*, **18**, 509-514. http://dx.doi.org/10.1097/ICU.0b013e3282f0ab33

[8] Rasheed, K. and Rabinowitz, Y.S. (2000) Surgical Treatment of Advanced Pellucid Marginal Degeneration. *Ophthalmology*, **107**, 1836-1840. http://dx.doi.org/10.1016/S0161-6420(00)00346-8

[9] Nguyen, P. and Yiu, S.C. (2008) Ocular Surface Reconstruction: Recent Innovations, Surgical Candidate Selection and Postoperative Management. *Expert Review of Ophthalmology*, **3**, 567-584. http://dx.doi.org/10.1586/17469899.3.5.567

[10] Kim, H.K. and Park, H.S. (2009) Fibrin Glue-Assisted Augmented Amniotic Membrane Transplantation for the Treatment of Large Noninfectious Corneal Perforations. *Cornea*, **28**, 170-176. http://dx.doi.org/10.1097/ICO.0b013e3181861c54

[11] Ma, D.H., Wang, S.F., Su, W.Y. and Tsai, R.J. (2002) Amniotic Membrane Graft for the Management of Scleral Melting and Corneal Perforation in Recalcitrant Infectious Scleral and Corneoscleral Ulcers. *Cornea*, **21**, 275-283. http://dx.doi.org/10.1097/00003226-200204000-00008

[12] Rodriguez-Ares, M.T., Tourino, R., Lopez-Valladares, M.J. and Gude, F. (2004) Multilayer Amniotic Membrane Transplantation in the Treatment of Corneal Perforations. *Cornea*, **23**, 577-583. http://dx.doi.org/10.1097/01.ico.0000121709.58571.12

[13] Yildiz, E.H., Nurozler, A.B., Ozkan Aksoy, N., *et al.* (2008) Amniotic Membrane Transplantation: Indications and Results. *European Journal of Ophthalmology*, **18**, 685-690.

14

Evolution of Diabetic Maculopathy from Marked Exudation to Subretinal Fibrosis: Clinical and Spectral Domain Optical Coherence Tomography Features

Daniel S. Churgin, Jonathan H. Tzu, Harry W. Flynn

Department of Ophthalmology, Bascom Palmer Eye Institute, University of Miami Miller School of Medicine, Miami, FL, USA
Email: HFlynn@med.miami.edu

Abstract

Diabetic maculopathy with marked exudation may lead to subretinal fibrosis. Two patients observed over multiple years evolved from macular exudation into subretinal fibrosis with severe visual loss. Spectral domain optical coherence tomography and color photographs document the clinical changes.

Keywords

Diabetes Mellitus, Retinopathy, Subretinal Fibrosis, Exudate, OCT, Maculopathy

1. Introduction

Marked exudation in the macula center of patients with advanced diabetic retinopathy is associated with significant visual loss, which may not improve with currently available treatments [1]-[7]. This case series documented spectral domain optical coherence tomography (SD-OCT) diagnosis and clinical outcomes of two patients with diabetes-related severe macular exudation, which evolved into subretinal fibrosis.

2. Case Series

2.1. Case 1

A 66-year-old type II diabetic woman presented with a history of decreased vision of the left eye for 3 years.

The patient had previously received focal photocoagulation in the left eye. Initial best-corrected visual acuity (BCVA) was 20/40 in the right eye and 20/400 in the left eye. Examination showed advanced non-proliferative diabetic retinopathy in both eyes, and marked macular exudation in the left eye with foveal involvement (**Figure 1(a)**). SD-OCT showed distorted foveal contour, intraretinal fluid, and subretinal exudate (**Figures 1(b)-(d)**). The patient underwent multiple intravitreal injections of bevacizumab for macular edema in the left eye, which eventually resolved. However, the large area of macular exudation in the left eye contracted over the following two years, and evolved into subretinal fibrosis (**Figure 2(a)**). Repeat SD-OCT showed distorted foveal contour, trace intraretinal fluid, and subretinal fibrosis (**Figures 2(b)-(d)**).Visual acuity remained 20/200 in the left eye over four years.

2.2. Case 2

A 59-year-old patient with type II diabetes presented with a history of decreased vision of the right eye for 5 years. The patient had not previously received treatment for diabetic retinopathy. Initial best-corrected visual acuity (BCVA) was 5/200 E in the right eye and 20/100 in the left eye. Examination showed advanced non-proliferative diabetic retinopathy in both eyes, and marked macular exudation and edema in the right eye with foveal involvement (**Figure 3(a)**), and moderate macular exudation and edema in the left eye with foveal involvement. SD-OCT of the right eye showed distorted foveal contour, retinal atrophy, intraretinal fluid, and very early subretinal exudate (**Figures 3(b)-(d)**). The patient underwent multiple intravitreal injections of bevacizumab, aflibercept, and triamcinolone acetonide for macular edema of both eyes. The area of macular and foveal exudation of the right eye worsened over the following three years, and the patient developed subretinal fibrosis (**Figure 4(a)**). Repeat SD-OCT of the right eye showed thinned and distorted foveal contour, intraretinal fluid, and subretinal fibrosis (**Figures 4(b)-(d)**). Visual acuity remained 5/200 E in the right eye over two years, and appearance on fundus examination and OCT remained stable.

3. Discussion

Although infrequently described in the literature, diabetes-related macular exudates may evolve into subretinal

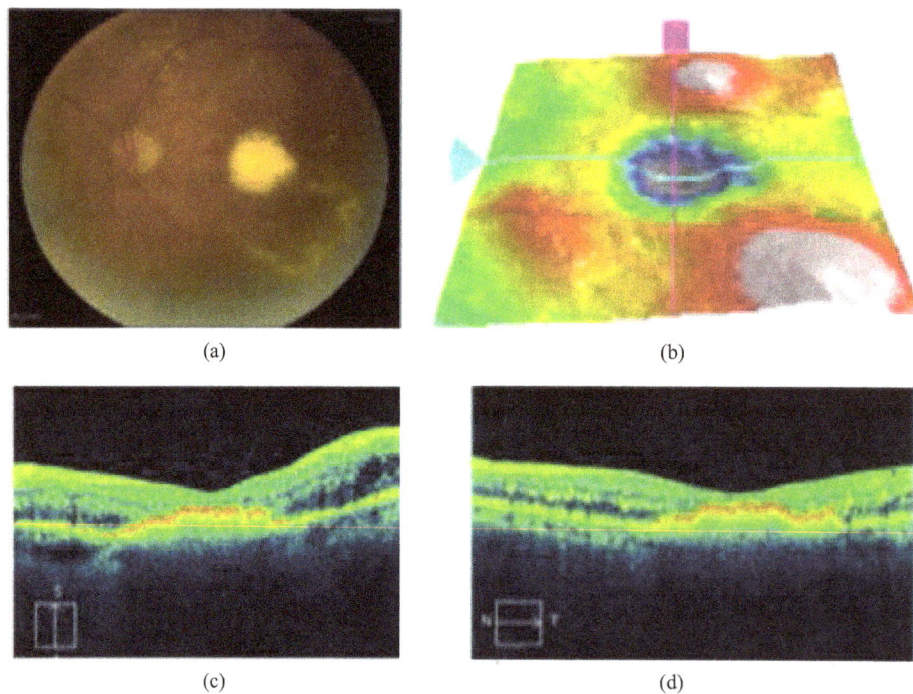

(a)   (b)

(c)   (d)

Figure 1. (a) At presentation, color image shows severe exudation with foveal involvement in the left eye. (b) SD-OCT topography map shows circinate rings of edema surrounding the macular center, which has relative thinning. (c) (d) SD-OCT demonstrates abnormal foveal contour, intraretinal fluid, and subfoveal exudation.

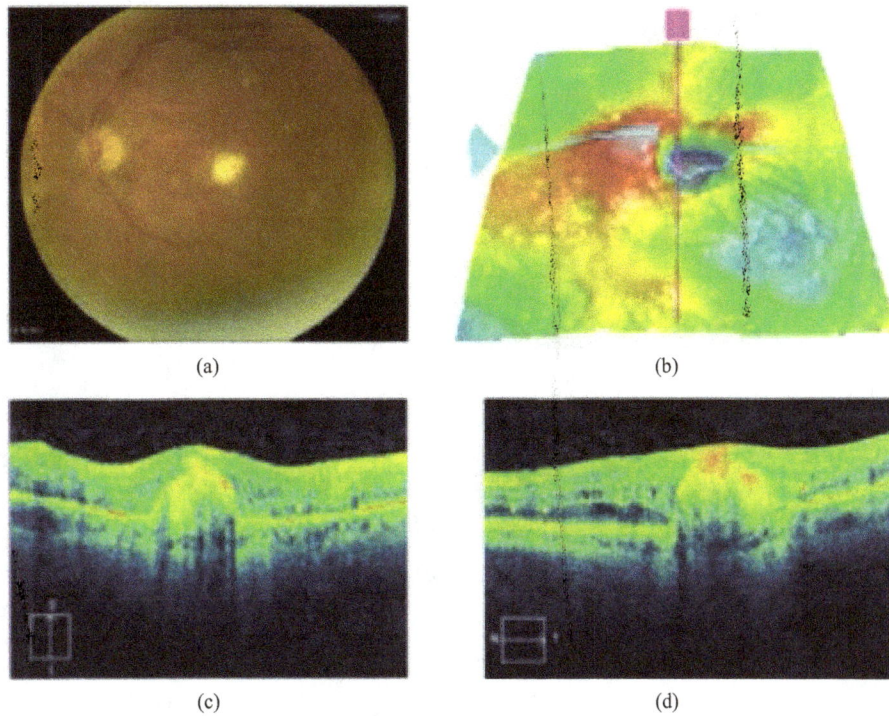

(a)   (b)

(c)   (d)

Figure 2. (a) Four years after initial presentation, color image shows contracted white subretinal fibrotic lesion. (b) Topography map shows persistent edema surrounding the macula center. (c) (d) SD-OCT shows persistent abnormal foveal contour, intraretinal fluid, and subretinal fibrosis involving the fovea.

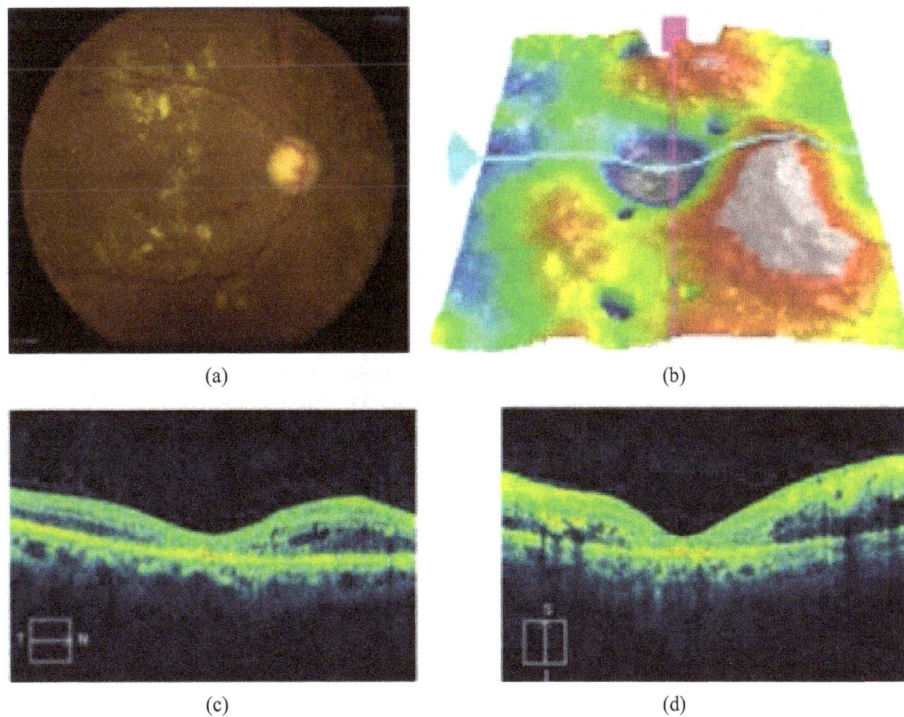

(a)   (b)

(c)   (d)

Figure 3. (a) At patient presentation, color image shows marked exudation with foveal involvement. (b) The topography map shows a large circinate ring of edema nasal to the fovea. (c) (d) SD-OCT demonstrates subfoveal exudate, intraretinal fluid, and relative thinning of the fovea.

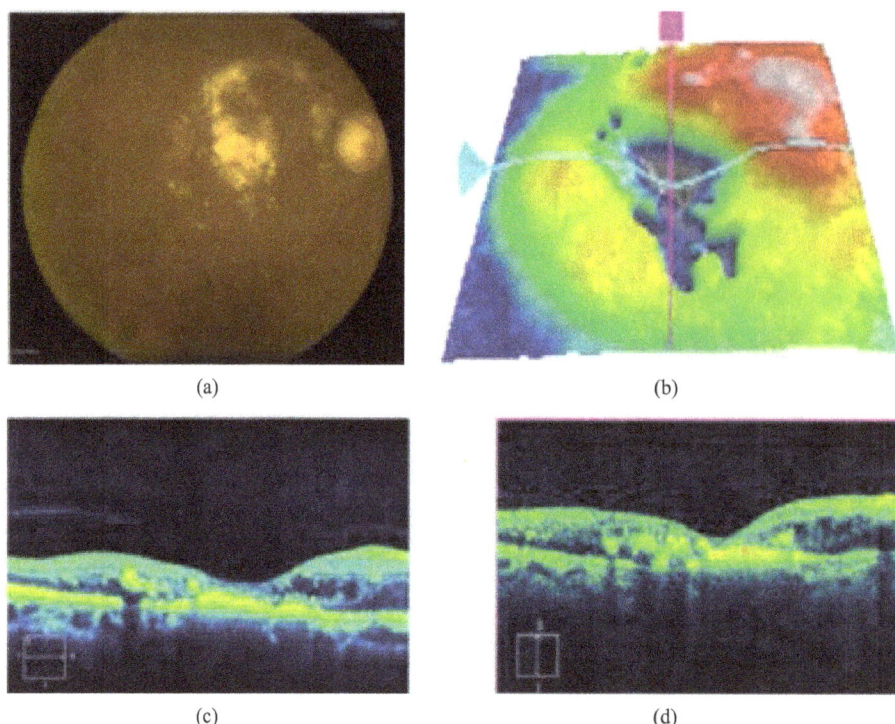

Figure 4. (a) Three years after initial presentation, color image shows worsened macular exudates. (b) Topography map shows persistent edema nasal to the fovea. (c) (d) SD-OCT shows foveal thinning, intraretinal fluid, and an organized plaque of subretinal fibrosis.

fibrosis. Clinicopathologic study of an organized plaque in exudative diabetic maculopathy was reported in 1976. In this case report, a poorly controlled diabetic patient was observed over the final years of the patient's life, during which time prominent macular exudates evolved into subretinal fibrosis. At autopsy, the authors observed diabetic microangiopathy, retinal degeneration and proliferation, and serous detachment of the pigment epithelium. The underlying Bruch's membrane and choriocapillaris were unaffected, suggesting that the origin of the subretinal fibrosis was from the retinal exudate. They theorized that cystoid macular edema and hard exudates disrupted the retina and later caused atrophy and degeneration, along with proliferation and serous separation of the pigment epithelium. The authors proposed that this space could then be filled in by fibrous tissue from both retinal and RPE origins [2]. In a later case series, the same authors further proposed that this large accumulation of exudates may incite metaplasia and over time, with resultant organization into a fibrotic scar [3]. In these five patients observed in these cases, vision was poor at presentation, and remained poor over long-term follow up [2] [3]. However, visual outcome for subretinal fibrosis may improve if the fovea is spared [4].

The largest case series of patients with subretinal fibrosis in the setting of diabetes was reported in the Early Treatment Diabetic Retinopathy Study (ETDRS) Report 23. The authors observed 5633 eyes with clinically significant macular edema (CSME) and no fibrotic changes, in contrast to 109 eyes with CSME and subretinal fibrosis. Of these 109 eyes with fibrosis, 74% of the eyes had very severe hard exudates in the macula before developing subretinal scarring [1]. Subretinal fibrosis has been described in association with higher burn intensity during focal photocoagulation [5]-[8], and the ETDRS authors also sought to discover whether focal photocoagulation was the root cause of subretinal fibrosis in diabetics. They observed that only 9 of the 109 eyes had focal photocoagulation adjacent to the subretinal fibrosis. In this study of 264 eyes with very severe hard exudates, 30.7% of these eyes showed the presence of subretinal fibrosis. The ETDRS study group concluded that although focal photocoagulation might be a risk factor for development of subretinal fibrosis, the strongest risk factor for development of subretinal fibrosis was the presence of very severe hard exudates in the macula. One important limitation of this study is that the study occurred prior to the use of OCT. Therefore, the exact location of the exudates could not be determined [1].

The patients in this case series add evidence to the body of literature that very severe diabetic macular exudation can evolve into subretinal fibrosis. In agreement with the ETDRS authors, it seems that the fibrosis develops in association with the severe exudation, as opposed to nearby focal laser scars. Vision remained poor but stable in these patients, and the disease followed a predictable course, evolving over time into subretinal fibrosis. In this era of anti-vascular endothelial growth factor widespread availability, both patients underwent multiple intravitreal injections of anti-vascular endothelial growth factor agents in order to treat CSME. There was no alteration in visual acuity or change in the natural course of this disease with these agents. Surgical removal of large foveal hard exudates has been reported, but visual improvement was minimal [9]. One small case series described the improvement of less severe exudates with the use of intravitreal triamcinolone [10]. A larger prospective study using SD-OCT would be needed to evaluate the course of prominent macular exudates undergoing frequent anti-VEGF or steroid injections. In addition, improved blood glucose control, blood pressure optimization, and control of serum lipids may improve the clinical course in these patients.

References

[1]   Fong, D.S., Segal, P.P., Myers, F., Ferris, F.L., Hubbard, L.D. and Davis, M.D. (1997) Subretinal Fibrosis in Diabetic Macular Edema. ETDRS Report 23. Early Treatment Diabetic Retinopathy Study Research Group. *Archives of Ophthalmology*, **115**, 873-877. http://dx.doi.org/10.1001/archopht.1997.01100160043006

[2]   Begg, I.S. and Rootman, J. (1976) Clinico-Pathological Study of an Organized Plaque in Exudative Diabetic Maculopathy. *Canadian Journal of Ophthalmology*, **11**, 197-202.

[3]   Sigurdsson, R. and Begg, I.S. (1980) Organised Macular Plaques In Exudative Diabetic Maculopathy. *British Journal of Ophthalmology*, **64**, 392-397. http://dx.doi.org/10.1136/bjo.64.6.392

[4]   Dobree, J.H. (1970) Simple Diabetic Retinopathy. Evolution of the Lesions and Therapeutic Considerations. *British Journal of Ophthalmology*, **54**, 1-10. http://dx.doi.org/10.1136/bjo.54.1.1

[5]   Lewis, H., Schachat, A.P., Haimann, M.H., *et al.* (1990) Choroidal Neovascularization after Laser Photocoagulation for Diabetic Macular Edema. *Ophthalmology*, **97**, 503-510, Discussion: 510-501.

[6]   Berger, A.R. and Boniuk, I. (1989) Bilateral Subretinal Neovascularization after Focal Argon Laser Photocoagulation for Diabetic Macular Edema. *American Journal of Ophthalmology*, **108**, 88-90.
http://dx.doi.org/10.1016/S0002-9394(14)73271-4

[7]   Han, D.P. Mieler, W.F. and Burton, T.C. (1992) Submacular Fibrosis after Photocoagulation for Diabetic Macular Edema. *American Journal of Ophthalmology*, **113**, 513-521. http://dx.doi.org/10.1016/S0002-9394(14)74722-1

[8]   Guyer, D.R., D'Amico, D.J. and Smith, C.W. (1992) Subretinal Fibrosis after Laser Photocoagulation for Diabetic Macular Edema. *American Journal of Ophthalmology*, **113**, 652-656.

[9]   Takagi, H., Otani, A., Kiryu, J. and Ogura, Y. (1999) New Surgical Approach for Removing Massive Foveal Hard Exudates in Diabetic Macular Edema. *Ophthalmology*, **106**, 249-256, Discussion: 256-247.

[10]   Ciardella, A.P., Klancnik, J., Schiff, W., Barile, G., Langton, K. and Chang, S. (2004) Intravitreal Triamcinolone for the Treatment of Refractory Diabetic Macular Oedema with Hard Exudates: An Optical Coherence Tomography Study. *British Journal of Ophthalmology*, **88**, 1131-1136. http://dx.doi.org/10.1136/bjo.2004.041707

15

Comparison of the Normal, Preperimetric Glaucoma, and Glaucomatous Eyes with Upper-Hemifield Defects Using SD-OCT

Fusako Fujimura[1]*, Nobuyuki Shoji[1,2], Kazunori Hirasawa[1], Kazuhiro Matsumura[2], Tetsuya Morita[2], Kimiya Shimizu[2]

[1]Department of Rehabilitation, Orthoptics and Visual Science Course, School of Allied Health Sciences, Kitasato University, Tokyo, Japan
[2]Department of Ophthalmology, School of Medicine, Kitasato University, Tokyo, Japan
Email: *f-fujimu@kitasto-u.ac.jp, nshoji@ahs.kitasato-u.ac.jp, hirasawa@kitasato-u.ac.jp, kazu-m@dd.iij4u.or.jp, tamosace@gmail.com, ks-secre@kitasato-u.ac.jp

Abstract

Purpose: We compared the thickness of circumpapillary retinal nerve fiver layer (cpRNFL) and macular ganglion cell layer with inner plexiform layer (GCL + IPL) using Cirrus HD-OCT (Ver.6.0: Carl Zeiss). Materials and Methods: This study included 12 eyes of normal controls, 10 eyes of preperimetric glaucoma (PPG) with loss of RNFL either in superior or in inferior hemisphere without visual field defects, and 22 eyes of glaucoma eyes with visual field defects restricted to upper hemifield (UHFD: early 10 eyes, severe 12 eyes). The cpRNFL thickness analyzed from disk center by dividing into 12 sectors. The GCL + IPL thickness analyzed from central fovea by dividing into six sectors. Both compared between normal eye group and other 3 groups using the average value of each sectors. Result: The cpRNFL and the GCL + IPL thickness were obviously thin as compared with normal eyes. Conclusion: Even if it is in the state where abnormalities are not detected using the Humphrey field Analyzer, it is suggested that the early structural change of glaucoma has already arisen.

Keywords

Glaucoma, Ganglion Cell Layer, Inner Plexiform Layer, Retinal Nerve Fiver Layer, SD-OCT

---

*Corresponding author.

1. Introduction

Glaucoma is an optic neuropathy characterized by loss of retinal ganglion cell (RGC) and thinning of retinal nerve fiber layer (RNFL), and diagnosed by a characteristic alteration of optic nerve head, loss of retinal nerve fiber, defect of visual field. However, when detected abnormal by the funduscopy or visual field testing, 20% to 40% of RGC has already disappeared [1] [2]. Earlier studies have shown that the thickness of circumpapillary retinal nerve fiver layer (cpRNFL) begins to decrease before visual field loss [3] [4]. It is difficult to detect the point of disappearance of RGC, or the thinning of RNFL correctly by traditional funduscopy diagnosis and visual field test. There is an issue that a glaucomatous detection is overdue. It is thought required for a glaucomatous early checkup to evaluate quantitatively the structural change of RGC and RNFL. Recently, the spectral domain optical coherent tomography (SD-OCT) is progressing, so it becomes possible to observe and analyze thickness of ganglion cell layer (GCL) and RNFL easily. By using SD-OCT, for glaucomatous eyes, the structure of macula and optic nerve head are examined, and Ganglion Cell Complex (GCC) and the cpRNFL are used as a measurement parameter. The GCC is the sum of RNFL, RGC, inner plexiform layer (IPL) at macular regions. In glaucomatous eyes, the GCC and the cpRNFL are thinner than normal eyes, so, these are useful for the diagnosis of glaucoma [5]-[7]. However, the GCL has been reported to be the early site of glaucomatous damage compared with RNFL and IPL, as shown in experimental model [8]. In the thickness analysis of GCC including RNFL, a possibility that is guessed we miss an early glaucomatous structural change. As opposed to this, the Cirrus HD-OCT (Ver6.0: Carl Zeiss) added the Ganglion Cell Analysis to the existing Glaucoma OU Analysis which was program of the analysis for the cpRNFL. The Ganglion Cell Analysis analyzes the thickness of two layers (GCL + IPL) which excluded RNFL from traditional GCC (RNFL + GCL + IPL). By using this Ganglion cell Analysis, we can consider a possibility to detect an early structural change of glaucoma more sensitively. In this study, we compared the thickness of the cpRNFL and the GCL + IPL using Cirrus HD-OCT (Ver.6.0: Carl Zeiss) in normal eyes, preperimetric glaucoma (PPG) eyes with loss of RNFL in the superior or inferior hemisphere without visual field defects, and glaucoma eyes with visual field defects restricted to the upper hemifield defect (UHFD).

2. Materials and Methods

This study protocol adhered to the tenets of the Declaration of Helsinki, and informed consent was obtained from each subjects.

The subjects were 44 eyes of 32 patients (18 eyes of males, 26 eyes of females) who receive regular outpatient treatment for glaucoma or undergo examination for glaucoma suspicion (mean age: 61.2 ± 10.5 years, mean equivalent refractive error: $-2.04 \pm 2.65D$). The visual field was examined by the Humphrey Visual Field Analyzer 740 (Carl Zeiss) using Swedish Interactive Threshold Algorithm 30-2 SITA Standard program. From the obtained result, we judged that their visual fields are normal or abnormal based on the judging standard of Anderson Patella [9]. Moreover, upper visual hemifield defects in glaucomatous eyes were defined that three points of probability symbols were not contiguous in the total deviation plot of the inferior hemifield, and the extent classified based on the Hodapp-Anderson-Parrish classification [7]. Then we divided the subjects into four groups, normal eyes, PPG eyes, early UHFD eyes, severe UHFD eyes. The glaucoma diagnosis was determined by checking glaucomatous defects of optic disk and RNFL with an ophthalmoscopic examination and a fundus photograph, and having a corresponding abnormal visual field. As a result, normal eyes were 12 eyes, PPG eyes were 10 eyes, early UHFD eyes were 10 eyes, severe UHFD eyes were 12 eyes. The age, gender, intra ocular pressure by Goldmann applanation tonometer, spherical equivalent refractive error, mean deviation (MD) value, pattern standard deviation (PSD) value of each group were shown in the **Table 1**. There were significant differences in MD value and PSD value among 4 groups ($p < 0.0001$: one-way ANOVA). There were no differences with age, gender, intraocular pressure, and equivalent refractive error significant among 4 groups (one-way ANOVA, gender: chi-square test). In addition, we gave sufficient explanation about the purport of this research, and after obtaining consent, we performed the following measurement. The cpRNFL and the GCL + IPL thickness measured by Cirrus HD-OCT (Ver.6.0: Carl Zeiss). The 6 mm square area (200 A-can × 200 A-scan) focusing on the optic disk was measured using the Optic Disk Cube 200 × 200 scan protocol. The circumference of 1.73 mm from center of optic nerve disk was divided automatically into 12 sectors using Glaucoma OU Analysis, and the cpRNFL thickness of each sector was analyzed. We used the average value of each sector for examination. In addition, we assigned 12 sectors to the 12th sector clockwise by making into the 1st sector the 1:00 direction which is a clock. The direction of 11, 12 and 1:00 were decided to superior side, the direction of 2,

Table 1. Background of subjects.

	Normal eyes (n = 12)	PPG eyes (n = 10)	early UHFD eyes (n = 10)	severe UHFD eyes (n = 10)	p-value
Age (year)	64.8 ± 10.2	55.2 ± 9.6	61.8 ± 10.0	59.4 ± 9.0	0.1453
Gender (M / F)	4/8	4/6	5/5	5/7	0.6330
IOP (mHg)	15.8 ± 3.3	16.0 ± 6.5	14.3 ± 3.5	13.2 ± 2.0	0.1608
Equivalent refractive error (D)	−0.54 ± 1.48	−2.24 ± 2.05	−3.30 ± 3.34	−2.38 ± 2.51	0.0696
MD value (dB)	1.45 ± 0.85	0.63 ± 1.67	−2.49 ± 0.80	8.50 ± 2.60	<0.0001
PSD value (dB)	1.68 ± 0.33	1.80 ± 0.30	−7.14 ± 3.35	13.07 ± 3.56	<0.0001

PPG eyes: preperimetric glaucoma eyes; UHFD eye: glaucomatous upper-hemifield defect eyes; MD value, PSD value were measured using Humphrey Visual Field Analyzer 740 (Carl Zeiss) using Swedish Interactive Threshold Algorithm 30-2 SITA Standard program one-way ANOVA, gender: chi- square test.

3 and 4:00 were decided to nasal side, the direction of 5, 6 and 7:00 were decided to inferior side, the direction of 8, 9 and 10:00 were decided to temporal side (**Figure 1**). The 6 mm square area (200 A-can × 200 A-scan) focusing on the macula was measured using the Macular Cube 200 × 200 scan protocol. The ellipse of 4.0mm long × 4.8 mm side from center of fovea (excluding ellipse of long 1.0 mm × wide 1.2 mm) was divided automatically into 6 sectors(superior-nasal sector: SN, superior sector: S, superior-temporal sector: ST, inferior-nasal sector: IN, inferior sector: I, inferior-temporal sector: IT) using the Ganglion Cell Analysis, and the GCL + IPL thickness of each sector was analyzed. We used the average value of each of sector for examination (**Figure 2**). However, in order to be equivalent for UHFD eye, we carry out an up-and-down inversion which is the result of four PPG eyes with RNFL defect in only superior hemisphere, and we added it to six PPG eyes with RNFL defect in only inferior hemisphere, and used it for examination. We compared the cpRNFL thickness and the GCL + IPL thickness between normal eye group and other three groups. Dunnett's test was used statistical analysis, p-values less than 0.05 were accepted as statistically significant.

3. Results

In inferior hemisphere that was equivalent to visual field defects, the cpRNFL thickness was significantly thinner than normal eyes, the early UHFD eyes were decrease in sector 5, 6, 7 (total 3 sectors), the severe UHFD eyes were decrease in sector 5, 6, 7, 8 (total 4 sector), the PPG eyes were decrease in sector 5, 6, 7 (total 3 sectors). In superior hemisphere that was equivalent to normal visual field, the cpRNFL thickness was significantly thinner than normal eyes, the early UHFD eyes were decrease in sector 11, 12, 1 (total 3 sectors), the severe UHFD eyes were decrease in sector 11, 12, 1, 2 (total 4 sector), the PPG eyes were decrease in sector 1 (**Table 2**; **Figure 3**).

In inferior hemisphere, the GCL + IPL thickness was significantly thinner than normal eyes, the early UHFD eyes were decrease in 3 sector (sector IT, I, IN), the severe UHFD eyes were decrease in 3 sector (sector IT, I, IS), the PPG eyes were decrease in 1 sector (sector I). In superior hemisphere, the GCL + IPL thickness was significantly thinner than normal eyes, the early UHFD eyes were decrease in 1 sector (sector SN), the severe UHFD eyes were decrease in 3 sector (sector SN, S, ST), the PPG eyes were decrease in 2 sector (sector SN, ST) (**Table 3**; **Figure 4**).

4. Discussion

Recently, the examination of RGC and RNFL in glaucoma eye has piled up using remarkable developed OCT. Tan *et al.* had used the Time-domain OCT and SD-OCT showed that glaucoma leads to thinning of macular nerve fiver, ganglion cell, inner prexiform layers, which was apparent even before visual field changes were detected [10] [11]. Lee *et al.* had reported that the cpRNFL thickness measured by a SD-OCT was thinner in glaucoma eyes, and the cpRNFL thickness correlated with visual sensitive defects [12]. Moreover, Wu *et al.* accepted abnormalities by a frequency doubling technology (FDT) in the normal visual field with hemifield defect of glaucoma eye measured by Humphrey Visual Field Analyzer [13]. Takagi *et al.* reported that the cpRNFL thick-

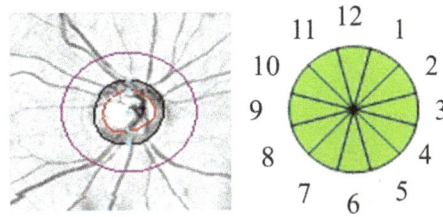

Figure 1. Measurement/Analysis of the cpRNFL. The 6 mm square area (200 A-can × 200 A-scan) focusing on the optic disk was measured using the Optic Disk Cube 200 × 200 scan protocol. The circumference of 1.73 mm from center of optic nerve head was divided automatically into 12 sectors using Glaucoma OU Analysis, and the cpRNFL thickness of each sector was analyzed. We assigned 12 sectors to the 12th sector clockwise by making into the 1st sector the 1:00 direction which is a clock. The direction of 11, 12 and 1:00 were decided to superior side, the direction of 2, 3 and 4:00 were decided to nasal side, the direction of 5, 6 and 7:00 were decided to inferior side, the direction of 8, 9 and 10:00 were decided to temporal side.

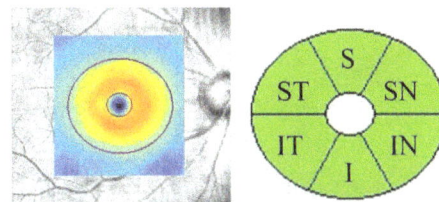

Figure 2. Measurement/Analysis of the GCL + IPL. The 6 mm square area (200 A-can × 200 A-scan) focusing on the macula was measured using the Macular Cube 200 × 200 scan protocol. The ellipse of 4.0 mm long × 4.8 mm side from center of fovea (excluding ellipse of long 1.0 mm × wide 1.2 mm) was divided automatically into 6 sectors (superior-nasal side: SN, superior side: S, superior-temporal side: ST, inferior-nasal side: IN, inferior side: I, inferior-temporal side: IT) using Ganglion Cell Analysis, and the GCL + IPL thickness of each sector was analyzed.

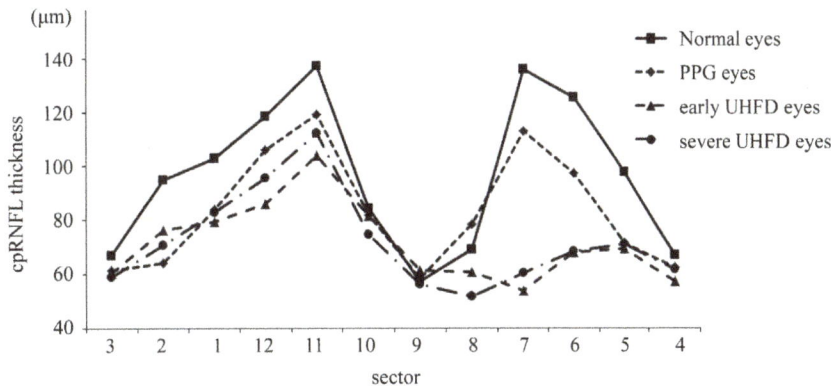

Figure 3. Results or the cpRNFL thickness. In inferior hemisphere that was equivalent to visual field defects, the cpRNFL thickness was significantly thinner than normal eyes, the early UHFD eyes were decrease in 3 sectors, the severe UHFD eyes were decrease in 4 sectors, the PPG eyes were decrease in 3 sectors. In superior hemisphere that was equivalent to normal visual field, the cpRNFL thickness was significantly thinner than normal eyes, the early UHFD eyes were decrease in 3 sectors, the severe UHFD eyes were decrease in 4 sectors, the PPG eyes were decrease in 1 sector. The results of statistical analysis were shown in **Table 2**.

ness, the GCC (RNFL + GCL + IPL) thickness of normal and abnormal hemisphere with the glaucomatous hemifield visual defect were thinner than normal eyes [5]. For these reasons, the normal hemifield with glaucomatous hemifeild defect measured by a static perimetry was regarded as a preceding state which glaucomatous

Table 2. Results of the cpRNFL thickness (μm).

sector		Normal eyes	PPG eyes	early UHFD eyes	severe UHFD eyes
superior	11	137.1 ± 25.9	119.2 ± 22.7	103.8 ± 14.2**	112.3 ± 24.4*
	12	118.6 ± 18.9	106.0 ± 14.3	85.8 ± 24.4*	95.8 ± 23.9**
nasal	1	102.8 ± 14.4	83.7 ± 11.0*	79.2 ± 15.6**	82.8 ± 18.5*
	2	94.8 ± 26.4	64.0 ± 10.7	76.1 ± 25.4**	70.6 ± 11.4**
	3	66.8 ± 9.7	61.3 ± 5.5	60.4 ± 18.1	59.0 ± 10.1
	4	66.8 ± 7.1	62.4 ± 7.3	57.2 ± 12.1	61.6 ± 10.8
inferior	5	97.8 ± 21.7	71.5 ± 18.2**	69.3 ± 19.5**	70.9 ± 9.4**
	6	125.3 ± 25.1	97.5 ± 17.0**	67.9 ± 13.6***	68.4 ± 18.4***
	7	135.8 ± 23.7	112.8 ± 25.5*	53.6 ± 14.8***	60.3 ± 9.8***
temporal	8	68.8 ± 12.3	78.5 ± 19.5	60.5 ± 11.3	51.8 ± 10.7**
	9	57.2 ± 11.3	58.2 ± 9.8	61.2 ± 6.9	56.3 ± 12.3
	10	84.3 ± 17.9	81.8 ± 18.3	81.3 ± 12.3	74.6 ± 13.3

PPG eyes: preperimetric glaucoma eyes; UHFD eye: glaucomatous upper-hemifield defect eyes; *: $p < 0.05$; **: $p < 0.01$; ***: $p < 0.001$, Dunnett's test.

Table 3. Result of the GCL + IPL thickness (μm).

sector	Normal eyes	PPG eyes	early UHFD eyes	severe UHFD eyes
SN	85.6 ± 7.8	76.8 ± 4.6*	75.2 ± 10.0*	76.2 ± 8.7*
S	84.0 ± 6.7	76.2 ± 3.1	73.8 ± 14.7	71.2 ± 14.6*
ST	81.9 ± 6.3	74.3 ± 5.3**	76.1 ± 5.9	71.3 ± 5.2***
IT	82.3 ± 6.7	76.9 ± 5.8	58.6 ± 6.4***	54.8 ± 4.0***
I	81.3 ± 5.7	73.2 ± 5.6*	66.3 ± 8.9***	57.9 ± 5.2***
IN	82.8 ± 6.7	75.0 ± 4.2	71.0 ± 11.6*	69.3 ± 8.3***

*: $p < 0.05$; **: $p < 0.01$; ***: $p < 0.001$; Dunnett's test superior-nasal side: SN, superior side: S, superior-temporal side: ST, inferior-nasal side: IN, inferior side: I, inferior-temporal side: IT.

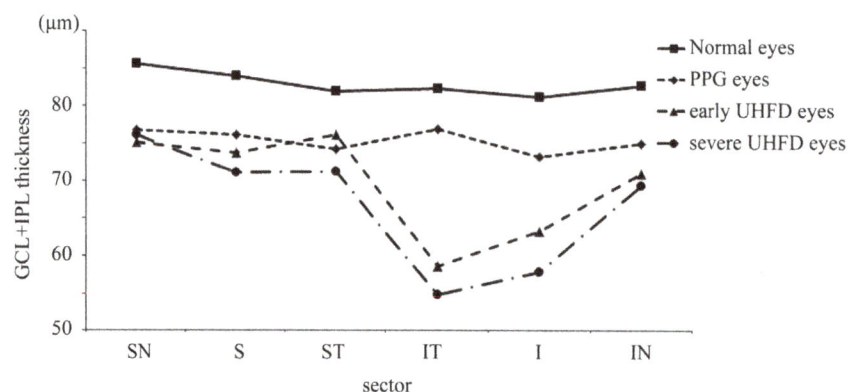

Figure 4. Results of the GCL + IPL thickness. In inferior hemisphere, the GCL + IPL thickness was significantly thinner than normal eyes, both the early and the severe UHFD eyes were decrease in 3 sectors, the PPG eyes were decrease in 1 sector. In superior hemisphere, the GCL + IPL thickness was significantly thinner than normal eyes, the early UHFD eyes were decrease in 1 sector, the severe UHFD eyes were decrease in 3 sectors, the PPG eyes were decrease in 2 sectors. The results of statistical analysis were shown in **Table 3**.

visual field change produces.

In this study, we compared the thickness of the cpRNFL and the GCL + IPL using Cirrus HD-OCT (Ver.6.0: Carl Zeiss) in normal eyes, PPG eyes, UHFD eyes (early and severe). As a result, also not only in the abnormality side but the normal side of UHFD eyes, the thickness of the cpRNFL and the GCL + IPL were significantly less than in normal eyes, we consider that it was able to detect that the glaucomatous structural change has arisen in the normal visual field with a glaucomatous visual hemifield defect the same as the past reports. In addition, in this study, the cpRNFL thickness and the GCL + IPL thickness of PPG eyes were significant thinner than normal eye, so it is suggested that in the state with the RNFL deficit, the structural change of glaucoma has developed the same as UHFD eye, even if there are no abnormalities in the result of the Humphrey Visual Field Analyzer. Considering the circumstances mentioned above, it is suggested that the result of measurement by the SD-OCT can be one of the important diagnostic views in progress observation of not only glaucoma eyes but also PPG eyes.

In the past report using the SD-OCT, the GCC which is the sum of the thickness of macular RNFL, GCL, IPL was adopted. Anatomically, the human retina contain more than 1 million RGCs, with substantial inter individual variability; approximately 50% of the cell are concentrated within 4.5 mm of fovea, and there is no variability in the RGC population in this small parafoveal area than the RNFL population [14]. Furthermore, the axons of not only macular RGCs but also those of some peripheral RGCs outside of macular pass through the macular area to reach optic nerve head, so it is difficult to separate and evaluate the change of macular RGC and a circumference part from the cpRNFL thickness. Moreover, in the recent reports, the cpRNFL thickness was influenced by age, ethnicity, axial length, optic disc size, and it was obviously that the result of the cpRNFL thickness has brought errors [15] [16]. It is suggested that the quantitative evaluation of the macular structure is the more sensitive method to detect a structure changes of the early glaucoma. However, the GCL has been reported to be the early site of glaucomatous damage, as shown in experimental models [7]. In the past examinations, it is guessed the macular GCC including the RNFL is without high ability to detect a glaucomatous structural change.

The Ganglion Cell Analysis in the Cirrus HD-OCT is the program to analyze only two layers thickness (GCL and IPL) excluding RNFL. Compared with evaluation of GCC, it is thought that the GCL + IPL analysis (Ganglion cell Analysis) has potential to be useful for glaucoma early detection. Mwanza *et al.* reported that the ability of macular GCIPL parameters to discriminate normal eyes and early glaucoma eyes is high and comparable to that of the best cpRNFL and ocular nerve head parameters [17]. In this study, we have not carried out comparison of the power to detect of the GCL + IPL, and the GCC (RNFL + GCL + IPL) and the cpRNFL. It needs future developments.

5. Conclusion

In this study, we compared the thickness of the cpRNFL and the GCL + IPL using Cirrus HD-OCT (Ver.6.0: Carl Zeiss) in normal eyes, PPG eyes, UHFD eyes. As a result, not only in the abnormality side of UHFD eyes but also in the normal side of UHFD eyes and PPG eyes, the thickness of the cpRNFL and the GCL + IPL were significantly less than in normal eyes. It is suggested that in the state with RNFL deficit, the structural change of glaucoma has developed, even if there are no abnormalities in the result of the Humphrey Visual Field Analyzer.

Institutional Review Board

This study was approved by the Institutional Review Board at Kitasato University Hospital (number B13-152, 2013) and followed the tenets of the Declaration of Helsinki.

Acknowledgements

The authors report no conflicts of interest. The authors alone are responsible for the content and writing of the paper.

References

[1]   Quigley, H.A., Dunkelberger, G.R. and Green, W.R. (1989) Retinal Ganglion Cell Atrophy Correlated with Automated Perimetry in Human Eyes with Glaucoma. *American Journal of Ophthalmology*, **107**, 453-464.

[2]   Kerrigan-Baumrind, L.A., Quigley, H.A., Pease, M.E., *et al.* (2000) Number of Ganglion Cells in Glaucoma Eyes Compared with Threshold Visual Field Tests in the Same Persons. *Investigative Ophthalmology & Visual Science*, **41**, 741-748.

[3]   Kanamori, A., Nakamura, M., Escano, M.F., *et al.* (2003) Evaluation of the Glaucomatous Damage on Retinal Nerve Fiber Layer Thickness Measured by Optical Coherence Tomography. *American Journal of Ophthalmology*, **135**, 513-520. http://dx.doi.org/10.1016/S0002-9394(02)02003-2

[4]   Wollstein, G., Ishikawa, H., Wang, J., *et al.* (2005) Comparison of Three Optical Coherence Tomography Scanning Areas for Detection of Glaucomatous Damage. *American Journal of Ophthalmology*, **139**, 39-43. http://dx.doi.org/10.1016/j.ajo.2004.08.036

[5]   Takagi, S.T., Kita, Y., Yagi, F., *et al.* (2012) Macular Retinal Ganglion Cell Complex Damage in the Apparently Normal Visual Field of Glaucomatous Eyes with Hemifield Defects. *Journal of Glaucoma*, **21**, 318-325. http://dx.doi.org/10.1097/IJG.0b013e31820d7e9d

[6]   Rao, H.L., Zangwill, L.M., Weinreb, R.N. *et al.* (2010) Comparison of Different Spectral Domain Optical Coherence Tomography Scanning Areas for Glaucoma Diagnosis. *Ophthalmology*, **117**, 1692-1699.

[7]   Huang, J.Y., Pekmezci, M., Mesiwala, N., *et al.* (2010) Diagnostic Power of Optic Disc Morphology, Peripapillary Retinal Nerve Fiber Layer Thickness, and Macular Inner Retinal Layer Thickness in Glaucoma Diagnosis with Fourier-Domain Optical Coherence Tomography. *Journal of Glaucoma*, **20**, 87-94. http://dx.doi.org/10.1097/IJG.0b013e3181d787b6

[8]   Desatnik, H., Quigley, H.A. and Glovinsky, Y. (1996) Study of Central Retinal Ganglion Cell Loss in Experimental Glaucoma in Monkey Eyes. *Journal of Glaucoma*, **5**, 46-53.

[9]   Anderson, D.R. and Patella, V.M. (1990) Automated Static Perimetry. 2nd Edition, St. Louis: Mosby, 121-190.

[10] Tan, O., Li, G., Lu, A.T., *et al.* (2008) Mapping of Macular Substructures with Optical Coherence Tomography for Glaucoma Diagnosis. *Ophthalmology*, **115**, 949-956.

[11] Tan, O., Chopra, V., Lu, A.T., *et al.* (2009) Detection of Macular Ganglion Cell Loss in Glaucoma by Fourier-Domain Optical Coherence Tomography. *Ophthalmology*, **116**, 2305-2314.

[12] Lee, J.R., Jeoung, J.W., Choi, J., *et al.* (2010) Structure-Function Relationships in Normal and Glaucomatous Eyes Determined by Time Domain and Spectral Domain Optical Coherence Tomography. *Investigative Ophthalmology & Visual Science*, **51**, 6424-6430. http://dx.doi.org/10.1167/iovs.09-5130

[13] Wu, L.L., Suzuki, Y., Kunimatsu, S., *et al.* (2001) Frequency Doubling Technology and Confocal Scanning Ophthalmoscopic Optic Disc Analysis in Open-Angle Glaucoma with Hemifield Defects. *Journal of Glaucoma*, **10**, 256-260. http://dx.doi.org/10.1097/00061198-200108000-00002

[14] Curcio, C.A. and Allen, K.A. (1990) Topography of Ganglion Cells in Human Retina. *Journal of Comparative Neurology*, **300**, 5-25. http://dx.doi.org/10.1002/cne.903000103

[15] Bendschneider, D., Tornow, R.P., Horn, F.K., *et al.* (2010) Retinal Nerve Fiber Layer Thickness in Normals Measured by Spectral Domain OCT. *Journal of Glaucoma*, **19**, 475-482. http://dx.doi.org/10.1097/IJG.0b013e3181c4b0c7

[16] Budenz, D.L., Anderson, D.R., Varma, R., *et al.* (2007) Determinants of Normal Retinal Nerve Fiber Layer Thickness Measured by Stratus OCT. *Ophthalmology*, **114**, 1046-1052. http://dx.doi.org/10.1016/j.ophtha.2006.08.046

[17] Mwanza, J.C., Durbin, M.K., Budenz, D.L., *et al.* (2012) Glaucoma Diagnostic Accuracy of Ganglion Cell-Inner Plexiform Layer Thickness: Comparison with Nerve Fiber Layer and Optic Nerve Head. *Ophthalmology*, **119**, 1151-1158. http://dx.doi.org/10.1016/j.ophtha.2011.12.014

16

Atrophy and Fibrosis of Extra-Ocular Muscles in Anti-Acetylcholine Receptor Antibody Myasthenia Gravis

Sean M. Gratton[1], Angela Herro[2], Jose Antonio Bermudez-Magner[2], John Guy[2]

[1]Truman Medical Center, Department of Neurology and Cognitive Neuroscience, University of Missouri—Kansas City School of Medicine, Kansas City, USA
[2]Bascom Palmer Eye Institute, University of Miami Miller School of Medicine, Miami, USA
Email: Sean.Gratton@tmcmed.org

Abstract

Myasthenia gravis (MG) is an autoimmune disorder involving the neuromuscular junction that frequently affects the extra-ocular muscles (EOMs). It has been described as a very rare cause of bilateral EOM atrophy, but histological analysis of such cases is lacking. A 66-year-old man presented with two months of right eyelid drooping and vertical diplopia. Examination showed bilateral ophthalmoparesis and complete right ptosis. The remainder of his exam was normal, and an MRI showed small EOMs. Acetylcholine receptor antibodies were elevated, establishing the diagnosis of MG. Oral corticosteroids and pyridostigmine followed by azathioprine improved his ptosis, but not his ophthalmoparesis. One year later he had surgical correction of his diplopia, and the resected superior rectus muscle showed complete replacement of EOM by connective tissue. MG can rarely cause bilateral EOM atrophy, which is characterized histologically by fibrosis in the muscle itself. Atrophy in the EOMs of a myasthenic patient may indicate a poor response to medical management alone.

Keywords

Myasthenia Gravis, Oculomotor Muscles, Muscular Atrophy

1. Introduction

Myasthenia gravis (MG) is an autoimmune disease of the neuromuscular junction most often caused by autoantibodies targeting the post-synaptic acetylcholine receptor (AChR). While the primary site of pathology in MG is the neuromuscular junction, muscle changes also occur. Lymphocyte infiltrates and muscle fiber atrophy are the most commonly described changes in the muscle of patients with MG [1]-[4]. While modern diagnostic techniques have made muscle biopsy obsolete in the diagnosis of MG, an understanding of the spectrum of muscle pathology in MG can still be pertinent to clinical practice. We present a case of anti-AChR antibody positive myasthenia gravis with atrophic and fibrotic extra-ocular muscles (EOMs) who had a poor response to medical therapy.

2. Case Report

A 66-year-old man presented with two months of right eyelid drooping and vertical binocular diplopia, both worse in the evening. Examination showed almost complete ophthalmoplegia of the right eye. The left eye also had limited abduction and depression. He had complete right upper lid ptosis. Digital forced ductions were normal indicating no mechanical restriction in moving the eye upwards. His pupils were 4.5 mm and equally reactive. The remainder of his exam was normal.

MRI showed uniformly small EOMs in both eyes (**Figure 1**). An intravenous edrophonium test was deferred due to elevated blood pressure (194/107). Serum AChR-binding antibodies were found to be elevated; therefore a diagnosis of myasthenia gravis was made.

The patient was treated with oral corticosteroids and pyridostigmine, followed by the addition of azathioprine. While his ptosis improved, he continued to have constant diplopia. One year later he opted for surgical correction of the diplopia. The resected superior rectus muscle specimen was sent for histopathological analysis. H&E stain showed fibrocellular material replacing muscle tissue, and modified trichrome stain revealed near-complete replacement of muscle by connective tissue (**Figure 2**). This was later confirmed using other stains such as desmin. There were no ragged red fibers.

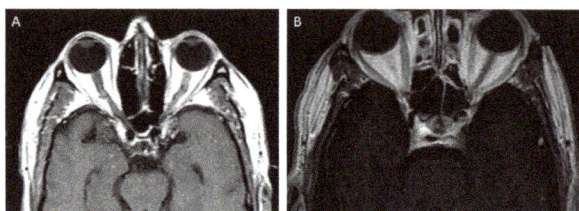

Figure 1. MRI brain of patient and control. (A) T1 axial post-gadolinium MR image of our patient at presentation showing uniformly atrophic extra-ocular muscles; (B) T1 axial post-gadolinium MR image of a healthy age-matched control patient to serve as a comparison for extra-ocular muscle size.

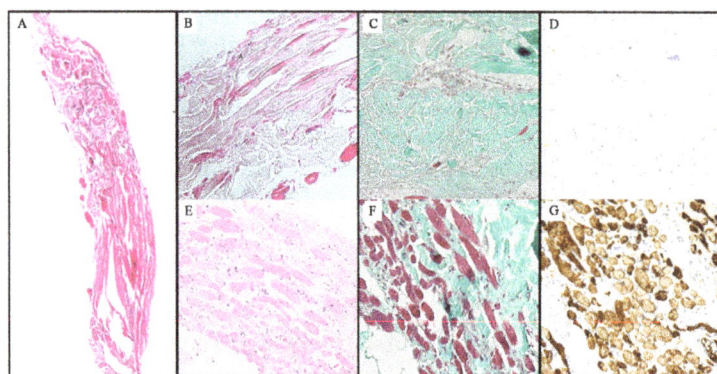

Figure 2. Extra-ocular muscle histopathology from patient ((A) 4× magnification; (B)-(D) 20× magnification and control; (E)-(G) 20× magnification). (A) Low-power H & E stain of the superior rectus muscle specimen showing fibrocellular tissue; (B) H & E stain at higher power showing fibrocellular tissue; (C) Modified trichrome stain showing near complete absence of muscle tissue replaced by collagen and no ragged red fibers; (D) Desmin stain with only trace staining consistent with absence of muscle tissue; (E) H & E stain of control muscle showing normal EOM fibers; (F) Modified trichrome highlights collagen around muscle fibers; (G) Desmin stain highlights muscular tissue.

3. Discussion

Bilateral EOM atrophy is a rare entity that has been described in mitochondrial myopathies, myotonic dystrophy, and congenital fibrosis syndromes [5]. MG has also been reported as an extremely rare cause of such atrophy. In a case series of seven patients with bilateral EOM atrophy, three patients had MG while the remainder had mitochondrial myopathies. One of the patients with MG in this series had anti-AChR antibodies [6]. Chan and Orrison reported the case of a 49-year-old man with anti-MuSK antibody positive MG who also had "severe wasting" of EOMs bilaterally [5]. All four of these MG patients with EOM atrophy received appropriate treatment, but none had significant improvement.

In the early part of the 20th century, muscle biopsy was used as an aid to the diagnosis of myasthenia gravis. In 1953, Russell published a landmark paper describing muscle findings in MG, including inflammatory changes and simple fiber atrophy [1]. In subsequent years, others would elaborate on these findings. Notably, Fenichel reported that the simple fiber atrophy described by Russell occurred in a "grouped" fashion, typical of denervation. The presence of both denervation changes and inflammation in the muscle itself led Fenichel to surmise that "the possibility that myasthenia may be a syndrome secondary to a primary abnormality on either side of the synapse is real" [2]. We now know that the primary abnormality in MG localizes to the synapse itself. Antibody-mediated inflammation leads to lymphocytic infiltration of the neuromuscular junction and surrounding tissue. Eventually the inflammatory response so damages motor endplates that the muscle is effectively denervated, resulting in atrophy.

Given the evolution of our knowledge about MG, and in particular the discovery of pathogenic autoantibodies in the disease, muscle biopsy is no longer performed as an aide to its diagnosis. Because our patient opted to undergo strabismus surgery, we had the unique opportunity to perform a histological examination of the affected muscle. To our knowledge this is the first report of histopathology in a patient with MG and EOM atrophy. This examination revealed abundant collagen deposition consistent with fibrosis that essentially replaced all of the muscle tissue. This fibrosis is consistent with a chronic process, most likely from chronic inflammation at the neuromuscular junction that has subsequently become dormant due to the absence of healthy AChR to serve as an autoantigen.

As was the case in the four previously reported patients with MG and EOM atrophy, our patient had a poor response to medical treatment. The histological findings in our patient provide a straightforward explanation for these outcomes: there simply isn't enough functioning EOM tissue left to effect muscle contraction even with appropriate treatment. Because of these findings, the clinician should be aware that MG can cause bilateral EOM atrophy, and that the presence of atrophic EOMs may portend a worse prognosis to medical therapy.

References

[1]   Russell, D. (1953) Histological Changes in the Striped Muscles in Myasthenia Gravis. *The Journal of Pathology and Bacteriology*, **65**, 279-289. http://dx.doi.org/10.1002/path.1700650202

[2]   Fenichel, G. (1966) Muscle Lesions in Myasthenia Gravis. *Annals of the New York Academy of Sciences*, **135**, 60-67. http://dx.doi.org/10.1111/j.1749-6632.1966.tb45463.x

[3]   Fenichel, G. and Shy, G. (1963) Muscle Biopsy Experience in Myasthenia Gravis. *Archives of Neurology*, **9**, 237-243. http://dx.doi.org/10.1001/archneur.1963.00460090043004

[4]   Oosterhuis, H. and Bethlem, J. (1973) Neurogenic Muscle Involvement in Myasthenia Gravis. A Clinical and Histopathological Study. *Journal of Neurology, Neurosurgery Psychiatry*, **36**, 244-254. http://dx.doi.org/10.1136/jnnp.36.2.244

[5]   Chan, J. and Orrison, W. (2007) Ocular Myasthenia: A Rare Presentation with MuSK Antibody and Bilateral Extraocular Muscle Atrophy. *British Journal of Ophthalmology*, **91**, 842-843. http://dx.doi.org/10.1136/bjo.2006.108498

[6]   Okamoto, K., Ito, J., Tokiguchi, S. and Furusawa, T. (1996) Atrophy of Bilateral Extraocular Muscles: CT and Clinical Features of Seven Patients. *Journal of Neuro-Ophthalmology*, **16**, 286-288. http://dx.doi.org/10.1097/00041327-199612000-00012

17

Exudative Retinal Detachment Associated with Complicated Retrobulbar Anesthesia

Volkan Yaylalı[1,2], Ibrahim Toprak[3*]

[1]Department of Ophthalmology, Faculty of Medicine, Pamukkale University, Denizli, Turkey
[2]Private Yaylalı Eye Hospital, Denizli, Turkey
[3]Department of Ophthalmology, Servergazi State Hospital, Denizli, Turkey
Email: volkanyaylali@yahoo.com, *ibrahimt@doctor.com

Abstract

Retrobulbar anesthesia (block) is used for many ocular surgeries, whereas it is well known that this procedure has complications such as for retrobulbar hemorrhage, globe perforation, optic nerve injury and brain stem anesthesia. In this report, we present a unique case in the literature of isolated exudative retinal detachment (RD) secondary to iatrogenic retrobulbar hemorrhage. A 73-year-old woman underwent retrobulbar block for combined phaco-vitrectomy. Immediately after the injection, progressive proptosis was recognized. The globe was decompressed and she underwent combined phaco-vitrectomy after stabilization of the eye on the same day. At the beginning of the vitrectomy, a dome shaped serous RD was observed in the infero-temporal quadrant. Peripheral exploration was performed, whereas there was no retinal tear or hole. On the first day postoperatively, serous RD was disappeared. In conclusion, this report suggests that increased intraorbital pressure secondary to iatrogenic retrobulbar hemorrhage might lead exudative RD.

Keywords

Retrobulbar Anesthesia, Retrobulbar Hemorrhage, Exudative Retinal Detachment

1. Introduction

Topical anesthesia is widely used for elective phaco surgery, whereas in complicated cases and posterior segment surgeries, surgeons prefer retrobulbar block, which provides a deeper anesthesia [1]. Injection of local anesthetic agents into retrobulbar space carries risks for many local and systemic complications such as subcon-

---

*Corresponding author.

junctival hemorrhage, chemosis, retrobulbar hemorrhage, extraocular muscle injury, globe perforation, optic neuropathy, retinal artery occlusion, seizures, transient blindness, cardiopulmonary collapse, III cranial nerve palsy and brainstem anesthesia [1]-[7].

Retrobulbar hemorrhage is a relatively common complication of retrobulbar block with an incidence of 0.1% - 3% [1] [2]. The sharp needle causes vascular injury and bleeding, which results in progressive proptosis, elevated intraocular pressure (IOP), chemosis and swelling of the eyelids. Immediate IOP lowering therapy such as intravenous mannitol infusion and lateral canthotomy are generally needed to prevent permanent visual damage [1] [2]. To best of our knowledge, this is the first study to report a case with isolated exudative retinal detachment following retrobulbar hemorrhage as a complication of retrobulbar block.

2. Case Report

A 73-year-old woman presented with visual deterioration in both eyes. A complete ophthalmological examination was performed. Best-corrected visual acuity (BCVA) was 0.6 and 0.2 (Snellen chart) in the right and left eyes (respectively). Slit-lamp biomicroscopy and dilated fundoscopy revealed bilateral senile cataract and epimacular membrane in the left eye. The patient was informed and combined phacoemulsification and pars plana vitrectomy (PPV) surgery was planned for the left eye.

On the operation day, the patient underwent retrobulbar anesthesia and three milliliters of local anesthetic agent was injected into the left retrobulbar space using *Atkinson needle* (25-gauge × 32 mm) at inferolateral orbital region as commonly described [1]. Immediately after the injection, dramatic proptosis, chemosis and eyelid edema were observed. Lateral canthotomy was performed urgently and intravenous mannitol infusion (300 cc 20%) was administered. The patient had no signs of systemic complications of retrobulbar block. Arterial blood pressure, heart rate, electrocardiography and pulse oximetry values were within normal limits. In an hour, marked proptosis and eyelid edema regressed, and IOP returned to normal. Phacoemulsification and 23-gauge PPV were performed in the same session.

At the beginning of the vitrectomy, a localized, dome shaped serous retinal detachment (RD) with a smooth surface was observed in the infero-temporal quadrant incidentally, which was not present in preoperative fundus examination (**Figure 1**). Peripheral retinal exploration was performed under scleral indentation, whereas we found no retinal break or signs of globe perforation. The operation was completed without any complication. On the first day postoperatively, dilated fundus examination revealed no serous retinal detachment or retinal tear in the left eye. During the postoperative follow up, ocular examinations were non-specific and the patient had a BCVA of 0.8 (Snellen) in the left eye.

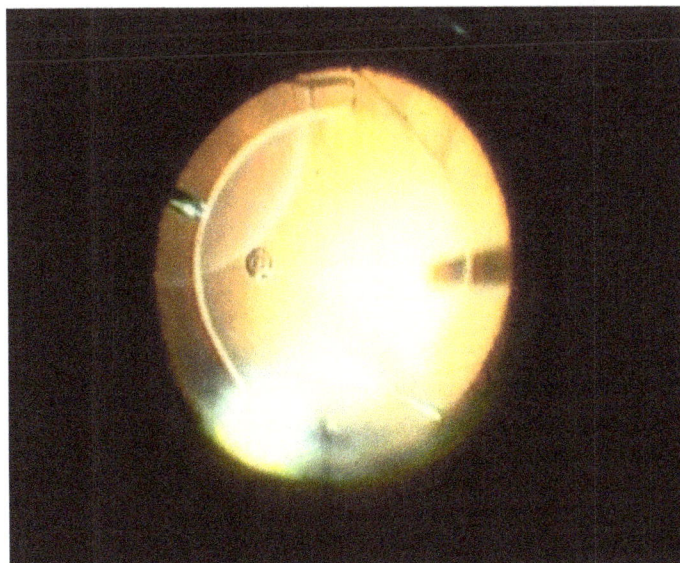

Figure 1. Intraoperative fundus image demonstrates infero-temporal quadrant located and dome shaped exudative retinal detachment (this image was captured from intraoperative video record and loss of resolution is related with intraoperative lighting conditions).

3. Discussion

The current literature comprises cases with common complications of retrobulbar block and RD related to iatrogenic globe perforation. However, there are a few numbers of case-reports presenting localized RD as a complication of retrobulbar anesthesia. Mieler *et al.* [2] presented a case with localized RD and coexisting central retinal artery and vein occlusion due to possible injection of the anesthetic agent into the optic nerve [2]. They reported that the patient showed no acute neurological symptoms, whereas visual loss was severe and permanent. Another study by Mameletzi *et al.* [8] reported a 78-year-old female with severe vision loss (light perception), multiple retinal arterial emboli, localized RD and magnetic resonance imaging (MRI) findings of optic neuritis in her left eye a day after uneventful cataract surgery, which was performed under retrobulbar anesthesia. They reported that retina was reattached after administration of IOP lowering therapy and intravenous methylprednisolone (1 g/day for three days), whereas visual acuity did not change [8].

In our study, isolated exudative RD might be due to compression of ocular venous drainage system like a vortex vein by retrobulbar hematoma and elevated intraorbital pressure [9] [10]. Under normal conditions, fluid is transported from vitreous to the choroid by active pumping function of retinal pigment epithelium and hydrostatic gradient. Deterioration in inflow-outflow balance leads to accumulation of fluid in the subretinal area and exudative RD develops [9] [10].

Herein, retrobulbar hematoma or/and increased intraorbital pressure might cause obstruction of venous outflow. However, quadrantic localization of the exudative RD might suggest vortex vein compression or damage as in nanophthalmic eyes and eyes underwent scleral buckling surgery [9] [10]. Rapid spontaneous resolution of exudative RD postoperatively can be explained with normalization of the intraorbital pressure.

4. Conclusion

In conclusion, our study might add exudative RD into the current literature as a complication of retrobulbar block.

Acknowledgements

This study was performed in adherence to the tenets of the Declaration of Helsinki. No author has a financial or proprietary interest in any product, material, or method mentioned. No financial support was received for this study.

References

[1]   Jaichandran, V. (2013) Ophthalmic Regional Anaesthesia: A Review and Update. *Indian Journal of Anaesthesia*, **3**, 7-13. http://dx.doi.org/10.4103/0019-5049.108552

[2]   Mieler, W.F., Bennett, S.R., Platt, L.W. and Koenig, S.B. (1990) Localized Retinal Detachment with Combined Central Retinal Artery and Vein Occlusion after Retrobulbar Anesthesia. *Retina*, **10**, 278-283. http://dx.doi.org/10.1097/00006982-199010000-00010

[3]   Tappeiner, C. and Garweg, J.G. (2011) Retinal Vascular Occlusion after Vitrectomy with Retrobulbar Anesthesia-Observational Case Series and Survey of Literature. *Graefe's Archive for Clinical and Experimental Ophthalmology*, **249**, 1831-1815. http://dx.doi.org/10.1007/s00417-011-1783-9

[4]   Gross, A. and Cestari, D.M. (2014) Optic Neuropathy Following Retrobulbar İnjection: A Review. *Seminars in Ophthalmology*, **29**, 434-439. http://dx.doi.org/10.3109/08820538.2014.959191

[5]   Naik, A.A., Agrawal, S.A., Navadiya, I.D. and Ramchandani, S.J. (2014) Management of Macular Epiretinal Membrane Secondary to Accidental Globe Perforation during Retrobulbar Anesthesia. *Indian Journal of Ophthalmology*, **62**, 94-95.

[6]   Spire, M., Fleury, J., Kodjikian, L. and Grange, J.D. (2007) Retinal Detachment Caused by Ocular Perforation during Periocular Anesthesia: Three Case Reports. *Journal Francais d'Ophtalmologie*, **30**, e16.

[7]   Aranda Calleja, M.A., Martínez Pueyo, A., Bellido Cuellar, S. and García Ruiz, P. (2011) III Cranial Nerve Palsy and Brainstem Disfunction Following Retrobulbar Anaesthesia. *Neurologia*, **26**, 563-564. http://dx.doi.org/10.1016/j.nrl.2011.04.013

[8]   Mameletzi, E., Pournaras, J.A., Ambresin, A. and Nguyen, C. (2008) Retinal Embolisation with Localised Retinal Detachment Following Retrobulbar Anaesthesia. *Klinische Monatsblätter für Augenheilkunde*, **225**, 476-478. http://dx.doi.org/10.1055/s-2008-1027268

[9]   Krohn, J. and Seland, J.H. (1998) Exudative Retinal Detachment in Nanophthalmos. *Acta Ophthalmologica Scandinavica*, **76**, 499-502. http://dx.doi.org/10.1034/j.1600-0420.1998.760421.x

[10] Takahashi, K. and Kishi, S. (2000) Remodeling of Choroidal Venous Drainage after Vortex Vein Occlusion Following Scleral Buckling for Retinal Detachment. *American Journal of Ophthalmology*, **129**, 191-198. http://dx.doi.org/10.1016/S0002-9394(99)00425-0

The Prevalence of Blindness, Visual Impairment and Cataract Surgery in Tuoketuo and Shangdu Counties, Inner Mongolia, China

Baixiang Xiao[1,2*], Jinglin Yi[1], Hans Limburg[3], Guiseng Zhang[4], Richard Le Mesurier[5], Andreas Müller[6], Nathan Congdon[2], Beatrice Iezzi[5]

[1]Affiliated Eye Hospital of Nanchang University, Nanchang City, China
[2]Zhongshan Ophthalmic Center, Guangzhou City, China
[3]London School of Hygiene & Tropical Medicine, London, United Kingdom
[4]Inner Mongolia Red Cross Chaoju Eye Hospital, Hohhot, China
[5]The Fred Hollows Foundation, Sydney, Australia
[6]World Health Organization, Western Pacific Regional Office, Manila, Philippines
Email: *xiaobaixiang2006@126.com

Abstract

Aim: A population-based survey was conducted in Tuoketuo and Shangdu Counties in Inner Mongolia Autonomous Region, China, in the Autumn of 2010, to assess the prevalence and causes of blindness and visual impairment of people aged 50 years and over. Methods: Random cluster sampling was used to select 82 clusters of 50 residents in the 2 counties. Each survey team included an ophthalmologist, a nurse and a coordinator, who went to door to door in each cluster to identify eligible people. A torch, direct ophthalmoscope and portable slit lamp were used for eye examination. Visual acuity (VA) was tested for each eye of every subject. Those with VA below 6/18 in either eye were examined and causes identified. Results: The survey identified a prevalence of blindness in people aged 50+ in Tuoketuo of 1.2% (95% Confidence Interval: 0.7% - 1.7%) and in Shangdu of 1.4% (95% CI: 1.0% - 1.9%). Cataract was identified as the leading cause of blindness (BL) and severe visual impairment (SVI), and uncorrected refractive errors were the major causes of moderate visual impairment (MVI) in both counties. Over two thirds of blindness, SVI and MVI were identified as avoidable. Conclusions: The prevalence of blindness in people aged 50+ in Tuoketuo and Shangdu was low compared to other studies conducted in China [1] [2]. The prevalence of blindness of people aged 50 years and over could be reduced by up to two thirds

---

*Corresponding author.

through better eye services in the two study areas.

Keywords

RAAB, Prevalence of Blindness, Cataract, Cataract Surgical Coverage, Survey, Inner Mongolia, China

1. Introduction

The World Health Organization (WHO) estimated that in 2010, there were 39 million blind people and another 245 million visually impaired globally [3]. 90% of people with visual impairment live in developing countries and over 80% of visual impairment is avoidable or treatable [4]. China has a total population of 1.4 billion in 2009, of whom an estimated 8.248 million were blind [3]—the largest of any country in the world for its number of population, and accounting for 20.9% of the world's blind. China is also estimated to have the world's most rapidly ageing population [5]. By 2020, the country's elderly population over 60 years is expected to increase by 90% and reach 240 million people nationwide. As the population ages, it is expected that more people will suffer from cataract. Despite this fact, the cataract surgical rate (CSR) in China is comparatively low, less than 800 in 2010 [6].

The Inner Mongolia Autonomous Region is located in northern China, and is geographically the third largest province in the country. Internationally, it borders Mongolia and Russia. The population density is among the lowest in China, and the geography is high altitude, relatively infertile and drought-prone. Administratively, the region is equivalent to a province, and is divided into 9 alliances (equivalent to prefectures in other provinces), approximately 87 counties, and 13 city-districts.

The population in Inner Mongolia was 24 million (2010), of which 53% lived in rural areas, and 52% were male. Life expectancy in Inner Mongolia was 70.7 years in 2005 [7]. Tuoketuo County is located in about 2 - 3 hours drive distance south west of Hohhot, the region's capital city. Shangdu County is at about 6 hours drive way east of Hohhot—closer to Beijing.

In Inner Mongolia, there were about 400 eye doctors. Although the ration of eye doctors per population is 1/60,000 and therefore within WHO's recommendations, less than 20% could independently conduct cataract surgeries. They were mostly working in urban Provincial/prefecture level hospitals. At county level in Inner Mongolia, cataract surgeries were mostly done by the visiting surgeons from Hohhot, or Beijing at the time when this survey conducted.

The most recent blindness prevalence data for the region was from the Chinese National Eye Study of 1992 [8]. It was estimated by the Regional Bureau of Health that in Inner Mongolia the annual number of cataract surgery was about 10,000 in 2010, while there were about 50,000 cataract blindness backlog in the region. In huge contrast, in the 16 years from 1988 to 2004, on average less than 7000 cataract surgeries were performed annually in Inner Mongolia. The estimated CSR was 435 in Inner Mongolia in 2009.

Tuoketuo County Hospital serves 200,000 people. It was the only one with an independent eye department amongst all the hospitals in the county. The 3 eye doctors in the department without other paramedical staff, were doing less than 20 cataract surgeries a year before the non-government organization started a project in August 2010. Shangdu County Hospital serves 342,000 people. There were 4 eye doctors in the EENT department without any nurses, or optometrists. One doctor was doing few cataract surgeries without knowing the results in 2010. There were no outreach activities from the hospital. Doctors from Beijing were invited to do one to two days cataract surgeries annually in the recent years.

The survey was designed to assess the prevalence of blindness, visual impairment and cataract service delivery situation in these two areas as the baseline data collection of a prevention of blindness project, supported by an international non-government organization and the local health authorities in Inner Mongolia.

2. Methods

2.1. Ethical Approval

Ethical approval for the survey was attained from all local project partners, including the Inner Mongolia Red

Cross Chaoju Eye Hospital-Hohhot, Tuoketuo County Hospital and Shangdu County Hospital. Verbal consent was obtained from every study subject before eye examinations were undertaken. Survey teams were trained to demonstrate respect and kindness towards the local villagers while conducting the survey. All the cataract eyes with VA < 6/60 found during this study were offered free surgeries one month after the survey, subsidized partially through the NGO project.

2.2. Sample Size and Selection

The latest RAAB software (version 4.03—in multi-language including Chinese) was used to calculate sample size. As the RAAB methodology required a population of 50,000 to 2,000,000, both Counties were treated as one district for sample size calculation. The Census data from the local bureau of police from the previous year was used to estimate the population of people aged 50 years and older in the two counties, and local eye care professionals provided an estimated prevalence of blindness for people aged 50 years and over (3.5%). Based on these inputs, a sample size of 4100 participants (82 clusters of size 50) was calculated to have enough power with a variation of 20% or less and confidence of 95%, assuming a non-compliance of 10%.

Although the total population of Shangdu County was almost double that of Tuoketuo County, Census data indicated that Tuoketuo County has a much older age structure than that in Shangdu and therefore the number of people aged 50 years and over was very similar in both Counties—59,000 in Tuoketuo and 55,000 in Shangdu Counties. As the RAAB only includes people aged 50 years and over, the distribution of sample clusters was therefore similar between the two counties—42 of the 82 clusters were selected from Tuoketuo and the remaining 40 from Shangdu.

2.3. Training of the Study Teams

There were four study teams (two per County) for the RAAB, simultaneously undertaking data collection. Each team consisted of an ophthalmologist, a nurse, an administrator and a driver. The four teams received five days training together in Hohhot immediately prior to the survey. The training covered: the background and principles of RAABs; calculation of sample size; selection of clusters; inter-observer variation (IOV); how to complete the survey form; examination of subjects and practice in the field. Variations identified during IOV were examined and the junior doctors were supervised by more experienced doctors during the first week of field work, to ensure RAAB implementation was consistent with the training and theory. The training was conducted by an international trainer (Dr. Hans Limburg) with Chinese interpretation and simultaneous English and Chinese slide shows.

Prior to data collection, the heads or party secretaries from all survey villages w were invited for a half day meeting to be briefed on the purpose of the study and cooperation needed from the villagers. In consultation with these village leaders, a schedule for data collection was established and clear protocol for contact and informing selected participants.

2.4. Ophthalmic Examination

The village leader was contacted again the day prior to data collection in the selected village, and a refresher provided by the study team on the purpose and concepts of the RAAB. The village leader then acted as guide for the study team in the village. A random start-point was selected by the study team, who then moved from house to house in one direction. A spinning bottle was used to choose the direction at each turn of the road. In each of the 82 survey villages, house visits continued until 50 people aged 50 years and over were examined (one cluster). If the study subjects were not at the house, other family members or neighbors were asked to help arrange examination appointments for later in the day. The subjects were treated as missed cases only if the team had made three home visits or were certain the study subjects were not available.

The WHO's definition of blindness (BL), severe visual impairment (SVI) and moderate visual impairment (MVI) were used for the study [9]. Blindness is defined as VA < 3/60 in the better eye with pinhole correction (Best Corrected Vision Acuity—BCVA). SVI is VA ≥ 3/60 - <6/60, MVI is VA ≥ 6/60 - <6/18. A tumbling "E" chart was used at 6 meters/3 meters or closer to measure the VA in good illumination by a trained nurse.

The tools used in the eye examination were torch, ophthalmoscope and portable slit lamp. Respondents with VA below 6/18 in either eye were examined again inside the house by the ophthalmologist, and causes were identified according to the WHO's eye diseases classification. In some cases, the pupil was dilated to increase the quality of assessment. For all respondents who had already undergone cataract surgery (including those with VA above 6/18), details such as the cataract surgical time, place, lens type (intraocular or other) and the result were assessed. Respondents who were assessed as needing cataract surgery but had not received the surgery were asked for the reasons.

2.5. Data Input and Analysis

Data were double entered into the Chinese version RAAB software each day after completion of one survey cluster, by the team ophthalmologist and nurse. Consistency checks and data cleaning were completed by the study coordinator (BX). The reports were generated automatically from the RAAB software. Confidence intervals were calculated using "Excel 2007" software.

3. Results

The examination rate was high in both counties, 96.4% (1976 out of 2050) in Tuoketuo and 98.8% (1975 out of 2000) in Shangdu. Of those missed, in Tuoketuo, 68 (3.3%) were not available, 1 (0.05%) refused and 5 (0.2%) were not capable of being examined, while in Shangdu, with a higher examination rate, there were only 19 (0.95%) not available, 6 (0.3%) were not capable and no subjects refused.

Age and gender composition in the sample population generally represented that of the survey area in Tuoketuo and Shangdu (**Table 1**).

The prevalence of bilateral blindness (BCVA) in both Tuoketuo and Shangdu was low, 1.2% (95% CI: 0.7% - 1.7%) and 1.4% (95% CI: 1.0% - 1.9%) respectively (**Table 2**). Prevalence of SVI in both counties was almost equal to that of blindness, while the MVI prevalence (4.4% and 4.6% respectively in Tuoketuo and Shangdu) was three times higher than the blindness rate in both counties. X^2-test found no significant difference ($p > 0.5$) between male and female blindness prevalence rates in Tuoketuo, or SVI and MVI in both counties, although the teams found more females were blind, SVI or MVI in the study.

Results were extrapolated to identify the age and gender adjusted prevalence of blindness and visual impairment in the two Counties. In Tuoketuo it was estimated that there were approximately 1543 people aged 50 years old or above were bilaterally blind; 1696 with severe visual impairment and 4696 with moderate visual impairment. In Shangdu, it was estimated that there were 851 blind people aged 50 or above, 1103 with severe visual impairment and 2438 with moderate visual impairment.

Cataract was still the leading cause of blindness (62.5% in Tuoketuo and 46.7% in Shangdu respectively) and SVI in both counties (**Table 3**). Uncorrected refractive error was the major cause of MVI, 50.6% in Tuoketuo and 46.2% in Shangdu, followed by cataract. Of all the blindness, SVI and MVI, 76.5% to 95.8% were treatable or preventable (avoidable) in both counties.

About half of all people with VA < 6/60 requiring cataract surgery had received surgeries (**Table 4**). If Cataract Surgical Coverage (CSC) was calculated on eyes, less than one third of the eyes that needed surgery had

Table 1. Age and gender composition of survey area and sample population.

| Age group (years) | Tuoketuo | | | | Shangdu | | | |
| | Survey area | | Sample | | Survey area | | Sample | |
	n = 1976	%	n = 55,050	%	n = 1975	%	n	%
50 - 54	296	15.0%	14,294	26.0%	336	17.0%	13,782	23.4%
55 - 59	450	22.8%	9934	18.0%	447	22.6%	15,327	26.0%
60 - 64	345	17.5%	9541	17.3%	392	19.8%	8997	15.3%
65 - 69	238	12.0%	8518	15.5%	268	13.6%	5765	9.8%
70 - 74	261	13.2%	6427	11.7%	279	14.1%	5779	9.8%
75 - 79	261	13.2%	3891	7.1%	173	8.8%	5470	9.3%
80 - 99	125	6.3%	2445	4.4%	80	4.1%	3772	6.4%

Table 2. Sample prevalence of blindness, SVI and MVI in Tuoketuo and Shangdu County-unadjusted.

Tuoketuo county	Male (n = 939)			Female (n = 1037)			Total (n = 1976)		
	n	%	95%CI	N	%	95%CI	n	%	95%CI
Blindness (pinhole correction)									
All bilateral blindness (BCVA < 3/60)	8	0.9%	(0.3% - 1.4%)	16	1.5%	(0.8% - 2.3%)	24	1.2%	(0.7% - 1.7%)
All blind eyes	56	3.0%	(1.9% - 4.1%)	85	4.1%	(2.9% - 5.3%)	141	3.6%	(2.8% - 4.4%)
Severe visual impairment (SVI)									
All bilateral SVI (BCVA<6/6/60, ≥3/60)	9	1.0%	(0.3% - 1.6%)	11	1.1%	(0.4% - 1.7%)	20	1.0%	(0.6% - 1.5%)
All SVI eyes	27	1.4%	(0.7%- 2.2%)	39	1.9%	(1.1% - 2.7%)	66	1.7%	(1.1% - 2.2%)
Moderate VI (pinhole)									
All bilateral MVI (VA < 6/18, ≥6/60)	34	3.6%	(2.4% - 4.8%)	53	5.1%	(3.8% - 6.5%)	87	4.4%	(3.5% - 5.3%)
All MVI eyes	93	5.0%	(3.6% - 6.3%)	129	6.2%	(4.8% - 7.7%)	222	5.6%	(4.6% - 6.6%)
Shangdu county	**Male (n = 980)**			**Female (n = 995)**			**Total (n = 1975)**		
Blindness (pinhole correction)									
All bilateral blindness (BCVA < 3/60)	9	0.9%	(0.3% - 1.5%)	19	1.9%	(1.1% - 2.8%)	28	1.4%	(1.0% - 1.9%)
All blind eyes	58	3.0%	(1.9% - 4.0%)	90	4.5%	(3.2% - 5.8%)	148	3.7%	(2.9% - 4.6%)
Severe visual impairment (SVI)									
All bilateral SVI (PVA < 6/6/60, ≥3/60)	16	1.6%	(0.8% - 2.4%)	24	2.4%	(1.5% - 3.4%)	40	2.0%	(1.4% - 3.4%)
All SVI eyes	40	2.0%	(1.2% - 2.9%)	49	2.5%	(1.5% - 3.4%)	89	2.3%	(1.6% - 2.9%)
Moderate VI (pinhole)									
All bilateral MVI (VA < 6/18, ≥6/60)	36	3.7%	(2.5% - 4.9%)	55	5.5%	(3.1% - 7.0%)	91	4.6%	(3.7% - 5.5%)
All VI eyes	97	4.9%	(3.6% - 6.3%)	129	6.5%	(5.0% - 8.0%)	226	5.7%	(4.7% - 6.7%)

Table 3. Causes of bilateral blindness and bilateral visual impairment with available correction.

	Tuoketuo						Shangdu					
	Blindness		SVI		MVI		Blindness		SVI		MVI	
	n = 24		n = 20		n = 87		n = 30		n = 40		n = 91	
Refractive error	0	0.0%	5	25.0%	44	50.6%	2	6.7%	7	17.5%	42	46.2%
Aphakia, uncorrected	0	0.0%	0	0.0%	0	0.0%	0	0.0%	0	0.0%	1	1.1%
Cataract, untreated	15	62.5%	10	50.0%	28	32.2%	14	46.7%	13	32.5%	23	25.3%
Total treatable	**15**	**62.5%**	**15**	**75.0%**	**72**	**82.8%**	**16**	**53.3%**	**20**	**50.0%**	**66**	**72.5%**
Other corneal opacity	1	4.2%	0	0.0%	1	1.1%	6	20.0%	3	7.5%	2	2.2%
Myopic retinopathy	3	12.5%	2	10.0%	4	4.6%	0	0.0%	10	25.0%	8	8.8%
Total preventable	**4**	**16.7%**	**2**	**10.0%**	**5**	**5.7%**	**6**	**20.0%**	**13**	**32.5%**	**10**	**11.0%**
Cataract surgical complications	2	8.3%	1	5.0%	2	2.3%	0	0.0%	1	2.5%	1	1.1%
Glaucoma	2	8.3%	0	0.0%	1	1.1%	1	3.3%	1	2.5%	0	0.0%
Diabetic retinopathy	0	0.0%	0	0.0%	0	0.0%	0	0.0%	0	0.0%	2	2.2%
Total avoidable	**23**	**95.8%**	**18**	**90.0%**	**80**	**92.0%**	**23**	**76.7%**	**35**	**87.5%**	**78**	**85.7%**
ARMD	0	0.0%	0	0.0%	3	3.4%	0	0.0%	1	2.5%	6	6.6%
Other posterior segment	1	4.2%	1	5.0%	3	3.4%	5	16.7%	4	10.0%	7	7.7%
Globe abnormality/CNS	0	0.0%	1	5.0%	1	1.1%	2	6.7%	0	0.0%	0	0.0%

Table 4. Cataract surgical coverage in Tuoketuo and Shangdu County.

		Tuoketuo			Shangdu		
		Male	Female	Total	Male	Female	Total
Blindness	Persons (%)	57.1%	50.0%	**51.7%**	66.7%	42.9%	**52.2%**
	Eyes (%)	25.6%	31.3%	**29.1%**	43.2%	19.6%	**30.1%**
SVI	Persons (%)	36.4%	44.0%	**41.7%**	54.5%	37.5%	**44.4%**
	Eyes (%)	19.2%	27.0%	**23.8%**	34.0%	15.0%	**23.4%**
MVI	Persons (%)	21.1%	28.9%	**26.3%**	47.4%	22.6%	**32.0%**
	Eyes (%)	11.8%	19.2%	**15.9%**	23.2%	9.4%	**15.2%**

been operated for all blindness, SVI and MVI in the two counties. These indicators showed the backload of cataract in the Counties.

In both counties, approximately half of the cataract operated eyes had good results (VA > 6/18), but over one in five cataract operated eyes had poor visual outcome (**Table 5**). These results were far below the WHO's recommended quality cataract surgical outcome, which recommends the proportion of good outcome (presenting VA) being over 85%, increased to 95% by correction. In both study counties, with pinhole correction, visual outcomes could be slightly improved, mainly in the eyes with IOLs implanted.

Of the poor cataract surgical outcomes, 59.6% in Tuoketuo County were due to surgical complication and over half in Shangdu County were due to sequelae.

Those with VA of less than 6/18 caused by cataract in the better eye were asked the reasons of not being operated (**Table 6**). In Tuoketuo, half responded that they felt no need, and a quarter said they were unaware of treatment was possible. Cost accounted for 12.9% of the barriers to surgery in the County. In Shangdu, 55.6% of the un-operated cataract patients were unaware of treatment possible, and cost was a barrier for 14.8%. A further of 14.8% potential patients were denied treatment by the provider in Shangdu. This was discussed with the local doctors and answers were that because the local surgeons were not confident with the operations and had to wait for visiting surgeons. That would lead to mutual misunderstanding between the doctors and patients. In both counties, fear of surgery was an important barrier to respondents seeking treatment (5.6% and 9.3% respectively in Tuoketuo and Shangdu).

4. Discussion

The rapid assessment of avoidable blindness (RAAB) in Tuoketuo and Shangdu Counties in Inner Mongolia, China, in August and September 2010, documented a lower than expected prevalence of blindness, severe visual impairment and moderate visual impairment. The major cause of blindness and SVI was cataract, and the leading cause of MVI was uncorrected refractive errors in both study areas.

Cataract surgical coverage was low in both Counties, especially when calculated on eyes (compared to respondents) and amongst respondents with SVI and MVI. The cataract surgical outcome rate was well below than that recommended by WHO. These findings should attract much attention to the eye surgical quality control in the study areas, although the results included both recent surgeries and those performed long before current microsurgery was available. Those operated over 10 years before had worse results because of technical and facility limitations.

Eye care public health promotion and health education in these two Counties have the potential to increase access to cataract surgeries by addressing the main barriers to surgery—being unaware of the services available, and not feeling that the surgery is needed. Cost was also one of the major barriers to potential patients in the study counties, although this will become less an issue as the new Chinese rural cooperation medical insurance scheme will cover 75% of the medical cost if the service is provided at County hospital level.

After training by expert (HL), the purpose and methodology of the study were clear to everyone so that the study teams went to the field for data collection without difficulties. The study coordination was conducted by an International Non-government Organization with good eye health survey experiences. The study had also gained great support from local eye care professionals as well as the bureau of health. These all ensured the

Table 5. Cataract surgical outcome in sample with corrections.

	Tuoketuo						Shangdu					
	IOLs eyes		Non IOLs eyes		All eyes		IOLs eyes		Non IOLs eyes		All eyes	
	n	%	n	%	n	%	n	%	n	%	n	%
Available corrected												
Good	12	70.6%	2	15.4%	14	46.7%	13	76.5%	1	12.5%	14	56.0%
Borderline	2	11.8%	3	23.1%	5	16.7%	2	11.8%	3	37.5%	5	20.0%
Poor	3	17.6%	8	61.5%	11	36.7%	2	11.8%	4	50.0%	6	24.0%
Best corrected												
Good	12	70.6%	2	15.4%	14	46.7%	14	82.4%	1	12.5%	15	60.0%
Borderline	3	17.6%	3	23.1%	6	20.0%	1	5.9%	3	37.5%	4	16.0%
Poor	2	11.8%	8	61.5%	10	33.3%	2	11.8%	4	50.0%	6	24.0%

Note: Good result: Can see 6/18, Borderline: Cannot see 6/18, can see 6/60; Poor: Cannot see 6/60.

Table 6. Barriers to cataract surgery, as indicated by persons in sample, with VA < 6/60.

	Tuoketuo				Shangdu			
Barriers	Bilateral		Unilateral		Bilateral		Unilateral	
	n	%	n	%	n	%	n	%
Need not felt	12	57.14%	27	50.00%	1	4.76%	2	3.70%
Fear	0	0.00%	3	5.56%	3	14.29%	5	9.26%
Cost	5	23.81%	7	12.96%	4	19.05%	8	14.81%
Treatment denied by provider	1	4.76%	3	5.56%	1	4.76%	8	14.81%
unaware treatment is possible	2	9.52%	14	25.93%	11	52.38%	30	55.56%
Cannot access treatment	1	4.76%	0	0.00%	0	0.00%	0	0.00%
Local reason	0	0.00%	0	0.00%	1	4.76%	1	1.85%
All barriers	**21**	**100.00%**	**54**	**100.00%**	**21**	**100.00%**	**54**	**100.00%**

quality of the study. Because the study method was for rapid assessment of blindness in the field, time and equipment limited better diagnosis and adequate categorization of posterior causes of visual impairment. Another limitation of this study was that interview on causes of cataract patients not coming for surgeries might not be accurate because of time constraints because of the team moving quickly in the villages.

The survey established the baseline data was generally consistent with some other surveys in China [1] [10] in the recent years. Prevalence of blindness and visual impairment were lower than that of studies conducted many years ago [8] [11]. Prevalence established was lower than the findings from similar study in Yunan Province in 2006 (bilateral blindness prevalence was 3.7% (95% CI: 2.8% - 4.6%) [12]. It was also lower than the study results from most of provinces, but similar to that in Beijing from the China Nine-Province Eye Survey [2] in 2006. The estimates were close to the study results in Jiangxi Province in 2007, which showed prevalence of blindness was from 1.4% to 1.8% in the three study areas [1]. The Beijing Eye Study and Handan Eye study estimated lower prevalence of blindness in people of younger age group [13] [14]. This study findings were consistent of the findings from other similar eye studies in China and had been used for prevention of blindness planning tools in Inner Mongolia.

The RAAB gave robust evidence of blindness, MVI and SVI baseline, the cataract surgical coverage and outcomes, the barriers to cataract services. The information gives the local blindness prevention policy makers and interested INGOs good program intervention references. The whole survey could be done involving local professionals through proper training of the study teams.

5. Conclusion

The rapid assessment of avoidable blindness (RAAB) in Inner Mongolia estimated a comparatively low prevalence of blindness and over 75% of them were avoidable. This indicates eye services capacity including eye care education should be still improved in the study areas. Better planning and targeting should be set from the findings for both government and service suppliers.

Acknowledgements

The authors acknowledge Dr. Junzhen Liu, Dr. Ping Huang, Dr. Jianhua Ding, the nurses and other staff from Tuoketuo and Shangdu County for their contribution to the field data collection, and substantial support in the administration arrangements for the survey.

Funding

The study received full finance support from The Fred Hollows Foundation.

Conflicts of Interest

None of the authors have any proprietary interests or conflicts of interest in relation to this submission.

References

[1]   Xiao, B., Kuper, H., Guan, C.h., Bailey, C. and Limburg, H. (2010) Rapid Assessment of Avoidable Blindness in Three Counties, Jiangxi Province, China. *British Journal of Ophthalmology*, **94**, 1437-1442. http://dx.doi.org/10.1136/bjo.2009.165308

[2]   Zhao, J.L., Ellwein, L.B., *et al.* (2010) Prevalence of Vision Impairment in Older Adults in Rural China, the China Nine-Province Survey. *The American Academy of Ophtalmology*, **117**, 409-416. http://dx.doi.org/10.1016/j.ophtha.2009.11.023

[3]   Pascolini, D. and Mariotti, S.P. (2012) Global Estimates of Visual Impairment: 2010. *The British Journal of Ophthalmology*, **96**, 614-618. http://dx.doi.org/10.1136/bjophthalmol-2011-300539

[4]   World Health Organization (2011) The Fact Sheet No. 282. *Bulletin of the World Health Organization*, April 2011.

[5]   (2010) Program and Policy Implications, Today's Research on Aging. Issue 20.

[6]   http://www.nhfpc.gov.cn/

[7]   Inner Mongolia Year Book 2005.

[8]   Zhang, S.Y., *et al.* (1992) National Epidemiological Survey of Blindness and Low Vision in China. *Chinese Medical Journal*, **105**, 603-608.

[9]   World Health Organization (1988) Coding Instruction for the WHO/PBL Eye Examination Record (Version III), Geneva; WHO. WHO Document, **PBL/88.1**.

[10] Zhao, J., *et al.* (2010) Prevalence and Outcomes of Cataract Surgery in Rural China the China Nine-Province Survey. *Ophthalmology*, **117**, 2120-2128. http://dx.doi.org/10.1016/j.ophtha.2010.03.005

[11] Zhao, J.L., Jia, L.J., Sui, R.F. and Ellwein, L.B. (1998) Prevalence of Blindness and Cataract Surgery in Shunyi County, China. *American Journal of Ophthalmology*, **126**, 506-514. http://dx.doi.org/10.1016/S0002-9394(98)00275-X

[12] Wu, M., Yip, J.L. and Kuper, H. (2008) Rapid Assessment of Avoidable Blindness in Kunming, China. *Ophthalmology*, **115**, 969-974. http://dx.doi.org/10.1016/j.ophtha.2007.08.002

[13] Liang, Y.B., *et al.* (2008) Prevalence and Causes of Low Vision and Blindness in a Rural Chinese Adult Population: The Handan Eye Study. *Ophthalmology*, **115**, 1965-1972. http://dx.doi.org/10.1016/j.ophtha.2008.05.030

[14] Xu, L., *et al.* (2006) Prevalence of Visual Impairment among Adults in China: The Beijing Eye Study. *American Journal of Ophthalmology*, **141**, 591-593. http://dx.doi.org/10.1016/j.ajo.2005.10.018

19

Treatment of Conjunctival Malignant Melanoma with Topical Interferon Alpha-2a

Naser Salihu[1], Belinda Pustina[1], Brigita Drnovšek-Olup[2]

[1]Department of Ophthalmology, University Clinical Center of Kosova, Prishtina, Kosova
[2]Eye Clinic, University Medical Center Ljubljana, Ljubljana, Slovenia
Email: belindapustina@gmail.com

Abstract

Conjunctival malignant melanoma (CMM) is a potentially lethal neoplasm with a high rate of recurrence. The modality of treatment includes a wide surgical excision, cryotherapy, topical mitomycin C and Interferon alpha 2b (INF α 2b). The aim of the study is to present the treatment of a case with CMM using topical Interferon alpha 2a. We present a 38-year-old female with diffuse bulbar dark pigmentation of the conjunctiva that arises from previously primary acquired melanosis (PAM). Biopsy resulted positive for CMM and further investigations were negative for any metastasis. Treatment with topical interferon alpha 2a was started immediately and after three months melanoma disappeared. One year after follow-up there was no sign of recurrence in regional lymph nodes or distant metastasis.

Keywords

Conjunctival Malignant Melanoma, Interferon Alpha 2a

1. Introduction

CMM is a rare but potentially lethal neoplasm with a high rate of recurrence and accounts for about 2% of all ocular malignancies [1]. It usually arises from PAM in 75% of cases and 20% from conjunctival pre-existing nevus or de novo. The modality of treatment includes a wide "no touch" surgical excision with adjuvant double freeze cryotherapy and tumor free margins of 4 mm, cryotherapy or topical chemotherapy with mitomycin C and INF α 2b. The overall mortality is about 12% at 5 years and 25% at 10 years [2] [3].

We report a case of CMM treated with topical interferon alpha 2a.

2. Case Presentation

A 38-year-old lady presented with diffuse bulbar dark pigmentation of the conjunctiva in her right eye. There was no history of any surgical treatment in the eye or otherwise.

Slit-lamp examination showed the dark colored lesion in her right eye that involved complete bulbar conjunctiva in superior and inferior nasal quadrants, perilimbal parts of cornea and caruncula (**Figure 1**).

Other examinations included visual acuity 1.0 (Snellen), intraocular pressure 13.0 mmHg AP, and a normal fundus. US-B scan resulted with no intraocular extension of the mass. The orbit and brain MRI, chest X-ray and an ultrasound of the abdomen and pelvis were normal. All blood examination results were also within normal limits.

No metastases were detected in regional lymph nodes or in distant organs.

Diagnosis was verified by histopathological examination. Immunohistochemistry was positive for HMB 45, Ki 67, CD 68 and AEI/3.

The left eye was normal.

After discussions with the patient, with her consent, we started the treatment with topical INF α-2a, 1 MIU/ml, qid. To our knowledge, this subtype of interferon alpha was never used before in the treatment of CMM. The treatment comprised of three sessions over a month. The changes started disappearing immediately after the first session and completely withdrew after the third (**Figure 2**). We didn't notice any local or systemic side effects during the treatment. The patient will undergo continuous monthly check-ups.

There was no evidence of local recurrence or distant metastasis one year after treatment.

3. Discussion

CMM are relatively rare tumors, but their importance lies in their potential to cause death. Early detection is

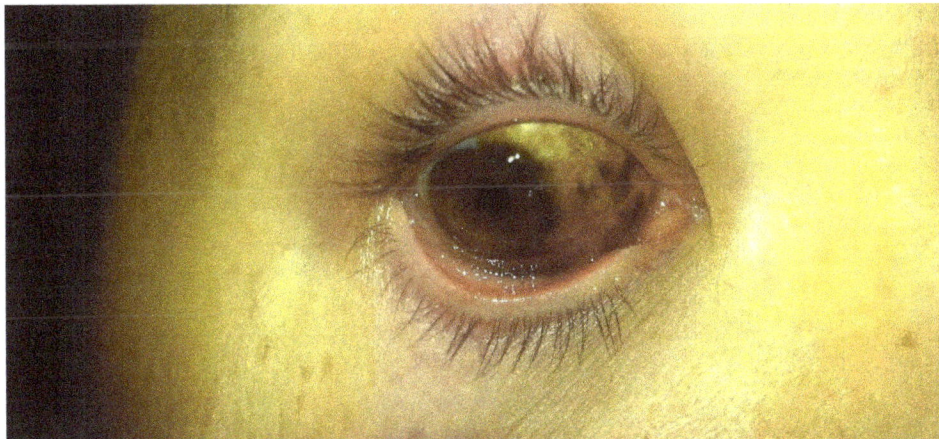

Figure 1. Right eye: pigmented nodules of nasal bulbar conjunctiva, cornea and caruncula.

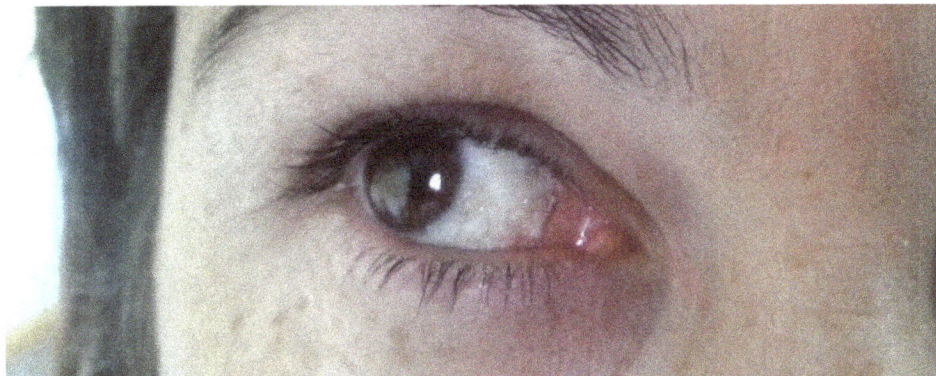

Figure 2. Right eye: after treatment with topical interferon alpha 2a.

very critical in initiating treatment and in preventing a lethal course.

Management of CMM is by surgical excision. Topical treatment has been taken in consideration lately especially in cases with wide conjunctival involvement. One of the topical drugs used in the treatment of CMM is INF [4].

INF is a natural multifunctional protein. Depending on the molecular structure they are classified as alpha, beta or gamma INF.

Antiproliferative activity of human IFN-α is deemed to consist of direct and indirect activities. Direct activity occurs through cancer cell growth inhibition by cell cycle arrest, apoptosis or differentiation. Indirect activity occurs through activation of immune cells such as T cells and natural killer cells, inhibition of vascularization (antiangiogenesis), and induction of cytokines [5].

The treatment of CMM with IFN alpha-2b is known. We have no evidence of someone reporting having used IFN apha-2a. We used INF alpha 2a because it was the only one available in our institution. The topical application of INF α-2a proved to be highly efficacious in our case. No local or systemic side effects were encountered during the treatment. There is no evidence of local recurrence or distant metastasis one year after the treatment. A year is certainly a small period of time to conclude on the efficacy of this treatment in one case. However, we are continuously monitoring the patient regarding long-term effects, the results of which we intend to publish later.

4. Conclusion

Topical INF α-2a, 1 MIU/ml qid for 3 months has been shown to be beneficial in treating CMM. No evidence of recurrence was noticed one year after follow-up. Further studies are required to assess the long-term safety in treating CMM.

References

[1]   Misra, S., Misra, N., Gogri, P., Reddy, V. and Bhandari, A. (2013) A Case of Conjunctival Malignant Melanoma with Local Recurrence. *Australasian Medical Journal*, **6**, 344-347. http://dx.doi.org/10.4066/AMJ.2013.1728

[2]   Shields, C.L., Kels, J.G. and Shields, J.A. (2015) Melanoma of the Eye: Revealing Hidden Secrets, One at a Time. *Clinics in Dermatology*, **33**, 183-196. http://dx.doi.org/10.1016/j.clindermatol.2014.10.010

[3]   Kanski, J.J. and Bowling, B. (2011) Clinical Ophthalmology: A Systematic Approach. 7th Edition, Elsevier Saunders, Edinburgh, 482-483.

[4]   Finger, P.T., Sedeek, R.W. and Chin K.J. (2008) Topical Interferon Alfa in the Treatment of Conjunctival Melanoma and Primary Acquired Melanosis Complex. *American Journal of Ophthalmology*, **145**, 124-129. http://dx.doi.org/10.1016/j.ajo.2007.08.027

[5]   Ningrum, R.A. (2014) Human Interferon Alpha-2b: A Therapeutic Protein for Cancer Treatment. *Scientifica*, **2014**, Article ID: 970315, 8 p.

20

Eye Rubbing as a Possible Cause of Clinical Progressive Keratoconus in a Forme Fruste Keratoconic Family

George D. Kymionis[1,2], Konstantinos I. Tsoulnaras[1*], Stella V. Blazaki[1], Michael A. Grentzelos[1]

[1]Vardinoyiannion Eye Institute of Crete (VEIC), Faculty of Medicine, University of Crete, Heraklion, Crete, Greece
[2]Department of Ophthalmology, Bascom Palmer Eye Institute, University of Miami, Miami, FL, USA
Email: *tsoulnarask@yahoo.gr

Abstract

We report a case of a 21-year-old male patient who underwent corneal cross-linking (CXL) due to bilateral progressive keratoconus. Topographical screening of his family members was performed for the detection of possible familial keratoconus and showed abnormal topographical patterns resembling to Forme Fruste Keratoconus (FFK) in all the members of his family. The reported keratoconic patient that underwent CXL was the only individual of this family that referred eye rubbing in his personal ocular history; ocular and medical history of the other family members was clear. Eye rubbing could be a possible adjuvant risk factor that contributes to conversion of FFK to clinical progressive keratoconus.

Keywords

Eye Rubbing, Family, Forme Fruste, Keratoconus, Topography

1. Introduction

Although keratoconus appears as an independent and isolated disorder, there are many keratoconic cases related with atopy, connective tissue disorders, referred eye rubbing and contact lens intolerance [1]. Despite the fact that etiology of keratoconus is not yet elucidated, inheritance and environmental factors seem to contribute to its pathogenesis [1]. Previous studies have already shown that familial pattern of keratoconus is possible and the in-

---

*Corresponding author.

cidence of familial keratoconus in keratoconic patients is estimated at 6% - 8% [2]. In these cases familial keratoconus inheritance follows the autosomal dominant and/or recessive pattern [2].

Eye rubbing is deemed a significant predictor for keratoconus progression and it is considered abnormal in
connection with frequency, intensity and duration [3]. McMonnies maintained that rubbing could cause thermal
effect to cornea that might increase collagenase activation [3]. It is also supported that rubbing-related mechanical
epithelial trauma is responsible for the release of inflammatory mediators, which contribute to keratoconus pathogenesis [3].

In this case we present a keratoconic patient's family in which all members (including the two parents and their
four children) are affected by Forme Fruste Keratoconus (FFK) documented by Dual-Scheimpflug topography.
Clinical progressive keratoconus was evident in the only family member that reported eye rubbing.

2. Case Report

A 21-year-old male with recently diagnosed bilateral progressive keratoconus referred to our institute with
gradually decreased visual acuity during the last six months. He had never used any spectacles or contact lenses
(CL). Medical history was negative for any keratoconus-associated disease; however he mentioned chronic allergic conjunctivitis and bilateral eye rubbing. Uncorrected distance visual acuity (UDVA) was 20/100 and 10/150
in his right and left eye, respectively. Best spectacle corrected visual acuity (BSCVA) was 20/25 with manifest
refraction of +0.25 − 3.50 × 70° in his right eye not improving with rigid gas permeable (RGP) CL trial, while
BSCVA was 20/40 with manifest refraction of +1.50 − 6.50 × 110° in his left eye improving to 20/25 with RGP CL
trial. Keratometry readings (Galilei dual-Scheimpflug analyzer, Ziemer Ophthalmic Systems AG, Port, Switzer-
land) were 47.79D/44.29D and 52.81D/46.56D in the right and left eyes, respectively. Minimum corneal thickness (MCT) measured by ultrasound pachymetry (Sonogage Corneo Gage Plus, Cleveland, Ohio) was 451 μm
and 429 μm for the right and left eyes, respectively. Slit lamp examination showed no other anterior or posterior
abnormalities. The patient underwent uneventful corneal cross-linking (CXL) [4].

As part of an ongoing research protocol of our institute concerning topographical screening of keratonic patients' families, all of the patient's family members were recruited to undergo slit lamp examination and topographical analysis of their eyes for the detection of FFK [5]. Institutional Review Board approval was obtained
and all members were appropriately informed before their participation in the current study, and they gave written
informed consent in accordance with institutional guidelines, according to the Declaration of Helsinki. Ophthalmological and topographical data of the participants are shown in **Table 1**. Axial curvatures of the family
members are shown in the provided pedigree tree chart (**Figure 1**).

Table 1. Demographical, ophthalmological and topographical data of the family individuals.

*F/M	Age	Eye	†Ks (‡D)	§Kf (D)	‖Pachy (μm)	**I-S (D)	Eye rubbing	Allergy	††A/K class
A1	57	OD	43.75	42.29	472	1.64	-	-	‡‡FFK
		OS	43.04	42.64	474	0.92	-	-	FFK
A2	47	OD	44.40	43.81	513	1.09	-	-	FFK
		OS	44.58	43.61	504	2.21	-	-	FFK
B1	28	OD	45.97	44.81	465	2.85	-	-	FFK
		OS	46.29	44.28	470	2.69	-	-	FFK
B2	26	OD	42.63	42.09	485	3.33	-	-	FFK
		OS	44.75	43.04	483	2.59	-	-	FFK
B3	23	OD	44.71	43.38	474	1.08	-	-	FFK
		OS	43.95	43.45	466	2.06	-	-	FFK
B4	21	OD	47.79	44.29	451	10.40	+	-	1
		OS	52.81	46.56	429	15.67	+	-	2

*F/M = Family member; †Ks = Steep keratometric values; ‡D = diopters; §Kf = Flat keratometric values; ‖Pachy = Thinnest corneal pachymetry; **I-S
index = Inferior-Superior keratometric index; ††A/K class = Amsler-Krumeich classification stage; ‡‡FFK = Forme Fruste Keratoconus; OD = right
eye; OS = left eye.

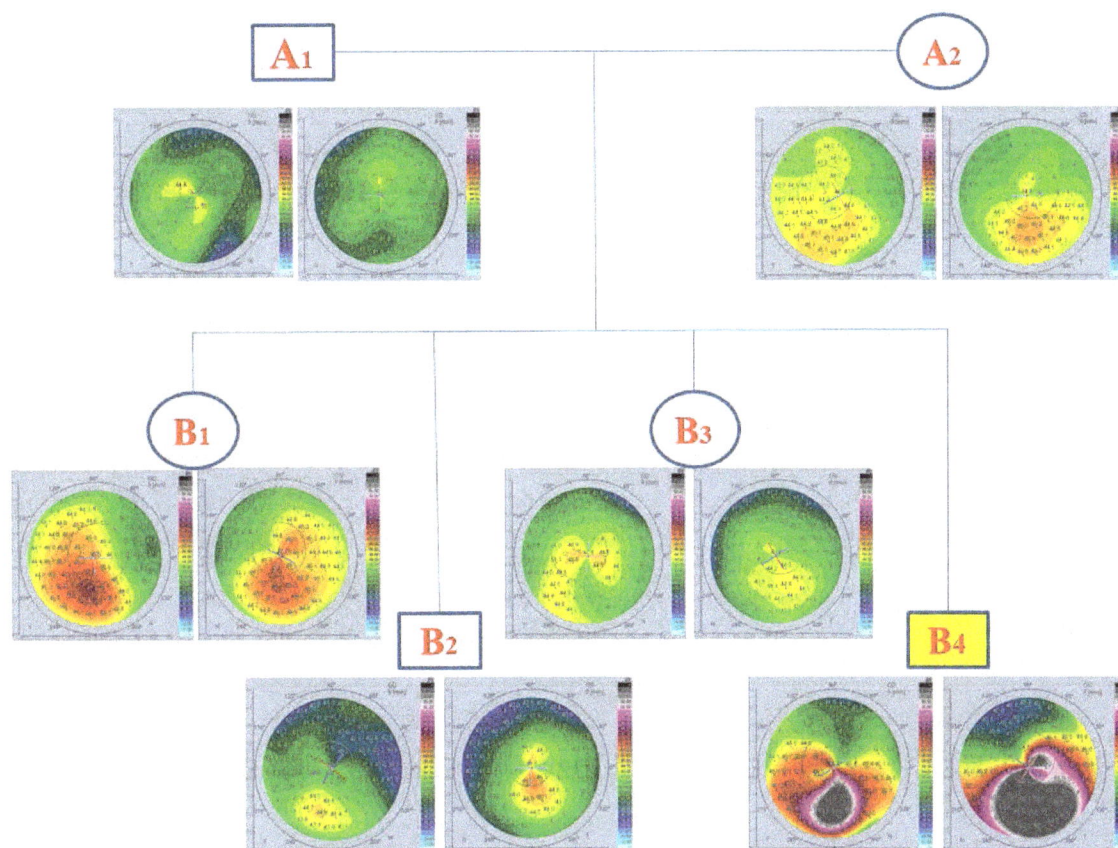

Figure 1. Pedigree tree chart of the keratoconic family; topographical axial curvatures are displayed below every family member. The highlighted B4 individual represents the CXL treated keratoconic patient.

Demographic and topographical data of the participants were collected in an Excel spreadsheet (Microsoft, Redmond, WA). SPSS software for Windows version 18.0 (SPSS, Inc, Chicago, IL) was used for statistical analysis of the results.

All family members' eyes were categorized as FFK, apart from the treated with CXL keratoconic patient; his right and left eye was classified with the Amsler-Krumeich classification as stage 1 and 2 respectively [6]. Mean age of family members was 33.67 ± 13.46. All members' eyes had clear cornea, with no clinical signs or symptoms of keratoconus. Slit lamp showed no sign of atopic disease (e.g. chronic allergic conjunctivitis) in all family members. None of the family members used any spectacles or contact lenses; none of them was aware of their possible refractive error. Past ocular history was negative for any ocular disease or previous ocular surgery in all family members; medical history was negative for any systemic disease possibly correlated with keratoconus (e.g. collagen tissue disorders and atopy). The keratoconic patient that underwent CXL was the only member of the family that reported chronic allergic conjunctivitis and eye rubbing in both eyes.

All eyes included in our case had abnormal topographic patterns. One eye had central-superior steepening, four eyes had inferior steepening and seven eyes had asymmetric bowtie with skewed radial axes and inferior steepening. Mean steep and flat keratometry values were 45.39D ± 2.74D and 43.69D ± 1.22D, respectively. Mean thinnest corneal pachymetry was 473.83 μm ± 22.04 μm. Mean Inferior-Superior asymmetric index was 3.88D ± 4.49D.

3. Discussion

There are many studies in the literature analyzing familial keratoconus [7]. Most of the currently published studies were performed for the detection of keratoconus genetic background [7]. Although genetic familial pattern of keratoconus has not been established yet, other environmental triggering factors (e.g. eye rubbing and atopy) have been also correlated with keratoconus development and progression [8].

FFK is characterized as subclinical form of keratoconus, which does not reveal any symptoms and remains unnoticed since corneal topography is undertaken (including asymmetric bowtie with a skewed radial axis) [6]. Visual acuity of 20/20 is also achievable with spectacle correction and there is absence of characteristic kerato-conic clinical signs while performing slit-lamp examination and corneal pachymetry [6]. According to kerato-conus classification based on disease evolution, it should be referred that FFK is a different condition from the early form of keratoconus in which corneal thinning is in progress while cornea scarring is not yet detectable [6].

In our case we present a keratoconic patient's family that all of its members diagnosed with FFK. The CXL-treated patient was the only member of this family that reported eye rubbing.

All family members had bilateral keratoconus according to the topographic findings, while mean thinnest corneal pachymetry was 473.83 ± 22.04 μm; therefore this family represents a model of familial FFK. The inheritance pattern of this family seems to be apparent dominant due to the fact that all the family members have diagnosed with a form of keratoconus. The unawareness of these family members about keratoconus disease and their refractive error strengthens the argument that there are many undetected individuals or even family members in the general population that will potentially develop keratoconus.

Rabinowitz reported that keratoconus prevalence is 0.1% and more than 6% in general population and relatives of keratoconic patients, respectively [1]. Considering that nowadays FFK is mainly detected in possible refractive candidates, it could be supposed that more individuals would have been ideally detected when general population was screened by corneal topography. Concerning the keratoconic patients' relatives, it is clarified that this subgroup of population should be topographically screened for the early detection and follow up of these undiagnosed keratoconic cases. Potential keratoconus progression could be managed by stabilization of their corneas with CXL treatment.

4. Conclusion

In conclusion, this is the first report of identification of a keratoconic patient's family that all of its members were diagnosed with FFK. Eye rubbing may converse FFK to clinical keratoconus.

Conflict of Interest

None of the authors has conflict of interest with the submission.

Funding

No financial support was received for the submission.

References

[1] Rabinowitz, Y.S. (1998) Keratoconus. *Survey of Ophthalmology*, **42**, 297-319. http://dx.doi.org/10.1016/S0039-6257(97)00119-7

[2] Steele, T.M., Fabinyi, D.C., Couper, T.A. and Loughnan, M.S. (2008) Prevalence of Orbscan II Corneal Abnormalities in Relatives of Patients with Keratoconus. *Clinical Experimental Ophthalmology*, **36**, 824-830. http://dx.doi.org/10.1111/j.1442-9071.2009.01908.x

[3] McMonnies, C.W. (2009) Mechanisms of Rubbing-Related Corneal Trauma in Keratoconus. *Cornea*, **28**, 607-6015. http://dx.doi.org/10.1097/ICO.0b013e318198384f

[4] Wollensak, G., Spoerl, E. and Seiler, T. (2003) Riboflavin/Ultraviolet-A-Induced Collagen Crosslinking for the Treatment of Keratoconus. *American Journal of Ophthalmology*, **135**, 620-627. http://dx.doi.org/10.1016/S0002-9394(02)02220-1

[5] Saad, A. and Gatinel, D. (2010) Topographic and Tomographic Properties of Forme Fruste Keratoconus Corneas. *Investigative Ophthalmology & Visual Science*, **51**, 5546-5555. http://dx.doi.org/10.1167/iovs.10-5369

[6] Amsler, M. (1946) KeratoconeClassiqueetKeratoconeFruste, Arguments Unitaires.Ophtalmologica. **111**, 96-101. http://dx.doi.org/10.1159/000300309

[7] Nielsen, K., Hjortdal, J., Pihlmann, M. and Corydon, T.J. (2013) Update on the Keratoconus Genetics. *Acta Ophthalmologica*, **291**, 106-113. http://dx.doi.org/10.1111/j.1755-3768.2012.02400.x

[8] Balasubramanian, S.A., Pye, D.C. and Willcox, M.D. (2013) Effects of Eye Rubbing on the Levelsof Protease, Protease Activity and Cytokines in Tears: Relevance in Keratoconus. *Clinical and Experimental Optometry*, **96**, 214-218. http://dx.doi.org/10.1111/cxo.12038

21

The Effect of Intraocular Pressure Lowering Medications on the Pressure Spike Associated with Intravitreal Injection

Olya Pokrovskaya[1]*, Ian Dooley[2], Salma Babiker[2], Catherine Croghan[2], Claire Hartnett[2], Anthony Cullinane[2]

[1]Department of Ophthalmology, Mater Misericordiae University Hospital, Dublin, Ireland
[2]Department of Ophthalmology, Cork University Hospital, Cork, Ireland
Email: *olya.pokrovskaya@gmail.com

Abstract

Aim: This study investigates whether the post intravitreal injection intraocular pressure (IOP) spike is modifiable with the use of prophylactic apraclonidine and dorzolomide. Methods: The study design was a prospective, randomised controlled trial. 80 eyes undergoing intravitreal injection of anti-VEGF agent were studied. A control group (n = 42) received no IOP lowering drops, and a study group (n = 38) received guttae apraclonidine and dorzolamide 30 to 40 minutes before the intravitreal injection. IOP measurements were taken in both groups using the Perkins tonometer at baseline, immediately before and after the injection, 5 minutes post-injection, and 15 minutes post-injection. Results: Mean IOP immediately post injection in the study group was 26.71 mmHg, and in the control group was 32.73. The main outcome measure was the area under the curve (AUC)—reflecting the trend of IOP post injection. The AUC was lower in the study group compared to the control group (Mann-Whitney U test, p = 0.046). Conclusions: The use of prophylactic apraclonidine and dorzolamide is effective in modifying the post-injection IOP spike. IOP lowering prophylaxis may be considered in patients with a high baseline IOP.

Keywords

Intraocular Pressure, Intravitreal Injection, Ranibizumab, Apraclonidine, Dorzolamide

---

1. Introduction

The most exciting and innovative advance in ophthalmology in recent years is the introduction of intravitreal in-

---

*Corresponding author.

jection of anti-VEGF drugs. These drugs have been shown to be sight-saving in a variety of retinal pathologies, including wet age-related macular degeneration and diabetic macular oedema [1]-[3]. One of the established side-effects of intravitreal injection is a temporary rise in the intraocular pressure (IOP) [4]-[6]. This has been attributed to volume expansion; however the exact mechanism remains unclear [7] [8]. Even a short-lived spike in the IOP can have potentially devastating consequences on an eye which is already compromised in terms of its vasculature. The Royal College of Ophthalmologists recommends routinely checking that the patient can see objects immediately after the injection, to ensure that the central retinal artery is patent (http://www.rcophth.ac.uk). Routine IOP measurement before and after injection is generally not necessary, however it should be considered in certain patients at risk of having a high IOP [9].

Several authors have addressed the issue of prophylaxis in reducing the post-injection IOP spike. Frenkel *et al.* carried out a retrospective study of 71 patients, which did not show any significant benefit of pressure-lowering medications [10]. El Chehab prospectively evaluated different regimens in 210 patients, and showed a significant reduction in the pressure spike with several topical medications but not with oral acetazolamide [11]. Theoulakis had a series of 88 patients and found a reduction of the pressure spike after the use of brimonidine/timolol [12]. To date, no prophylactic regimen has been established to be clearly effective and beneficial in patients undergoing intravitreal injection. Indeed, the question remains whether it is at all advantageous to use prophylactic pressure lowering medications prior to intravitreal injections, and if so, in which patients. The objective of our study is to determine whether the IOP spike is modifiable by the prophylactic use of the combination of dorzolamide and apraclonidine 1%. Both of these drugs are readily available in single dose units, which have useful infection control advantages.

2. Materials and Methods

A prospective, randomised controlled trial was performed between October 2011 and April 2012 in a single treatment centre. Ethical approval was obtained from the Clinical Research Ethics Committee of the Cork Teaching Hospitals.

80 consecutive patients due to undergo intravitreal injection of ranibizumab (0.5 mg/0.05ml) for a variety of retinal pathologies were included in the study. We selected patients based on specific inclusion and exclusion criteria. Inclusion criteria were patients aged 18 and over presenting for intravitreal anti-VEGF injections for the treatment of wet AMD, diabetic macular oedema, or macular oedema secondary to retinal vein occlusion. Exclusion criteria included a history of ocular hypertension or glaucoma, and intravitreal injection of agents other than ranibizumab. One eye only was included per patient. Written informed consent was obtained from all patients included in the study.

A random number generator assigned patients to either study or control group before the injection. The control group received no IOP lowering medications. The study group received guttae apraclonidine 1% (Iopidine, Alcon) and dorzolamide 2.0% (Trusopt, MSD) 30 to 40 minutes before the injection. IOP measurements were taken with the Perkins tonometer (Clement Clarke, Essex, United Kingdom) at baseline before the administration of drops (T-0). Subsequent measurements were 1 minute before injection (T-1), 2 minutes after injection (T-2), 5 minutes after injection (T-3), and 15 minutes after injection (T-4). To minimise inter-observer error, the same physician carried out all measurements for a given patient, (there were 4 such physicians over the 6 month period of data collection). Physicians were not blinded to the group of the patient. The IOP measurement technique and endpoint were clearly defined and standardised for all physicians involved prior to data collection. Identical injection technique of 0.05 ml of ranibizumab was used across all cases. A sterile cotton tip was applied to the injection site to prevent subconjuctival reflux. In between IOP measurements, the tonometer was made aseptic using alcohol swabs, and then dried using sterile gauze. Guttae chloramphenicol was administered after each IOP measurement.

The main outcome measure was the area under the curve (AUC) with respect to ground. This method is useful for detecting possible associations between repeated measures and other variables, over several time points [13]. We calculated this using a formula derived from the trapezoid formula [13].

$$AUC = \sum_{i=1}^{n-1} \frac{\left(m_{(i+1)} + m_i\right) \cdot t_i}{2}$$

AUC is area under the curve with respect to ground. m_i represents the mean IOP values for study and control groups from immediately before the injection (T-1) to 15 minutes after the injection (T-4). t_i denotes the individual time intervals between measurements. n is the total amount of measures.

Statistical analysis was carried out using SPSS version 18. Data was tested for normality using the Shapiro-Wilk test and the appropriate statistical tests used to compare means (Independent samples t test for parametric data, and Mann-Whitney U test for non-parametric data). A p value less than 0.05 was considered statistically significant.

3. Results

The study and control groups did not differ significantly in terms of baseline IOP, with a mean (±standard deviation) of 14.17 ± 3.82 mmHg in the study group, and 13.88 ± 3.83 mmHg in the control group (p = 0.77). The mean age was 72 years in the study group, and 71 years in the control group.

Thirty to forty minutes post administration of IOP lowering prophylaxis to the study group, these patients showed a mean IOP drop of 4.09 mmHg (**Figure 1**, **Table 1**). Immediately pre-injection the study group had a

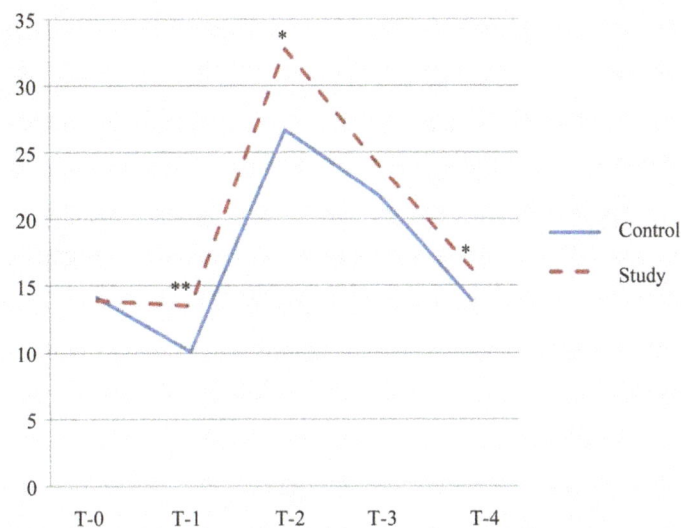

Figure 1. This figure illustrates the trend of IOP (intraocular pressure) over time in the study and control groups. The time intervals are baseline (T-0), immediately before the injection (T-1), immediately after the injection (T-2), 5 minutes after the injection (T-3), and 15 minutes after the injection (T-5). The IOP was significantly lower in the study group compared to the control group at T-1 (p < 0.01), at T-2 (p < 0.05) and at T-4 (p < 0.06); *p < 0.05; **p < 0.01.

Table 1. Mean IOP (mmHg) and difference between study and control groups.

Interval	Mean IOP (mmHg) ± SD		Mean Difference Between Groups (95% CI)	p Value*
	Study group	Control group		
T-0	14.17 ± 3.82	13.88 ± 3.83	0.29 (−1.68 to 2.27)	0.769
T-1	10.08 ± 3.61	13.53 ± 3.66	-3.44 (−5.32 to −1.56)	0.001
T-2	26.71 ± 10.36	32.73 ± 9.79	-6.02 (−11.29 to −0.74)	0.026
T-3	21.75 ± 8.42	24.95 ± 8.06	-2.30 (−6.61 to 2.01)	0.288
T-4	13.92 ± 3.35	16.20 ± 5.76	-2.28 (−4.56 to −0.01)	0.049

Table 1. This table summarises the mean IOP (intraocular pressure) in study and control groups at various time intervals—at baseline (T-0), immediately before the injection (T-1), immediately after the injection (T-2), 5 minutes after the injection (T-3), and 15 minutes after the injection (T-4). The groups are compared and significance levels shown. CI = Confidence interval; SD = Standard deviation; *Study versus control group, independent t test.

significantly different mean IOP of 10.08 mmHg, compared to the control group's mean IOP of 13.53 mmHg, with a *p* value of <0.001 (Independent samples t test).

The mean IOP immediately post injection in the study group was 26.71 mmHg, and in the control group it was 32.73. Using the mean values for study and control groups at T-1 to T-4 we constructed a curve and calculated the AUC. The values for AUC were not normally distributed (Shapiro-Wilke, p = 0.053), so we used non-parametric tests to compare the study and control groups (Mann-Whitney U test). The study group had a lower AUC than the control group (Mann-Whitney U test, p = 0.046).

A significant positive correlation was found between T-1 (IOP immediately pre-injection) and the AUC—Kendel's tau: r = 0.268; p < 0.001. Data on axial length was available for 15 patients. No significant correlation emerged between the IOP spike and the axial length (Pearson's correlation: r = −0.001; p = 0.997).

In both study and control groups, the IOP showed rapid normalisation post-injection. 79 of 80 eyes had an IOP of less than 30 mmHg within 15 minutes post injection. The patient who didn't was in the control group and achieved an IOP of 28 mmHg twenty minutes following injection.

4. Discussion

Acutely raised IOP in an eye which already has compromised vasculature is one of the most hazardous complications of intravitreal injection. Prophylactic IOP lowering medications are effective in preventing IOP spikes following procedures such as ALT-trabeculoplasty and nd:YAG laser capsulotomy [14]-[16]. To our knowledge, this is the first prospective, randomised controlled trial investigating the effect of dorzolamide and apraclonidine on the post intravitreal injection IOP spike.

In our study we used a single regimen—the combination of dorzolamide and apraclonidine. These agents are available in single-dose formulation and hence are a cost-effective method of reducing intraocular pressure when only a single administration is required in each patient. It is interesting to note the extent of IOP reduction recorded in our study with this combination, just 30 minutes after administration. The IOP was reduced from 14.17 mmHg to 10.08 mmHg—approximately a 28% reduction. Such a pronounced reduction in IOP at just 30 minutes is greater than previously expected. Perhaps this phenomenon was due to the concurrent administration of local anaesthetic drops and their effect on corneal permeability, however no firm evidence for this was found in the literature.

Our study suggests that a lower starting IOP pre-injection is associated with lower pressure following the injection. We excluded glaucoma and ocular hypertension patients from our study, as this would confound our results. Erratic diurnal IOP fluctuation is more common in eyes with glaucoma and ocular hypertension than in a healthy eye, and hence the IOP may be more likely to reach a higher peak post intravitreal injection [17]. To the patients included in our study, prophylaxis has little clinical advantage—data showed that in both study and control groups the IOP spike was transient, with the vast majority of patients returning to a pressure of less than 25 mmHg within 15 minutes post-injection. This finding is similar to that of other authors—El Chehab, Falkenstein, and several other authors all found the IOP spike to be short lived [4] [11] [18] [19]. Consistent with this, is our finding that the difference in IOP between study and control groups seemed less at 5 minutes and 15 minutes post injection, as oppose to immediately before and after injection. El Chehab and colleagues reported similar findings [11]. This may be due to the fact that IOP normalises rapidly post the immediate pressure spike. Within a few minutes of the injection, the difference between normal and control group IOP is less, as the IOP in both groups is rapidly returning to normal.

It is interesting that the post injection IOP spike was higher in Frenkel *et al*'s study than in our present study. This discrepancy may be partially explained by the high number of glaucoma patients included in Frenkel's study (36.6% in the pegaptanib group, 33.3% in the ranibizumab group, and 21.2% in the bevacizumab group). Furthermore, the volume of injection of pegaptanib is 0.09 ml, almost double the standard injection volume of ranibizumab and bevacizumab (0.05 ml) used both by Frenkel *et al*. and ourselves, so it is not surprising that the pegaptanib group had generally higher IOP spikes than the other two groups.

Why the post-injection IOP spike is much greater in some patients than others, is uncertain. Possible factors which influence the magnitude of the post-injection IOP spike include pre-existing glaucoma (excluded from this study), axial length, age, and reflux of synergetic vitreous/drug.

We postulated that the magnitude of the IOP spike post-injection may be related to the axial length, since the injection of 0.05 ml into a smaller, hyperopic eye would represent a greater proportion of the total ocular volume than in a larger emmetropic or myopic eye. Data on axial length was only available on 15 of our 80 participants, and did not show a significant correlation between magnitude of IOP spike and axial length. The phakic status of patients is also an interesting consideration—since during intravitreal injection in phakic patients the lens-iris diaphragm may shift forward and reduce aqueous outflow. El Chehab recorded the axial length and phakic status of patients, and did not find a significant correlation between the IOP spike and either of these variables [11].

We also considered the role of age as a confounding factor. Previous literature reports a positive correlation between ocular rigidity and age [20]. It is reasonable to suppose that older eyes may have less ocular compliance, and hence respond with a greater IOP spike to ocular volume increase. Interestingly, our data showed no such correlation.

Our trial's strengths and advantages lie largely in its prospective nature. Consistent technique is used for all injections and IOP measurements, lending reliability to the findings. Limitations include that greater patient numbers are needed to more accurately determine the possible factors leading to adverse IOP spikes. This was not a double-blind study, which allows for potential bias in the results. The study is subject to selection bias, and to measurement error and bias, as physicians were not blind to the status of the patient (study or control group). Our trial demonstrates the effect of relatively mild IOP prophylaxis, and we would be interested to see whether a greater effect on the IOP spike would be possible with other regimens.

Our study adds evidence that prophylaxis is unnecessary in those without glaucoma or ocular hypertension who are undergoing intravitreal injection of 0.05 ml. Given current evidence that the patients with glaucoma may have greater IOP fluctuations than those without glaucoma, and that the optic nerves of glaucomatous eyes are sensitive to these IOP fluctuation [17] [21]-[23], future studies should focus specifically on the magnitude, duration, modifiability and potential deleterious effects of the post-injection spike in glaucomatous eyes. A future trial could also examine the rate of visual field progression in patients with glaucoma who are also receiving serial intravitreal injections, versus those who are not.

5. Conclusion

Our study demonstrates that topical dorzolamide and apraclonidine can indeed modify the IOP spike associated with intravitreal injection. Clinicians may use this evidence when considering IOP lowering prophylaxis in patients with high baseline IOP or compromised vasculature.

Acknowledgements

Dr. Jean Saunders, consultant biostatistician, University of Limerick, Ireland.

References

[1]   Bloch, S.B., Larsen, M. and Munch, I.C. (2012) Incidence of Legal Blindness from Age-Related Macular Degeneration in Denmark: Year 2000 to 2010. *American Journal of Ophthalmology*, **153**, 209-213, e202.

[2]   Bressler, N.M., Doan, Q.V., Varma, R., *et al.* (2011) Estimated Cases of Legal Blindness and Visual Impairment Avoided Using Ranibizumab for Choroidal Neovascularization: Non-Hispanic White Population in the United States with Age-Related Macular Degeneration. *Archives of Ophthalmology*, **129**, 709-717.
http://dx.doi.org/10.1001/archophthalmol.2011.140

[3]   Skaat, A., Chetrit, A., Belkin, M., *et al.* (2012) Time Trends in the Incidence and Causes of Blindness in Israel. *American Journal of Ophthalmology*, **153**, 214-221, e211.

[4]   Falkenstein, I.A, Cheng, L. and Freeman, W.R. (2007) Changes of Intraocular Pressure after Intravitreal Injection of Bevacizumab (Avastin). *Retina*, **27**, 1044-1047. http://dx.doi.org/10.1097/IAE.0b013e3180592ba6

[5]   Wu, L. and Evans, T. (2010) [Immediate Changes in Intraocular Pressure after an Intravitreal Injection of 2.5 mg of Bevacizumab]. *Archivos de la Sociedad Espanola de Oftalmologia*, **85**, 364-369.
http://dx.doi.org/10.1016/j.oftal.2010.09.010

[6]   Sharei, V., Hohn, F., Kohler, T., *et al.* (2010) Course of Intraocular Pressure after Intravitreal Injection of 0.05 mL Ranibizumab (Lucentis). *European Journal of Ophthalmology*, **20**, 174-179.

[7]   Hariprasad, S.M., Shah, G.K. and Blinder, K.J. (2006) Short-Term Intraocular Pressure Trends Following Intravitreal Pegaptanib (Macugen) Injection. *American Journal of Ophthalmology*, **141**, 200-201.
http://dx.doi.org/10.1016/j.ajo.2005.07.053

[8]   Rosenfeld, P.J., Brown, D.M., Heier, J.S., *et al.* (2006) Ranibizumab for Neovascular Age-Related Macular Degenera-

tion. *The New England Journal of Medicine*, **355**, 1419-1431. http://dx.doi.org/10.1056/NEJMoa054481

[9] Aiello, L.P., Brucker, A.J., Chang, S., *et al.* (2004) Evolving Guidelines for Intravitreous Injections. *Retina*, **24**, S3-S19. http://dx.doi.org/10.1097/00006982-200410001-00002

[10] Frenkel, M.P., Haji, S.A. and Frenkel, R.E. (2010) Effect of Prophylactic Intraocular Pressure-Lowering Medication on Intraocular Pressure Spikes after Intravitreal Injections. *Archives of Ophthalmology*, **128**, 1523-1527. http://dx.doi.org/10.1001/archophthalmol.2010.297

[11] El Chehab, H., Le Corre, A., Agard, E., *et al.* (2012) Effect of Topical Pressure-Lowering Medication on Prevention of Intraocular Pressure Spikes after Intravitreal Injection. *European Journal of Ophthalmology*, **23**.

[12] Theoulakis, P.E., Lepidas, J., Petropoulos, I.K., *et al.* (2010) Effect of Brimonidine/Timolol Fixed Combination on Preventing the Short-Term Intraocular Pressure Increase after Intravitreal Injection of Ranibizumab. *Klinische Monatsblatter fur Augenheilkunde*, **227**, 280-284. http://dx.doi.org/10.1055/s-0029-1245201

[13] Pruessner, J.C., Kirschbaum, C., Meinlschmid, G., *et al.* (2003) Two Formulas for Computation of the Area under the Curve Represent Measures of Total Hormone Concentration versus Time-Dependent Change. *Psychoneuroendocrinology*, **28**, 916-931. http://dx.doi.org/10.1016/S0306-4530(02)00108-7

[14] Robin, A.L., Pollack, I.P., House, B., *et al.* (1987) Effects of ALO 2145 on Intraocular Pressure Following Argon Laser Trabeculoplasty. *Archives of Ophthalmology*, **105**, 646-650. http://dx.doi.org/10.1001/archopht.1987.01060050064039

[15] Barnes, S.D., Campagna, J.A., Dirks, M.S., *et al.* (1999) Control of Intraocular Pressure Elevations after Argon Laser Trabeculoplasty: Comparison of Brimonidine 0.2% to Apraclonidine 1.0%. *Ophthalmology*, **106**, 2033-2037. http://dx.doi.org/10.1016/S0161-6420(99)90420-7

[16] Ladas, I.D., Baltatzis, S., Panagiotidis, D., *et al.* (1997) Topical 2.0% Dorzolamide vs oral Acetazolamide for Prevention of Intraocular Pressure Rise after Neodymium:YAG Laser Posterior Capsulotomy. *Archives of Ophthalmology*, **115**, 1241-1244. http://dx.doi.org/10.1001/archopht.1997.01100160411003

[17] Wilensky, J.T., Gieser, D.K., Dietsche, M.L., *et al.* (1993) Individual Variability in the Diurnal Intraocular Pressure Curve. *Ophthalmology*, **100**, 940-944. http://dx.doi.org/10.1016/S0161-6420(93)31551-4

[18] Kim, J.E., Mantravadi, A.V., Hur, E.Y., *et al.* (2008) Short-Term Intraocular Pressure Changes Immediately after Intravitreal Injections of Anti-Vascular Endothelial Growth Factor Agents. *American Journal of Ophthalmology*, **146**, 930-934, e931.

[19] Hollands, H., Wong, J., Bruen, R., *et al.* (2007) Short-Term Intraocular Pressure Changes after Intravitreal Injection of Bevacizumab. *Canadian Journal of Ophthalmology*, **42**, 807-811. http://dx.doi.org/10.3129/i07-172

[20] Pallikaris, I.G., Kymionis, G.D., Ginis, H.S., *et al.* (2005) Ocular Rigidity in Living Human Eyes. *Investigative Ophthalmology & Visual Science*, **46**, 409-414. http://dx.doi.org/10.1167/iovs.04-0162

[21] Detry-Morel, M. (2008) Currents on Target Intraocular Pressure and Intraocular Pressure Fluctuations in Glaucoma Management. *Bulletin de la Societe belge d'ophtalmologie*, 35-43.

[22] Realini, T., Barber, L. and Burton, D. (2002) Frequency of Asymmetric Intraocular Pressure Fluctuations among Patients with and without Glaucoma. *Ophthalmology*, **109**, 1367-1371. http://dx.doi.org/10.1016/S0161-6420(02)01073-4

[23] Zeimer, R.C., Wilensky, J.T., Gieser, D.K., *et al.* (1991) Association between Intraocular Pressure Peaks and Progression of Visual Field Loss. *Ophthalmology*, **98**, 64-69. http://dx.doi.org/10.1016/S0161-6420(91)32340-6

22

Managing Macular Holes in a Developing Economy

Bassey Fiebai, Chinyere N. Pedro-Egbe

Department of Ophthalmology, University of Port Harcourt Teaching Hospital,
Port Harcourt, Nigeria
Email: bassief@yahoo.com

Abstract

Background: Macular holes are the common cause of visual impairment especially in the elderly and have a variety of etiological factors. The advances in the management of macular holes are encouraging and are now available in developing countries although scarce, where hitherto; patients seek attention outside their country. The need to understand this disease has therefore become pertinent in all retina clinics. Objective: To evaluate the pattern of presentation of macular holes and its management in a retina clinic in South South Nigeria. Methods: A 5 year retrospective, non comparative review of 24 consecutive cases presenting to a retinal clinic was carried out. Relevant information was extracted from the medical records and analyzed. Results: Three hundred and sixty four cases were seen between January 2009 and December 2013. Twenty four cases had macular holes and ten (41.7%) had bilateral presentation with a total of 34 eyes. The incidence of macular holes was 6.6%. The mean age was 46 years (SD ± 13.42) with a female preponderance, 5:1. Idiopathic holes formed the bulk of the cases 14(58.3%); others were trauma 4(16.7%), posterior uveitis 2, (8.3%), chemotherapy 2 (8.3%), Solar retinopathy and retinitis pigmentosa 1 (4.2%). Nineteen (55.9%) of the 34 eyes were visually impaired (BCVA <6/18). Nineteen eyes had full thickness holes (55.9%) requiring surgery, however only 3(12.5%) of these could afford to have surgery with one reoperation. Four patients (16.7%) had complications in form of retinal detachments at presentation. Conclusion: This study has shown that the incidence of macular holes in the developing world is significant and resources to manage these cases are grossly lacking. Specialist training, with government subsidizing costs will alleviate these difficulties and reduce visual loss from macular holes.

Keywords

Developing Economy, Macula Hole, Pattern, Management

1. Introduction

Macular holes are full thickness openings of the neurosensory retina in the centre of the fovea from the internal limiting membrane to the outer segment of the photoreceptor layer [1]. Since the fovea is replete with cones, this defect subsequently leads to a drop in central vision and metarmorphopsia [1] [2].

Even though macula holes were originally described by Knapp in relation to trauma [3], it is commoner to find them now in non traumatic settings [2]-[4]. Kunt was the first to describe non traumatic macular holes and this was buttressed by other studies showing that majority of macular holes are idiopathic, occurring in eyes with no previous pathology [4] [5].

Trauma related macular holes are believed to result from a transmission of concussive form in a contrecoup manner, while idiopathic holes are believed to result from focal shrinkage of the prefoveal cortical vitreous, with persistent adherence of the vitreous to the fovealregion [5] [6]. Other etiological factors that have been shown to cause macular holes include myopia, trauma, and solar retinopathy [1]. Macular holes have also been reported and presumed to be secondary to other conditions such as accidental laser burns, retinitis pigmentosa, complications of chemotherapy, posterior uveitis and branch retinal vein occlusion [7]-[11]. By and large, the pathogenesis is still incompletely understood and is believed to be an interplay between vitreomacular traction and some form of degenerative dissolution of inner retinal layers in the fovea [12].

The diagnosis and management of this condition have become more encouraging with the use of Optical coherence tomography (OCT) and the clinical staging of the disease by Gass. OCT affords the ophthalmologist a high resolution cross sectional examination of the macular and provides information concerning diagnosis, classification and aetiology of macular holes. The revolution in the management of macular hole with vitrectomy, cortical vitreous peeling by Kelly and Wendel, resulting in a good anatomical outcome, fovealreappositioning and a subsequent improvement in visual outcome further piqued the interest of retinal specialists globally and in the developing world [13].

Even though the excitement of ophthalmologists in developing countries towards these milestones is short lived, as these equipments are not readily available coupled with lack of the requisite expertise, the need to understand this disease entity, its pattern of presentation, diagnosis, management and prognosis has become pertinent in all retinal clinics as macular hole surgery is now available in Nigeria,

2. Materials and Methods

This study was a 5 year retrospective non comparative review of the medical records of 24 consecutive patients who presented to the retina clinic of the eye department of University of Port Harcourt Teaching Hospital between January 2009-December 2013. Data extracted included demographic data such as age and sex; others were best corrected visual acuity on presentation (BCVA) and other relevant clinical information. The diagnosis of a macula hole was made based on the history of the known risk factors and clinical findings of a macular lesion with biomicrsoscopy. Staging of the macular hole was done according to the Gass classification. Stage 1 was a macular cyst, stage 2; early full thickness macular hole, stage 3; fully developed macular hole with posterior vitreous attachment and stage 4; fully developed macular hole with complete vitreous separation. Fundal examinations were carried out with 90D stereoscopic lens, and a mydriatic fundus photograph. Optical coherence tomography (Stratus OCT, Carl Zeiss Meditec Inc., USA) was used to confirm the diagnosis, classification and complications of macular hole.

Information from each subject was entered into a spreadsheet using the Statistical Package for Social Sciences (SPSS) 11.0 for Windows statistical software and analysed. Bivariate analysis involved the use of chi-square test and Fisher exact test for testing the significance of associations between categorical variables. P values of 0.05 and below were considered statistically significant.

3. Results

A total of 24 subjects comprising 20 females and 4 males were seen over the 5 year period and diagnosed with macular holes. Ten subjects had bilateral holes (41.7%) as shown in **Table 1**. The mean age was 46 years (SD ± 13.42). Females were more affected with a ratio of 5:1. **Table 2** shows the age and gender distribution of the patients.

The hospital incidence of macular holes was 6.6%.

Table 1. Laterality of macula hole in the 24 patients.

Eye	Frequency	Percentage
BIL	10	41.7
LT	7	29.2
RT	7	29.2
Total	**24**	**100.0**

Bilateral—BIL, Left—LT, Right—RT.

Table 2. Age and gender distribution of patients with macular holes.

Age group (years)	Gender male	Total (%) female
1 (4.2)	2 (8.3)	3 (12.5)
0 (0.0)	5 (20.8)	5 (20.8)
0 (0.0)	4 (16.7)	4 (16.7)
2 (8.3)	6 (25.0)	8 (33.3)
1 (4.2)	3 (12.5)	4 (16.7)
4 (16.7)	20 (83.3)	24 (100.0)

Chi-square = 2.89; df = 4; p-value = 0.577 (p-value not significant (p > 0.05).

Table 1 shows that 10 (41.7%) out of the 24 cases had macular holes in both. eyes.

There were numerous etiological factors seen, but idiopathic presentation (58.3%) was the commonest as shown in **Table 3**. Others were trauma 4 (16.7%), posterior uveitis 2, (8.3%), chemotherapy 2 (8.3%), Solar retinopathy and retinitis pigmentosa 1 (4.2%). Nineteen (55.9%) of the 34 eyes were visually impaired (BCVA < 6/18). Nineteen eyes had full thickness holes (55.9%) requiring surgery, however only 3 (12.5%) of these could afford to have surgery with one reoperation. Four patients (16.7%) had complications in form of retinal detachments at presentation.

Table 4 shows that there was no statistically significant difference between risk factors and the age of the subjects.

Table 5 shows the distribution of visual acuity of the patients. Nineteen (55.9%) of the 34 eyes were visually impaired (BCVA < 6/18). Nineteen eyes had full thickness holes (55.9%) requiring surgery as shown in **Table 6**, however only 3 (12.5%) of these could afford to have surgery with one reoperation.

3 out of the 24 patients had the macular hole surgery.

As illustrated in **Table 7**, four patients (16.7%) had complications in form of retinal detachments at presentation.

4. Discussion

Twenty four cases of macular holes were seen in this study with ten (41.7%) cases presenting bilaterally (**Table 1**) giving a total of 34 eyes. This appears to be higher than what is recorded in other studies probably due to the late presentation and intervention which are common factors in the developing world [14] [15]. **Table 2** shows that the mean age was 46 years (SD ± 13.42) with a female preponderance. The mean age here is at variance with other studies where the mean age is higher because most of the available studies focused on idiopathic macular holes and other aetiological factors were not reported [15]. Females accounted for 83.3% of the study group with a female to male ratio of 5:1 [14]. This is consistent with other studies and lends credence to the postulations implicating hormonal changes [2] [14] [15]. The hospital incidence of macular holes was 6.6% of persons and 9.3% of eyes. There is a dearth of studies on incidence of macular holes. Most studies report prevalence [16]-[18]. However a population based incidence reported 7.8 persons and 8.69 eyes per 100,000 population [14]. Our incidence is quite significant considering that it is a hospital based study with a smaller

Table 3. Shows the risk factors at presentation of the 24 patients.

Risk Factors	Frequency	Percentage (%)
Idiopathic	14	58.3
Trauma	4	16.7
Posterior Uveitis	2	8.3
Chemotherapy	2	8.3
Solar Retinopathy	1	4.2
Retinitis Pigmentosa	1	4.2
Total	**24**	**100**

Table 4. Relationship between risk factor and age.

Risk Factors	Age Group					Total
	≤30	31 - 40	41 - 50	51 - 60	>60	
Ca Breast	0	1 (4.2)	0	0	0	1 (4.20)
Ca Prostate	0	0	0	0	1 (4.2)	1 (4.2)
RP	0	1 (4.2)	0	0	0	1 (4.2)
Idiopathic	1 (4.2)	0	4	6 (25.0)	3 (12.5)	14 (58.3)
Post Uveitis	1 (4.2)	0	0	1 (4.2)	0	2 (8.3)
Solar	1 (4.2)	0	0	0	0	1 (4.20)
Trauma	0	3 (12.5)	0	1 (4.2)	0	4 (16.7)
Total	**3 (12.5)**	**5 (20.8)**	**4 (16.7)**	**8 (33.3)**	**4 (16.7)**	**24 (100.0)**

Chi-square = 35.65; df=24; p-value = 0.0593.

Table 5. Best corrected visual acuity at presentation.

Visual acuity	Number (n = 34 eyes)	Percentage
<6/18	15	44.1
6/18 - 6/60	16	47.1
>6/60	3	8.8
Total	34	100

Table 6. Macula hole staging in 34 eyes.

Stage	Number (n = 34 eyes)	Percentage
0	7	20.6
1	3	8.8
2	4	11.8
3	8	23.5
4	7	20.6
Total	**34**	**100**

Table 7. Proportion of patients with complications.

Risk Factor	Frequency (%)	Complications-RD (%)
Idiopathic	14 (58.3)	3 (12.5)
Trauma	4 (16.7)	1 (4.2)
Posterior Uveitis	2 (8.3)	-
Chemotherapy	2 (8.3)	-
Solar Retinopathy	1 (4.2)	-
Retinitis Pigmentosa	1 (4.2)	-
Total	**24 (100)**	**4 (16.7)**

RD—Retinal detachment.

sample size. The commonest aetiological factor in this series was idiopathic macular holes just as reported widely (**Table 3**). Again there is very little documentation on other causes of macular holes as most studies focus on idiopathic holes [15]. Idiopathic macular hole commonly affects otherwise healthy individuals in their 6th or 7th decade and prefoveola traction have been widely accepted as the pathogenesis implicated in idiopathic macular hole [2].

Trauma contributed to 4 of the cases, while 2 of the cases resulted from poorly treated posterior uveitis resulting in vitreoretinal traction and retinal detachment. Photochemical changes in the retina with increased temperature while sun gazing is believed to cause macular damage [19] [20]. One case of solar retinopathy was seen in our study. Two cases were attributed to chemotherapy following breast cancer and prostate cancer. Tamoxifen retinopathy though rare has been reported to cause foveal cysts that could lead to macular holes [9]. The female patient who was on Tamoxifen therapy was 32 years old which ruled out a typical idiopathic etiology, while the other was male. Both had bilateral presentation which was a pointer to a systemic aetiology. **Table 4** shows that there was no statistically significant difference between the risk factors and age of subject in this study, a larger study however will most likely demonstrate this. Central vision loss is the commonest manifestation of macular holes and can be visually disabling. Out of the 34 eyes more than half, had low vision(<6/18) from macular hole (19 eyes (55.9%)) and presented with full thickness holes (**Table 5** and **Table 6**).

Retinal detachment is the most common complication following the development of macular hole as subretinal fluid insinuates between the neurosensory retina and retinal pigment epithelium through this defect to cause a detachment. In our study 4 patients had retinal detachment at presentation.

The management of macular holes was revolutionized by Kelly and Wendel with vitrectomy, internal limiting membrane peeling and tamponade. Though macular hole surgery is now available in a few private centers in Nigeria, majority who require this service, utilize the government health centers and have to travel long distances to access this specialized service at high costs.

The private centres were these services are available, are all located in the South West geopolitical zones. Rivers State is located in the South South geopolitical zone of the country with about 19 Ophthalmologists. There is only one ophthalmologist trained in Medical Retina and there are no facilities for vitrectomy in the state presently. Patients therefore have no option but to travel out of their state of residence to access this service with the attendant risks and heavy costs.

Even though 19 eyes in this series had full thickness holes that required surgery, only 3 patients could afford surgery, with one requiring reoperation. The direct cost of surgery and the fact that surgery had to be done outside the residence of abode were factors that militated against the take up of this service outside.

5. Conclusion

This study has shown that the incidence of macular holes in the developing world is significant and resources to manage these cases are grossly lacking. Specialist training, with government subsidizing costs will alleviate these difficulties and reduce visual loss from macular holes.

References

[1]   Oh, K.T. (2013) Macular Hole Treatment and Management. http://http:emedicine.medscape.com/article/1224320

[2]   Ezra, E. (2001) Idiopathic Full Thickness Macular Hole: Natural History and Pathogenesis. *British Journal of Ophthalmology*, **85**, 102-108.

[3]   Knapp, H. (1869) UeberIsolirtezerreissungen der aderhautinfolge von traumen auf augapfel. *Archives of Ophthalmology and Otology (Archiv für Augen- und Ohrenheilkunde)*, **1**, 6-29.

[4]   Kuhnt, H. (1900) Tber eineeigentumlicheveranderung der netzhautadmaculam (retinitis atrophicanssiverareficanscentralis). *Zeitschrift für Augenheilkunde*, **3**, 105.

[5]   Gass, J.D. (1988) Idiopathic Senile Macular Hole. Its Early Stages and Pathogenesis. *Archives of Ophthalmology*, **106**, 629-639. http://dx.doi.org/10.1001/archopht.1988.01060130683026

[6]   Aaberg, T.M. (1970) Macular Holes. A Review. *Survey of Ophthalmology*, **15**, 139-162.

[7]   Gao, L., Dong, F. and Chan, W. (2007) Traumatic Macular Hole Secondary to Nd: YAG Laser. *Eye*, **21**, 571-573.

[8]   García-Fernández, M., Castro-Navarro, J. and Bajo-Fuente, A. (2013) Unilateral Recurrent Macular Hole in a Patient with Retinitis Pigmentosa: A Case Report. *Journal of Medical Case Reports*, **7**, 69. http://dx.doi.org/10.1186/1752-1947-7-69

[9]   Eisner, A. and Luoh, S.W. (2011) Breast Cancer Medications and Vision: Effects of Treatments for Early-Stage Disease. *Current Eye Research*, **10**, 867-885.

[10] Bonnin, N., Cornut, P., Chaise, F., Labeille, E., Manificat, H., Feldman, A., Perard, L., Bacin, F., Chiambaretta, F. and Burillon, C. (2013) Spontaneous Closure of Macular Holes Secondary to Posterior Uveitis: Case Series and Literature Review. *Journal of Ophthalmic Inflammation and Infection*, **3**, 34. http://dx.doi.org/10.1186/1869-5760-3-34

[11] Leibovitch, I., Azmon, B., Pianka, P., Alster, Y. and Loewenstein, A. (2003) Macular Hole Secondary to Branch Retinal Vein Occlusion Diagnosed by Retinal Thickness Analyzer. *Ophthalmic Surgery, Lasers & Imaging*, **34**, 53-56.

[12] Smiddy, W.E. and Flynn Jr., H.W. (2004) Pathogenesis of Macular Holes and Therapeutic Implications. *American Journal of Ophthalmology*, **137**, 525-537. http://dx.doi.org/10.1016/j.ajo.2003.12.011

[13] Kelly, N.E. and Wendel, R.T. (1991) Vitreous Surgery for Idiopathic Macular Holes. Results of a Pilot Study. *Archives of Ophthalmology*, **109**, 654-659. http://dx.doi.org/10.1001/archopht.1991.01080050068031

[14] McCannel, C.A., Ensminger, J.L., Diehl, N.N. and Hodge, D.N. (2009) Population Based Incidence of Macular Holes. *Ophthalmology*, **116**, 1366-1369. http://dx.doi.org/10.1016/j.ophtha.2009.01.052

[15] Sen, P., Bhargava, A., Vijaya, L. and George, R. (2008) Prevalence of Idiopathic Macular Hole in Adult Rural and Urban South Indian Population. *Clinical and Experimental Ophthalmology*, **36**, 257-260. http://dx.doi.org/10.1111/j.1442-9071.2008.01715.x

[16] Klein, R., Klein, B.E., Wang, Q. and Moss, S.E. (1994) The Epidemiology of Retinal Membranes. *Transactions of the American Ophthalmological Society*, **92**, 403-425.

[17] Rahmani, B., Tielsch, J.M., Katz, J., Gottsch, J., Quigley, H., Javitt, J., et al. (1996) The Cause-Specific Prevalence of Visual Impairment in an Urban Population. Baltimore Eye Survey. *Ophthamology*, **103**, 1721-1726. http://dx.doi.org/10.1016/S0161-6420(96)30435-1

[18] Mitchell, P., Smith, W., Chey, T., Wang, J.J. and Chang, A. (1997) Prevalence and Associations of Epiretinal Membranes. The Blue Mountains Eye Study, Australia. *Ophthalmology*, **104**, 1033-1040. http://dx.doi.org/10.1016/S0161-6420(97)30190-0

[19] Comander, J., Gardiner, M. and Loewenstein, J. (2011) High-Resolution Optical Coherence Tomography Findings in Solar Maculopathy and the Differential Diagnosis of Outer Retinal Holes. *American Journal of Ophthalmology*, **152**, 413-419. http://dx.doi.org/10.1016/j.ajo.2011.02.012

[20] Macarez, R., Vanimschoot, M., Ocamica, P. and Kovalski, J.L. (2007) Optical Coherence Tomography Follow-Up of a Case of Solar Maculopathy. *Journal Français d'Ophtalmologie*, **30**, 276-280. http://dx.doi.org/10.1016/S0181-5512(07)89590-8

23

The Effect of Limbal Autograft in Recurrence of Pterygium

Suleyman Ciftci[1*], Eyup Dogan[1], Leyla Ciftci[2], Ozlem Demirpence[3]

[1]Department of Ophthalmology, Diyarbakır Training and Research Hospital, Diyarbakır, Turkey
[2]Department of Cardiology, Faculty of Medicine, Dicle University, Diyarbakır, Turkey
[3]Department of Biochemistry, Tunceli State Hospital, Tunceli, Turkey
Email: [*]ciftci1977@hotmail.com

Abstract

Background: Assessing the effect of limbal autograft shifting in recurrence of pterygium. Methods: This single-center study was carried out in a tertiary health facility. A review of data on consecutive patients who underwent pure limbal autografts shifting after pterygium resection was done. In all the cases, the pterygia extended at least 3 mm beyond the limbus. The resected each limbal grafts included a width of 1.5 mm and a length of 2 or 3 mm of limbus and a depth of 250 μm. Schmer test was performed at the eighth month postoperatively. Pterygium recurrence was accepted endpoint of the study. One patient had recurrent pterygium, whereas the others had primary pterygium. Patients with other ocular surface diseases or ocular pathology and, patients who discontinued follow-up visits were excluded from the study. Results: The study included 10 patients, with 5 males and 5 females. Median age of the patients was 40 (25 - 70). Follow-up was conducted for a minimum of 8 months for patients with recurrence and at least for 16 months for non-recurrent cases. Recurrence was observed in 6 patients out of 10, in one patient, atypia was reported and excluded from the study. Four recurrent patients experienced decreased levels of tears. The rest one patient with recurrence had not any tear abnormality. The remaining 4 patients responded well to the surgery. Because of the high recurrence rate, it was decided to terminate the study. Conclusions: Limbal autografts shifting alone is not an appropriate treatment for primary pterygium because of the high recurrence rate.

Keywords

Limbal Autograft, Recurrence, Pterygium

---

[*]Corresponding author.

Article Summary

Pterygium is a complex disease and the benefits of limbal graft are limited when working alone. As such, pterygium may be defined as a final common formation of some interactive instabilities that constitute fibrovascular tissue. Dysfunction of the limbus affects the results of this study favorably whereas without excised tenon's layer affect the results of this study unfavorably. Currently conjunctival-limbal autografts combining with tenon's layer removal seem to manage many factors that actively participate in the formation of pterygium.

This study has limited number of participants and lack of control group; however it proved several points and complimentary indications such as atypia, asymmetric dry eye, effects of limbus in recurrence and in multiple pterygium and effect of tenon's layer comparable to limbal stem cells. These are vital clues for the causes of recurrence.

1. Introduction

Pterygium represents a pathologic condition occurring more frequently in certain populations. Its incidence varies greatly with different geographical zones. A lot of factors such as genetic, environmental, ocular surface instability, limbal deficiency and atypia play an active role either individually or synergistically in the development of pterygium. In general, pterygium may be defined as an end-product of some interactive instabilities that constitute the fibrovascular tissue [1].

Some of the existing approaches to the treatment of pterygium were evolved on the basis of the knowledge acquired from recent etiopathogenetic and clinical studies that emphasized the role of limbus [2]-[5]. Therefore, especially conjunctival-limbal autograft became the more preferred surgery, with a relatively shorter operative time and a low rate of recurrence as well as comparable to adjuvants [6]-[15].

Conceptually, the number of recurrences of pterygium could possibly be reduced by including the limbus in the conjunctival autograft used in the surgical technique because conjunctival-limbal autografts make more physiological reparation [8]. However, there is no clear explanation on the additive successful result of conjunctival-limbal autograft that is ensured by interaction effect of the grafts with each other or is ensured by pure effect of limbal autograft [6]. Pure limbal autograft, as a technique for pterygium surgery appears to be an appropriate model to test the knowledge acquired from recent studies and to determine the utility of this technique in the management of all forms of pterygium (etc., primary or recurrent) clinically. Even, Shimazaki *et al.* experienced a similar technique in recurrent pterygium previously and reported favorable results [5]. They used limbal autograft transplantation. Superior limbal tissue was taken with conjunctival flap and transferred to the excised area. However, they attributed favorable results to limbal autograft. They used conjunctival flap conjunction with limbus. However, we know that autologous conjunctival transplantation has favorable impact on recurrence [6] [9] [10]. The main difference between our technique and Shimazaki's is that we balance favorable impact of conjunctiva by unexcised tenon's tissue.

In the preliminary study, the effect of pure limbus in recurrence of pterygium was assessed in order to understand the exact mechanism of success based upon limbal autograft coupled with decreased rates of recurrence.

2. Materials and Methods

This single-center study was carried out in a tertiary health facility. A review of data on consecutive patients who underwent pure limbal autografts shifting after pterygium resection during the period from May 2011 to August 2011 was done. The measurement of the rate of recurrence is the key factor of this study and pterygium recurrence was accepted endpoint of the study. A true recurrence was defined as a fibro-vascular ingrowth of 1.5 mm or more across the limbus with conjunctival drag [16].

Informed consent was obtained from all the patients who participated in this study. This study was approved by The Institutional Review Board of Batman State Hospital (Batman, Turkey). The tenets of the Declaration of Helsinki were followed. Patient consent was obtained for use of figures accompanying this paper. One of the patients had recurrent pterygium, whereas the others had primary pterygium. Patients with a clinically apparent ocular surface disease or ocular pathology, and patients who discontinued follow-up visits were excluded from the study. None of the patients had previously undergone any ocular procedures except for pterygium surgery in one of the patients.

In all the cases, the pterygia extended at least 3 mm beyond the limbus and in stage IV or V. All the operations were performed by the same surgeon who experienced in ocular surface surgery including limbal autografting and pterygium surgery. The surgical technique is shown in **Figure 1**. The surgeries were performed under sub-tenon's anesthesia with 2% lidocaine. After the injection of lidocaine under the conjunctiva in the body of the pterygium, dissection was performed from the head toward the body (**Figure 1**, top right and top left). The corneal defect was shaved for any residual tissue using a blade. The limbal grafts including stem cells were harvested from the upper and the lower adjacent healthy corneal limbus (**Figure 1**, bottom left). The resected each limbal grafts included a width of 1.5 mm and a length of 2 or 3 mm of limbus and a depth of 250 μm. The harvested limbal grafts' length was adjusted according to the excised pterygium size in the head portion which was between 4 or 6 mm. The adjacent episcleral and conjunctival tissue and tenon's layer in harvested limbal graft was maintained and both the adjacent conjunctiva and tenon's layer was released from episclera in superior and inferior portions behind the limbus. Once these grafts were shifted to the excised region of pterygium while maintaining limbus to limbus orientation, the adjacent tissue dislocated to the midline with the limbal graft. Then the grafts and adjacent episcleral and conjunctival tissue were secured with interrupted 10.0 nylon sutures. The conjunctiva was closed with 10.0 nylon sutures, leaving no bare sclera (**Figure 1**, bottom right). The donor site was left to epithelialize without closure of the defect. The duration of the procedure was approximately one hour. A bandage closure was applied postoperatively to all patients for a week. The specimens were sent for pathologic analysis. Sutures were removed after one month.

Postsurgically, oral analgesia was administered for the first day, topical dexamethasone solutions for at least 45 days on a tapered regimen until conjunctival injection resolved, moxifloxacin for two weeks and lubrication for one month. Schirmer test was performed at the eighth month postsurgery. Follow up was made in postoperative first day, first week, first month, and later every month. At each visit macrophotography of the eye and slit-lamp examination were undertaken. Patients who failed to return for the recommended follow-up appointments were telephoned to encourage compliance with follow-up.

3. Results

This study was conducted on a total of 10 patients, consisting of 5 males and 5 females. Median age of the patients was 40 (25 - 70). The details of the patients are presented in **Table 1**. Primary pterygium was found in eight patients, recurrent pterygium in one patient and multiple pterygium in one patient. All the patients were followed-up for a minimum period of eight months. In one of the patients (**Table 1**, Patient No. 6), atypia was reported in the pathology report, all other specimens were consistent with pterygium. In the patient whom atypia was reported recurrence was observed very early. According to methodology this patient was excluded from the study. All the other recurrences began to develop after three months and got completed in less than eight months.

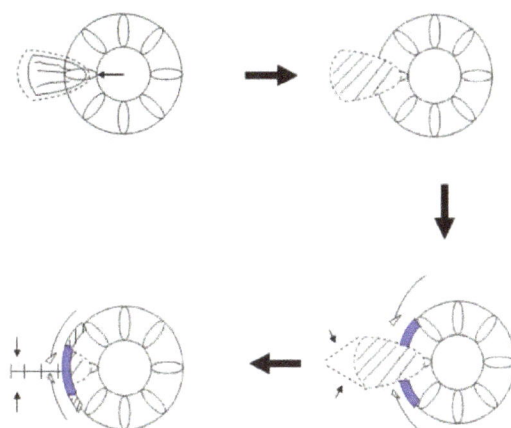

Figure 1. Top right. Dissection was continued from the head toward the body; top left. The corneal defect was shaved for any residual tissue using a blade; bottom left. The limbal grafts including stem cells were harvested from the upper and the lower adjacent healthy corneal limbus; bottom right. The grafts were shifted to the excised region of pterygium maintaining limbus to limbus orientation. The grafts were secured with interrupted 10.0 nylon and conjunctiva was closed with 10.0 nylon sutures, leaving no bare sclera.

Table 1. Clinical data of the patients.

Patient No.	Age (Yr)	Sex	Follow-Up (month)	Presentation	Recurrence and time (month)	Atypia	Schmer	Side
1	65	M	16	Multiple, primary	No	No	24/24	R
2	44	F	16	Primary	No	No	30/15	R
3	28	M	8	Primary	Yes, between 3 to 8	No	30/30	R
4	60	F	16	Recurrent	No	No	25/25	L
5	40	F	8	Primary	Yes, between 3 to 8	No	3/25	R
6	26	F	8	Primary	Yes, in 1,5	Yes	30/30	R
7	30	M	8	Primary	Yes, between 3 to 8	No	35/15	L
8	32	M	8	Primary	Yes, between 3 to 8	No	19/30	R
9	25	M	16	Primary	No	No	35/35	L
10	70	F	8	Primary	Yes, between 3 to 8	No	35/15	L

M; male, F; female, R, right; L, left; m, months.

Hence, the follow-up was limited to eight months among all the five recurrent cases. In total, recurrence was observed in five patients with a recurrence rate of 55.5%. In four of the recurrent cases, the quantity of tears decreased on the region of recurrence and one of these patients is presented in **Table 1** as fifth patient having dry eye. Artificial tear and cyclosporine were prescribed to the patients. After medical treatment these patients were free from eye complaint and declined further operation. Because the rate of recurrence following this surgical approach was high within the eight months of follow-up, the study was terminated and no new patients were enrolled to the study.

The follow-up period was extended to at least 16 months for 4 patients with no recurrence with a surgical success rate of 44.5%. One of these patients, presented in **Table 1** as fourth patient, had recurrent pterygium and had received conjunctival autograft. Recurrence developed one month after the surgery (**Figure 2**). In this patient, the previous recurrence appeared to be caused by dysfunction of the limbus. Another patient presented in **Table 1** as first patient had multiple pterygia and responded well to limbal shifting surgery. The cause of multiple pterygia in this patient appears to be due to dysfunction of the limbus.

4. Discussion

The effect of pure limbal autograft shifting in recurrence of pterygium was assessed in this retrospective study. It was found that the rate of recurrence of this technique was 55.5% in a sample size of 9 patients. Hence, it was concluded that the effect of limbus shifting in this study was not better than primary pterygium excision and, the enrollment of patients into the study was discontinued. In addition, no control group was formed for this study.

In accordance with the criteria set out by Singh, recurrences of pterygial growth necessitate an extended time, hence exact time of recurrence could not be determined [16]. Instead the time from the initial stage to the completion of pterygial recurrence was determined. Survival curve analysis indicated that there existed 50% chance of recurrence of pterygium within the first 120 days, and a 97% chance within 12 months of its removal [17]. Follow-up period was determined based on this information. Follow-up of the patients with recurrence was discontinued when full formation stage occurred and follow-up extended up to 16 months for patients without recurrence.

In this study, an alternative treatment for pterygium is not being proposed; hence the complications associated with the surgery were not reported. However, a new pterygium surgery technique to test the effect of pure limbal autograft in recurrence of pterygium was used. As determined in this study, treatment modalities in pterygium fail when a single reason is considered. Responding well to limbal shifting surgery in this study, the response of the two the patients: one with recurrent pterygium and the other with multiple pterygia is attributed to dysfunction of the limbus. Dysfunction of the limbus was found to affect the results of this study favorably. Results in dysfunction of the limbus were consistent with the findings of Shimazaki *et al.* [5]. Interestingly in four patients

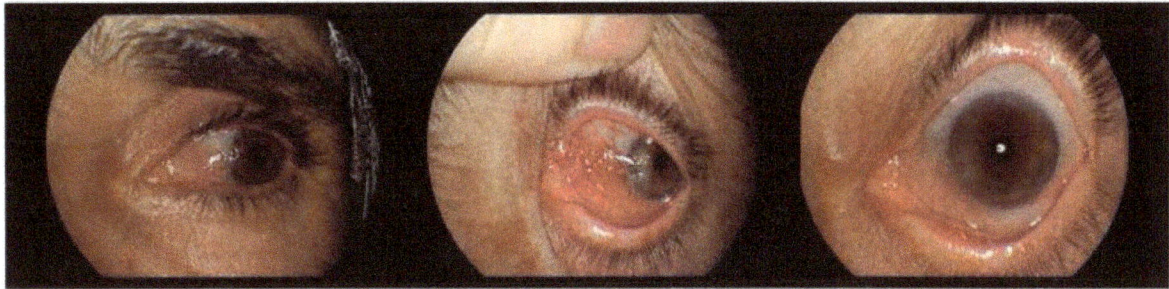

Figure 2. The clinical photograph of the patient are shown in Table 1 as fourth patient. Right, preoperative figure shows recurrent pterygium; Middle, early postoperative figure; Left, the eighth month postoperative figure.

with recurrences, schirmer test showed decreased tear secretion on the side of recurrence. All of four pterygiums were primary. However, tear secretion of the other side remained normal. Recurrence and asymmetric dry eyes disclosed an interesting association and raised some questions such as prevalence of asymmetric dry eye in pterygium so it needs of further investigation. Also atypia in one of the patient that resulted in very early recurrence is an interesting confirmation of Weinstein's report [18]. Although this study was conducted on limited number of participants, atypia was reported in one of the patients in the presented study that raises interesting questions such as the impact of atypia in recurrence of pterygium. It appears that ocular surface instability and atypia affected the outcome of this study unfavorably. However, no possible reason could be attributed to the recurrence observed in one patient (**Table 1**, third patient), who was young, aged twenty-eight years. An in-depth study of the VEGF isoforms may shed light onto the possible roles they play in recurrence. But conclusive evidence is still at large for this patient.

In analysing possible causes of high recurrence rate in this study, some questions can ensue such as inadequate post-operative medication, poor handling of limbal graft and in-appropriate size of the limbal graft. Yaisawang and Piyapattanakorn emphasized the importance of corticosteroids and encourage surgeons to use topical corticosteroids for enough time. Otherwise inadequate post-operative medication can cause high recurrence rate [19]. Clearly, we administered topical dexamethasone solutions for at least 45 days on a tapered regimen until conjunctival injection resolved and this regimen is definitely adequate. However Ti *et al.* emphasized that recurrence rates are inversely related to previous experience and simply poor handling of surgery can cause high recurrence rate [12], whereas it does not seems a causative factor of failing in hand of an experienced surgeon. We limited length of limbal graft according to the excised pterygium in head portion. Although the length between 4 or 6 mm and a width of 1.5 mm is a mini graft, it is an appropriate size for this technique because this size is enough large when compared with the component used in the limbal-conjunctival autograft so it can mimic the favorable effect of limbal component easily. Also we want to provide the effect of limbal stem cells in only the excised head portion. Besides to exclude the favorable impact of healthy conjunctiva on pterygium recurrence such as in conjunctival autograft that emphasized in some article, we did not excised tenon's layer from adjacent conjunctiva that dislocated to the midline [6] [11] [12]. Although limbal otograft, the adjacent tenon's layer may be the possible cause of high recurrence rate. This clue also mentioned in reports by Hirst [20]. He mentioned in his studies that transplantation of limbal stem cells was studiously avoided, seems to refute the need to deplete the superior limbus of their stem cells to achieve a low recurrence rate. The presented study confirms this suggestion from another way and in fact complements each other as such: he achieved low recurrence rate with extensive tenon's layer removal without transplantation of limbal stem cells whereas we failed in our technique by transplantation of limbal stem cells without tenon's layer removal [20].

As Hirst's mentioned the importance of extensive tenon's layer removal, it is well-known that the recurrence of pterygium is high when the underneath tenon's layer is not excised but this high recurrence rate was always shown in series without effect of limbal stem cells. The characteristic that distinguishes this work is that limbal stem cells on one side of pendulum whereas tenon's effect is on another side. So, the presented study proposes based on findings that tenon's layer is more determinative in recurrence than limbal stem cells, also widespread acceptance and high success of conjunctival autografting [9] [10] and/or limbal-conjunctival autograft probably due to excision of tenon's layer [7] [21] [22]. Limbal-conjunctival autograft results have been reported as successful as mitomycin C group [13] and Pulte reported conjunctiva-limbus autografts in pterygia have excellent efficacy against recurrence [21]. Probably conjunctival autograft adheres to episclera tightly and prevents fibro-vascular growth up to forward.

Although this study has limited number of participants and lack of control group, it proved several points and complimentary indications such as atypia, asymmetric dry eye, effects of limbus in recurrent and multiple ptery-gia and effect of tenon's layer comparable to limbal stem cells. These are vital clues for the causes of recurrence. In this respect this study is unique.

5. Conclusion

In conclusion, from the above observations, it appears that pterygium is a complex disease with several under-lying causative factors. The benefits associated with limbal graft are limited when applied alone. Instead, this study proposes a more comprehensive therapy into consideration. Conjunctival-limbal autograft, combining with extensive tenon's layer removal and if needed treatment for ocular surface instabilities, seems logical.

Funding/Support

None.

Financial Disclosures

None.

The Contributions of the Authors

The contributions of the authors are as follows: conception and design (SC, ED, LC, and OD), analysis and interpretation (SC, ED, LC, and OD), writing the article (SC), critical revision of the manuscript (SC, ED, LC, and OD), final approval of the manuscript (SC, ED, LC, and OD), data collection (SC), provision of the materials and patients (SC), literature search (SC), and administrative, technical, and logistical support (SC, ED, LC, and OD).

Acknowledgements

Suleyman Ciftci (SC): I had full access to all the data in the study, and take responsibility for the integrity of the data and the accuracy of the data analysis. Each of the coauthors (ED, LC, and OD) has seen and agrees with each of the changes made to this manuscript.

References

[1] Hirst, L.W. (2003) The Treatment of Pterygium. *Survey of Ophthalmology*, **48**, 145-180. http://dx.doi.org/10.1016/S0039-6257(02)00463-0

[2] Reid, T.W. and Dushku, N. (2010) What a Study of Pterygia Teaches Us about the Cornea? Molecular Mechanisms of Formation. *Eye Contact Lens*, **36**, 290-295. http://dx.doi.org/10.1097/ICL.0b013e3181eea8fe

[3] Kwok, L.S. and Coroneo, M.T. (1994) A Model for Pterygium Formation. *Cornea*, **13**, 219-224. http://dx.doi.org/10.1097/00003226-199405000-00005

[4] Dushku, N. and Reid, T.W. (1994) Immunohistochemical Evidence That Human Pterygia Originate from an Invasion of Vimentin-Expressing Altered Limbal Epithelial Basal Cells. *Current Eye Research*, **13**, 473-481. http://dx.doi.org/10.3109/02713689408999878

[5] Shimazaki, J., Yang, H.Y. and Tsubota, K. (1996) Limbal Autograft Transplantation for Recurrent and Advanced Pte-rygia. *Ophthalmic Surgery Lasers & Imaging*, **27**, 917-923.

[6] Al Fayez, M.F. (2013) Limbal-Conjunctival vs Conjunctival Autograft Transplant for Recurrent Pterygia: A Prospec-tive Randomized Controlled Trial. *JAMA Ophthalmology*, **131**, 11-16. http://dx.doi.org/10.1001/archophthalmol.2012.2599

[7] Gris, O., Güell, J.L. and del Campo, Z. (2000) Limbal-Conjunctival Autograft Transplantation for the Treatment of Re-current Pterygium. *Ophthalmology*, **107**, 270-273. http://dx.doi.org/10.1016/S0161-6420(99)00041-X

[8] Jaworski, C.J., Aryankalayil-John, M., Campos, M.M., *et al.* (2009) Expression Analysis of Human Pterygium Shows a Predominance of Conjunctival and Limbal Markers and Genes Associated with Cell Migration. *Molecular Vision*, **20**, 2421-2434.

[9] Vastine, D.W., Stewart, W.B. and Schwab, I.R. (1982) Reconstruction of the Periocular Mucous Membrane by Autologous Conjunctival Transplantation. *Ophthalmology*, **89**, 1072-1081. http://dx.doi.org/10.1016/S0161-6420(82)34681-3

[10] Kenyon, K.R., Wagoner, M.D. and Hettinger, M.E. (1985) Conjunctival Autograft Transplantation for Advanced and Recurrent Pterygium. *Ophthalmology*, **92**, 1461-1470. http://dx.doi.org/10.1016/S0161-6420(85)33831-9

[11] Riordan-Eva, P., Kielhorn, I., Ficker, L.A., McG Steele, A.D. and Kirkness, C.M. (1993) Conjunctival Autografting in the Surgical Management of Pterygium. *Eye*, **7**, 634-638. http://dx.doi.org/10.1038/eye.1993.146

[12] Ti, S.E., Chee, S.P., Dear, K.B. and Tan, D.T. (2000) Analysis of Variation in Success Rates in Conjunctival Autografting for Primary and Recurrent Pterygium. *British Journal of Ophthalmology*, **84**, 385-389. http://dx.doi.org/10.1136/bjo.84.4.385

[13] Güler, M., Sobaci, G., Ilker, S., Oztürk, F., Mutlu, F.M. and Yildirim, E. (1994) Limbal-Conjunctival Autograft Transplantation in Cases with Recurrent Pterygium. *Acta Ophthalmologica*, **72**, 721-726. http://dx.doi.org/10.1111/j.1755-3768.1994.tb04688.x

[14] Zheng, K., Cai, J., Jhanji, V. and Chen, H. (2012) Comparison of Pterygium Recurrence Rates after Limbal Conjunctival Autograft Transplantation and Other Techniques: Meta-Analysis. *Cornea*, **31**, 1422-1427. http://dx.doi.org/10.1097/ICO.0b013e31823cbecb

[15] Mutlu, F.M., Sobaci, G., Tatar, T. and Yildirim, E. (1999) A Comparative Study of Recurrent Pterygium Surgery: Limbal Conjunctival Autograft Transplantation versus Mitomycin C with Conjunctival Flap. *Ophthalmology*, **106**, 817-821. http://dx.doi.org/10.1016/S0161-6420(99)90172-0

[16] Singh, G., Wilson, M.R. and Foster, C.S. (1990) Long Term Follow up Study of Mitomycin Eye Drops as Adjunctive Treatment for Pterygia and Its Comparison with Conjunctival Autograft Transplantation. *Cornea*, **9**, 331-334. http://dx.doi.org/10.1097/00003226-199010000-00011

[17] Hirst, L.W., Sebban, A. and Chant, D. (1994) Pterygium Recurrence Time. *Ophthalmology*, **101**, 755-758. http://dx.doi.org/10.1016/S0161-6420(94)31270-X

[18] Weinstein, O., Rosenthal, G., Zirkin, H., Monos, T., Lifshitz, T. and Argov, S. (2002) Overexpression of p53 Tumor Suppressor Gene in Pterygia. *Eye*, **16**, 619-621. http://dx.doi.org/10.1038/sj.eye.6700150

[19] Yaisawang, S. and Piyapattanakorn, P. (2003) Role of Post-Operative Topical Corticosteroids in Recurrence Rate after Pterygium Excision with Conjunctival Autograft. *Journal of the Medical Association of Thailand*, **86**, 215-223.

[20] Hirst, L.W. (2008) Prospective Study of Primary Pterygium Surgery Using Pterygium Extended Removal Followed by Extended Conjunctival Transplantation. *Ophthalmology*, **115**, 1663-1672. http://dx.doi.org/10.1016/j.ophtha.2008.03.012

[21] Pulte, P., Heiligenhaus, A., Koch, J., Steuhl, K.P. and Waubke, T. (1998) Long-Term Results of Conjunctiva-Limbus Autografts in Patients with Pterygia. *Klinische Monatsblätter für Augenheilkunde*, **213**, 9-14. http://dx.doi.org/10.1055/s-2008-1034937

[22] Koch, J.M., Mellin, K.B. and Waubke, T.N. (1990) Initial Experience with Autologous Conjunctiva/Limbus Transplantation in Pterygium. *Klinische Monatsblätter für Augenheilkunde*, **197**, 106-109. http://dx.doi.org/10.1055/s-2008-1046250

24

Efficacy of 2 Drops versus 3 Drops Proparacaine 0.5% Ophthalmic Solution for Phacoemulsification Surgery: A Comparative Study

Tanie Natung, Jacqueline Syiem, Avonuo Keditsu, Nilotpal Saikia, Ranendra Hajong, Laura Amanda Lyngdoh

North Eastern Indira Gandhi Regional Institute of Health & Medical Sciences,
Shillong, India
Email: natungtanie@gmail.com

Abstract

Background and Aim: Phacoemulsification surgery with intraocular lens implantation is routinely done under topical anaesthesia in many centres. No comparative study on the efficacy of number of drops of topical anaesthetics effective for phacoemulsification surgery has been done. This study was conducted to compare the efficacy of 2 drops versus 3 drops proparacaine 0.5% ophthalmic solution for phacoemulsification surgery. Methods: Patients with uncomplicated cataract undergoing phacoemulsification surgery were randomised into two groups. Group 1 (n = 53) received 3 drops of proparacaine 0.5% whereas group 2 (n = 47) received 2 drops of the same solution before the start of surgery. All the patients underwent phacoemulsification with foldable intraocular lens implantation. Each patient's subjective experience of pain was measured using a 10 point Visual Analogue Pain Scale (VAS). Patient's cooperation during the surgery was assessed using a 3 point score. Both the evaluating resident doctor and patients were blinded. Results: In group 1, 73.6% patients scored 0, 20.8% scored 1 and 5.7% scored 2 of VAS respectively and in group 2, 89.4%, 6.4%, 4.3% patients scored 0, 1 and 2 of VAS respectively. In patient cooperation, 90.1% and 9.4% patients in group 1 scored 1 and 2 respectively whereas 87.2% and 12.8% patients scored 1 and 2 respectively in group 2. No statistically significant difference in the mean VAS (P = 0.0.55) and patient cooperation score (P = 0.597) was found between the two groups. The mean VAS score was 1.24 ± 0.534 and the mean patient cooperation score was 1.11 ± 0.314. The mean total surgical time was 25.11 ± 2.68 minutes. No additional drops were required for either group. Conclusions: Topical anaesthesia with both 2 drops and 3 drops proparacaine 0.5% ophthalmic solution is effective for phacoemulsification with intraocular lens implantation. Additional

anaesthesia may be unnecessary in these cases.

Keywords

Topical Anaesthesia, Proparacaine 5% Ophthalmic Solution, Phacoemulsification Surgery, Visual Analogue Pain Scale

1. Introduction

Clear corneal phacoemulsification with intraocular lens (IOL) implantation under topical anaesthesia is a standard practice today in many centres. However, prolonged doses of local anaesthetic agents can be toxic to the corneal epithelium. High or repeated doses can impair wound healing and cause corneal erosion [1]. Some patients may even be allergic to certain topical medications. Surgery under topical anesthesia may be rendered more difficult by repeated administration of topical medications which causes clouding of cornea [1]. Topical anaesthetic can also cause irritation to the eyes. Therefore, a minimal number of drops of topical anaesthetic agents effective for phacoemulsification surgery will help in reducing the toxicity.

Many studies on the effectiveness of anesthesia for cataract surgeries have been carried out using the Visual Analogue Pain Scale (VAS) [2]. Although No-anesthesia clear corneal phacoemulsification [3] and phacoemulsification with a single drop proparacaine hydrochloride [4] have been done, no comparative study on the efficacy of number of drops has been done to the best of our knowledge. Therefore, we conducted the present study to evaluate the efficacy of 2 drops versus 3 drops proparacaine 0.5% ophthalmic solution for phacoemulsification surgery.

2. Methods

The study was carried out in a medical college of Northeast India from April, 2013 to September, 2013. It was a prospective, randomised, comparative, interventional study. All the patients underwent anterior segment examination, refraction, applanation tonometry, biometry, dilated funduscopy and syringing of the lacrimal sacs. The inclusion criteria were patients with uncomplicated cataract. The exclusion criteria were patients with allergy to proparacaine, hard nuclear cataract ($\geq$Grade 5, Lens Opacification Classification III), uncooperative nature, difficulty in communication, non-dilating pupils, pseudoexfoliation syndrome, inability to understand the VAS and psychiatric disorders. Institute Ethics clearance was taken for the study. All the patients signed an informed written consent. We adhered to the tenets of the declaration of Helsinki.

Preoperatively, all the patients were explained in detail about the 10 point VAS, as used by Stevens in his study [2] (**Table 1**) and how they should respond according to their subjective experience to pain. Cases were randomised into two groups using computer generated random numbers. Group 1 (n = 53) received 3 drops of proparacaine 0.5% ophthalmic solution (Paracain, *Sunways P Ltd., Mumbai*) whereas group 2 (n = 47) received 2 drops of the same solution before the start of surgery. In group 1, one drop was put just before the cleaning and draping of the patient. The second drop was put after cleaning the conjunctival sac with betadine solution, just before the first corneal incision. The third drop was put after the completion of nucleotomy. In group 2, one drop was put just before the cleaning and draping of the patient. The second drop was put after cleaning the conjunctival sac with betadine solution, just before the first corneal incision. The flow chart of the comparative study design is given in **Flow Chart 1**. No intracameral or any other additional anesthesia was given. All the surgeries were performed by a single highly experienced and skilled faculty surgeon, who has the experience of performing hundreds of phacoemulsification surgeries with intraocular implantation. All the surgeries were done using clear corneal 2.8 mm main incision with 2 side ports, anterior continuous curvilinear capsulorrhexis, hydrodissection, phacoemulsification either with divide and conquer or stop and chop technique, irrigation and aspiration, both anterior and posterior capsular polishing, implantation of IOL with foldable lens (Acrysof IQ, Alcon Pvt. Ltd.), irrigation and aspiration again including underneath the IOL and stromal hydration of ports. All the surgeries were done using Laureate phacoemulsifier (Alcon Pvt. Ltd). One drop of preversative free moxifloxacin 0.5% eye drop (Vigamox®) was put at the end of the surgery before the removal of the speculum.

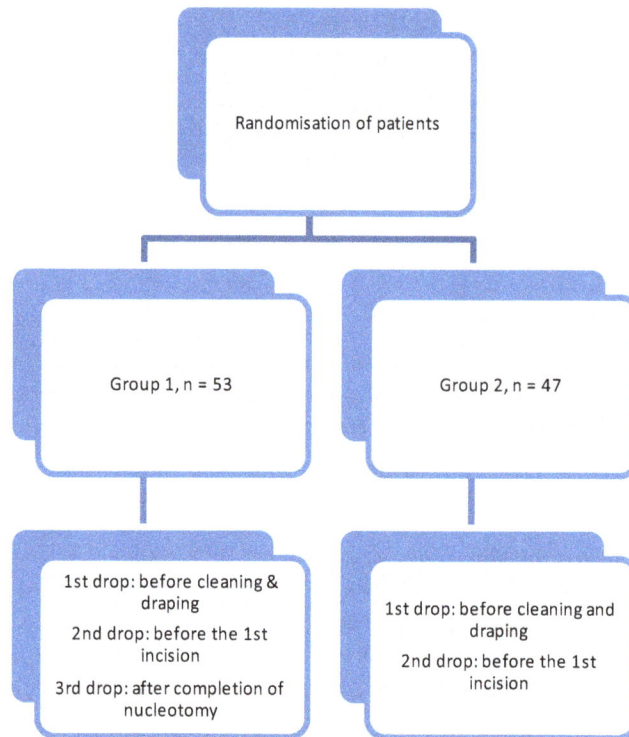

Flow Chart 1. Flow chart of the study design.

Table 1. Visual Analogue Pain Scale.

Numerical Scores	Descriptive Score
0	No Pain
1	Slight Discomfort
2	Slight Pain
3	Light Pain
4	Light to Moderate Pain
5	Moderate Pain
6	Moderate to Severe Pain
7	Severe Pain
8	Very Severe Pain
9	Excruciating Pain
10	Unbearable Pain

Adopted from Stevens JD[2].

Each patient's subjective experience of overall pain during the surgery was measured using a 10 point VAS [2], 10 minutes after the surgery by a senior resident doctor. Both the resident doctor and the patient were blinded from the number of drops. Patients' cooperation during the surgery was assessed using a 3 point score (Excellent = 1, Good = 2, Poor = 3) [5]. The total surgical time in minutes was taken as the duration between the first incision to the removal of speculum.

3. Statistical Analysis

Descriptive statistics was used to calculate the mean ± standard deviation and percentages. Mann Whitney test was used to compare the mean pain and patient cooperation scores between the two groups, between genders and between right or left eyes. Similarly, Independent-Samples t test was used to compare the mean surgical time between the two groups, between the genders and between right or left eyes. A P-value of less than 0.05 was considered significant. Statistical analysis was performed using the SPSS software package (SPSS for Windows, version 22.0; SPSS, Inc., Chicago, IL).

4. Results

Patient characteristics and scores are shown in **Table 2**. All the patients had uneventful surgery. In group I, 73.6% patients scored 0 (no pain), 20.8% scored 1 (slight discomfort) and 5.7% scored 2 (slight pain) using the VAS (**Figure 1**). In group II, 89.4%, 6.4%, 4.3% patients scored 0, 1 and 2 respectively (**Figure 2**). In patient cooperation, 90.1% and 9.4% patients in group 1 scored 1 and 2 respectively whereas 87.2% and 12.8% patients scored 1 and 2 in group 2 respectively. No statistically significant difference in the mean patient-reported pain scores for overall pain was found between the two groups (P = 0.055) (**Table 3**). Similarly, there was no statistically significant difference in the mean patient cooperation for surgery between the two groups (P = 0.597) (**Table 3**).

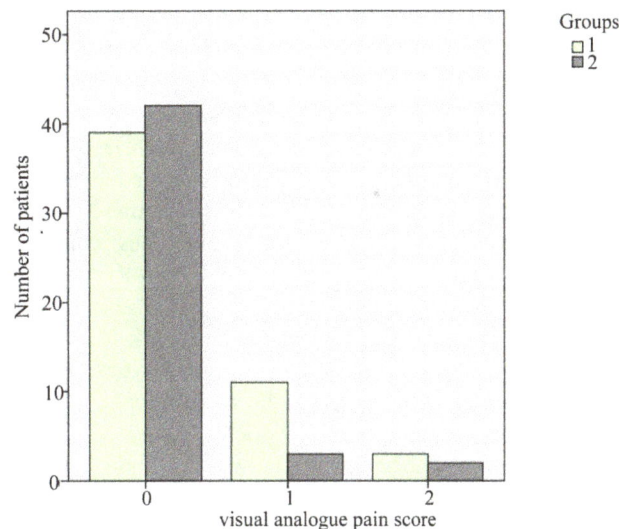

Figure 1. VAS scores recorded for the operative procedures in group 1 and 2.

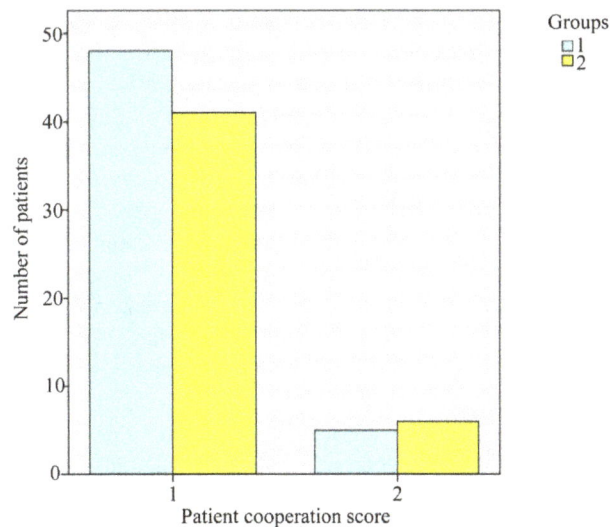

Figure 2. Patient cooperation scores during the procedure in group 1 and 2.

Table 2. Patient characteristics by groups.

Characteristics	Group 1	Group 2
Number of cases	53	47
Mean age ± SD (Years)	63.83 ± 12.22	57.79 ± 17.01
Male/Female	28/25	26/21
Mean total surgical time (minutes)	24.87 ± 2.85	25.06 ± 3.010

There was no statistically significant difference in the VAS score by gender (P = 0.500) and by right or left eyes (P = 0.124). Similarly, there was no statistically significant difference in the patient cooperation score by gender (P = 0.969) and by right or left eyes (P = 0.244) (**Table 3**).

The mean VAS score was 1.24 ± 0.534 and the mean patient cooperation score was 1.11 ± 0.314. The mean surgical time was 25.11 ± 2.68 minutes. No additional drops were required for either group.

The mean surgical time was 24.57 ± 2.85 and 25.06 ± 3.01 minutes in group 1 and 2 respectively. The difference was not statistically significant (P = 0.739) (**Table 3**). The pain scale core was weakly correlated with the duration of surgery (P = 0.655).

5. Discussion

Topical anesthesia in general has been found to be safe and effective for phacoemulsification surgery [4] [6]-[12]. It has many advantages. It eliminates the risks associated with retrobulbar and peribulbar blocks, as well as the risks associated with general anesthesia [13]. There is faster recovery of postoperative uncorrected visual acuity and the duration of surgery is shorter [11] [14]. It is also more economical as compared with peribulbar, subtenon or retrobulbar anaesthesia [11] [15]. Yet, the level of anesthesia is as good as that of subtenon anesthesia [16] [17]. No significant difference is found in their studies by Kim *et al.* and Sarkar *et al.* [16] [17].

Topical anesthesia alone without additional supplementation also has been established to be effective for cataract surgeries. Crandall *et al.* found that topical anesthesia alone was as good as topical anesthesia plus intracameral lidocaine in providing "good operative conditions for the surgeon and comfortable surgical circumstances for the patient" [18]. Also, there appears to be no difference by gender in the level of pain perception. Gupta *el al.* found that patients who underwent cataract surgery under topical anesthesia perceive comparable pain and discomforted irrespective of their sex [5]. However, although both topical and intracameral anesthesia appears to be safe for phacoemulsification surgery, they are not totally safe for the ocular structures [19]. Intracameral lignocaine supplement is known to be more effective in decreasing the level of pain, but detailed research is lacking in terms of its toxicity [11] [20]. During short term *in-vitro* exposure, lidocaine HCL appeared to be safe to both human and rabbit endothelium but further *in vivo* and *vitro* studies were suggested by Kim *el al.* to determine long-term effects of intraocular lidocaine on the corneal endothelium [21]. In a metanalaysis by Ezra *et al.*, it was found that intracameral lidocaine reduced intra-operative pain during cataract surgery under topical anaesthesia but possible adverse effects of intracameral lidocaine could not be excluded and they had reservations regarding recommending this additional intervention [22].

There have been many studies on the effectiveness and safety of topical anesthesia for phacoemulsification with intraocular lens implantation. However, there has been no comparative study on the number of drops adequate for the procedure. Therefore, our objective was to compare the efficacy of 2 versus 3 drops 0.5% eye drops for phacoemulsification surgery with intraocular lens implantation. In our study, there was no statistically significant difference in the mean patient-reported pain scores for overall pain between the two groups (P = 0.055). Similarly, there was no statistically significant difference in the mean patient cooperation for surgery between the two groups (P = 0. 597). The mean pain score was 1.24 ± 0.534 and the mean patient cooperation score was 1.11 ± 0.314. There was no difference in the VAS score by gender (P = 0.500). This is in agreement with Gupta *et al.* [5]. There was also no statistically significant difference in the mean VAS score between right and left eyes (P = 0.124). No additional drops were required for either group.

Different authors have used different anaesthetics for phacoemulsification in their studies and have got different VAS scores. The mean VAS score in the study by Pandey *et al.* was 1.44 ± 1.04 [3]. They used 4% Xylocaine. It was 4.19 ± 2.321 in the study by Tsoumani *et al.* [7]. They used 0.5% tetracaine. Similarly, the mean VAS scores were 1.53 ± 0.29 and 1.171 ± 1.50 in the study by Soliman *et al.* and Joshi RS respectively [4] [8].

Table 3. Parameters and scores.

Parameters	P values		
	By groups	By gender	By eye
Pain scale (0 - 10) [2]	0.055	0.500	0.124
Patient cooperation (0 - 3) [5]	0.597	0.969	0.244
Surgical time (minutes)	0.739	0.900	0.407

Table 4. Comparison of mean VAS scores and anaesthetics used in different studies.

Study	Mean VAS score	Anaesthetics used	Subjects (n)
Pandey et al. [3]	1.44 ± 1.04	4% Xylocaine drop, intracameral Xylocaine.	51
Tsoumani et al. [7]	4.19 ± 2.321	0.5% tetracaine, Lidocaine 2% gel.	90
Soliman et al. [8]	1.53 ± 0.29	Lido 2%, 0.5% bupivacaine, Benoxinate 0.4%.	295
Joshi RS [4]	1.171 ± 1.50	0.5% proparacaine drop, 0.5% intracameral Xylocaine.	75
Present study	1.24 ± 0.534	0.5% proparacaine drops.	100

Soliman *et al.* used 0.5% bupivacaine whereas Joshi used 0.5% proparacaine [4] [8]. In our study, we used 0.5% proparacaine which was similar to that of Joshi *et al.* The mean pain score in our study is comparable to the mean pain score found in these similar studies using different topical anesthetics (**Table 4**).

To conclude, our study has shown that topical anaesthesia with both 2 drops and 3 drops proparacaine 0.5% ophthalmic solution is effective for phacoemulsification with intraocular lens implantation and that 2 drops of proparacaine are adequate for this procedure. Topical anesthesia is a standard form of anesthesia accepted for phacoemulsification surgery but requires experienced surgeon and faster surgery. Therefore, the choice of anesthesia has to be individualised depending upon the surgeon's experience and operative comfort and taking into account patients' conditions and requirements. It is suggested that to minimise the amount of medication and its toxicity, 2 drops of 0.5% proparacaine HCL is adequate for phacoemulsification surgery with intraocular lens implantation in routine cases in expert hands. Intracameral anaesthesia or other additional form of anesthesia may be unnecessary in these cases.

References

[1] Malik, A., Fletcher, E.C., Chong, V. and Dasan, J. (2010) Local Anesthesia for Cataract Surgery. *Journal of Cataract & Refractive Surgery*, **36**, 133-152. http://dx.doi.org/10.1016/j.jcrs.2009.10.025

[2] Stevens, J.D. (1992) A New Local Anaesthesia Technique for Cataract Extraction by One Quadrant Sub-Tenon's Infiltration. *British Journal of Ophthalmology*, **76**, 670-674. http://dx.doi.org/10.1136/bjo.76.11.670

[3] Pandey, S.K., Wener, L. and Apple, D.J., *et al.* (2001) No-Anaesthesia Clear Corneal Phacoemulsification versus Topical and Topical plus Intracameral Anesthesia. Randomized clinical trial. *Journal of Cataract & Refractive Surgery*, **27**, 1643-1650. http://dx.doi.org/10.1016/S0886-3350(01)00793-3

[4] Joshi, R.S. (2013) A Single Drop of 0.5% Proparacaine Hydrochloride for Uncomplicated Clear Corneal Phacoemulsification. *Middle East African Journal of Ophthalmology*, **20**, 221-224. http://dx.doi.org/10.4103/0974-9233.114795

[5] Gupta, S.K., Kumar, A. and Agarwal, S. (2010) Cataract Surgery under Topical Anesthesia: Gender-Based Study of Pain Experience. *Oman Journal of Ophthalmology*, **3**, 140-144. http://dx.doi.org/10.4103/0974-620X.71893

[6] Duguid, I.G.M., Claque, C.M.P., Thamby-Rajah, Y., *et al.* (1995) Topical Anaesthesia for Phacoemulsification Surgery. *Eye*, **9**, 456-459. http://dx.doi.org/10.1038/eye.1995.106

[7] Tsoumani, A.T., Asproudis, I.C. and Damigos, D. (2010) Tetracaine 0.5% Eyedrops with or without Lidocaine 2% Gel in Topical Anesthesia for Cataract Surgery. *Journal of Clinical Ophthalmology*, **4**, 967-970. http://dx.doi.org/10.2147/OPTH.S11755

[8] Soliman, M.M., Macky, T.A. and Samir, M.K. (2004) Comparative Clinical Trial of Topical Anesthetic Agents in Cataract Surgery: Lidocaine 2% Gel, Bupivacaine 0.5% Drops and Benoxinate 0.4% Drops. *Journal of Cataract & Refractive Surgery*, **30**, 1716-1720. http://dx.doi.org/10.1016/j.jcrs.2003.12.034

[9]   Waheeb, S. (2010) Topical Anesthesia in Phakoemulsification. *Oman Journal of Ophthalmology*, **3**, 136-139. http://dx.doi.org/10.4103/0974-620X.71892

[10]   O'Brian, P.D., Fulcher, T., Wallace, D. and Power, W. (2001) Patient Pain during Different Stages of Phacoemulsification Using Topical Anesthesia. *Journal of Cataract & Refractive Surgery*, **27**, 880-883. http://dx.doi.org/10.1016/S0886-3350(00)00757-4

[11]   Hasan, S.A., Edelhauser, H.F. and Kim, T. (2001) Topical/Intracameral Anesthesia for Cataract Surgery. *Survey of Ophthalmology*, **46**, 178-181. http://dx.doi.org/10.1016/S0039-6257(01)00248-X

[12]   Patel, B.C., Burns, T.A., Crandall, A., Shomaker, S.T., Pace, N.L., van Eerd, A. and Clinch, T. (1996) A Comparison of Topical and Retrobulbar Anesthesia for Cataract Surgery. *Ophthalmology*, **8**, 1196-1203. http://dx.doi.org/10.1016/S0161-6420(96)30522-8

[13]   Oberg, T.J., Sider, S., Jorgensen, A.J. and Mifflin, M.D. (2012) Topical-Intracameral Anesthesia without Preoperative Mydriatic Agents for Descemet-Stripping Automated Endothelial Keratoplasty and Phacoemulsification Cataract Surgery with Intraocular Lens Implantation. *Journal of Cataract & Refractive Surgery*, **38**, 384-386. http://dx.doi.org/10.1016/j.jcrs.2011.12.025

[14]   Rizvi, Z., Rehman, T., Malik, S., Qureshi, A., Paul, L., Qureshi, K., *et al.* (2003) An Evaluation of Topical and Local Anesthesia in Phacoemulsification. *Journal of Pakistan Medical Association*, **53**, 167-170.

[15]   Monestam, E., Kusik, M. and Wachtmeister, L. (2001) Topical Anesthesia for Cataract Surgery: A Population-Based Perspective. *Journal of Cataract & Refractive Surgery*, **27**, 445-451. http://dx.doi.org/10.1016/S0886-3350(00)00637-4

[16]   Kim, M.J. and Jain, S. (2013) What Makes a Good Operation Great? Factors Determining Patient Satisfaction with Local Anaesthesia in Cataract Surgery. *Eye*, **27**, 1114. http://dx.doi.org/10.1038/eye.2013.125

[17]   Sarkar, S., Maiti, P., Nag, S., Sasmal, N.K. and Biswas, M. (2010) Changing Trends of Ocular Anaesthesia in Phacoemulsification Surgery. *Journal of Indian Medical Association*, **108**, 823-825.

[18]   Crandall, A.S., Zabriskie, N.A., Patel, B.C., Burns, T.A., Mamalis, N., Malmquist-Carter, L.A. and Yee, R. (1999) A Comparison of Patient Comfort during Cataract Surgery with Topical Anesthesia versus Topical Anesthesia and Intracameral Lidocaine. *Ophthalmology*, **106**, 60-66. http://dx.doi.org/10.1016/S0161-6420(99)90007-6

[19]   Shah, R. (2010) Anesthesia for Cataract Surgery: Recent Trends. *Oman Journal of Ophthalmology*, **3**, 107-108. http://dx.doi.org/10.4103/0974-620X.71881

[20]   Lofoco, G., Ciucci, F., Bardocci, A., Quercioli, P., De Gaetano, C., Ghirelli, G., *et al.* (2008) Efficacy of Topical plus Intracameral Anesthesia for Cataract Surgery in High Myopia: Randomised Controlled Trial. *Journal of Cataract Refractive Surgery*, **34**, 1664-1668. http://dx.doi.org/10.1016/j.jcrs.2008.06.019

[21]   Kim, T., Holley, B.S., Lee, J.H., Broocker, G. and Edelhauser, H.F. (1998) The Effects of Intraocular Lidocaine on the Corneal Endothelium. *Ophthalmology*, **105**, 125-130. http://dx.doi.org/10.1016/S0161-6420(98)91666-9

[22]   Ezra, D.G., Nambiar, A. and Allan, B.D. (2008) Supplementary Intracameral Lidocaine for Phacoemulsification under Topical Anesthesia: A Meta-Analysis of Randomized Controlled Trials. *Ophthalmology*, **115**, 455-487. http://dx.doi.org/10.1016/j.ophtha.2007.09.021

25

Exogenous Endophthalmitis Due to Illicit Drug Injection in an I.V. Drug User

Seyed Ali Tabatabaei, Mohammad Soleimani*, Mohammad Reza Mansouri, Mohammad Ebrahimi, Parisa Abdi, Mohammad Riazi Esfahani

Eye Research Center, Farabi Eye Hospital, Tehran University of Medical Sciences, Iran
Email: *Soleimani_md@yahoo.com

Abstract

Background: Drug abuse could cause complications; infection and overdose are the most prevalent of them. Unreliable history of addicted patients also makes the diagnosis difficult and leads to delayed treatment and poor prognosis. Early recognition and prompt treatment are required to minimize the destructive damage. To our knowledge, there is not any previous report of bilateral eye injection among drug abusers, causing traumatic endophthalmitis in the English literature and our report helps ophthalmologists to think about rare sources of endophthalmitis. Aim: The aim is to emphasize the importance of considering exogenous endophthalmitis in I.V. drug users who abuse drugs. Methods: A 40-year-old I.V. drug user man was referred complaining a history of the pain, redness and impaired vision of both eyes from three days ago. Perilimbal injection and anterior chamber cellular reaction were present in both eyes. Both corneas were hazy; corneal edema, abscess, sealed corneal lacerations and dull red reflex were visible in both eyes. Results: After an ultrasonography based on the suspicion of endophthalmitis, anterior chamber and vitreous aspiration and intravitreal injection of vancomycin 1 mg and ceftazidime 2.25 mg were performed. The right eye rapidly deteriorated and was eviscerated two days later and the left eye had a good response to medications. Conclusion: This report illustrates that the orbit can be a potential site of drug injection and endophthalmitis should be considered in individuals who abuse drugs.

Keywords

Endophthalmitis, IV Drug User, Addiction, Trauma

1. Introduction

Endophthalmitis is an ocular emergency potentially leading to poor prognosis. It is known as an intraocular in-

---

*Corresponding author.

fection and is classified to exogenous type due to ocular surgery or trauma, and endogenous type. Intravenous drug abuse is a known risk factor of endogenous endophthalmitis. Common organisms isolated in these patients are gram-positive cocci (streptococcus and staphylococcus), bacillus species and fungi. Early recognition of signs and symptoms and prompt treatment with systemic and intravitreal antibiotics and vitrectomy is required to minimize the destructive damage [1].

Drug abuse could cause many complications; infection and overdose are the most prevalent of them. Searching for new sites for injection could lead to uncommon complications of drug abuse. Unreliable history taken from addicted patients also makes the diagnosis difficult and leads to delayed treatment and poor prognosis.

2. Case Presentation

A 40-year-old I.V. male drug (heroin) abuser was referred to the emergency ward, complaining of a history of pain, redness and impaired vision of both eyes from three days ago. The patient denied any other drug use or trauma and his past medical history was negative according to his statements. The visual acuities in the right and left eyes were no light perception and counting fingers, respectively. Perilimbal injection and lid swelling were present in both eyes especially in the right eye. Both corneas were hazy; corneal edema and abscess as well as dull red reflex were visible in both eyes. Slit lamp examination demonstrated sealed corneal lacerations and scars in both eyes as signs of penetrating injury at the inferior site of both corneas. Cellular and fibrinous reaction was prominent in anterior chamber of both eyes. The left eye had a focal sealed anterior lens capsular rupture and localized traumatic cataract. There were vitreous opacities in both eyes and fundus examination was impossible (**Figure 1**). However the patient declared bilateral eye injections the day after admission.

After performing ultrasonography based on the suspicion of endophthalmitis, anterior chamber and vitreous aspiration was performed and intravitreal injection of vancomycin 1 mg and ceftazidime 2.25 mg was performed. Also the patient was admitted and intravenous antibiotics (vancomycin 1 gr twice a day and ceftazidime 1 gr three times a day) were administered. The smear of vitreous and AC aspiration were reported as gram-positive cocci and the culture showed the staphylococcus aureus growth, which was susceptible to the administered antibiotics. Other lab data were unremarkable. The right eye condition rapidly deteriorated and it was eviscerated two days later (following performing pars plana vitrectomy showing numerous abscesses in vitreous the day before) and the left eye had a good response to medications and the patient was discharged because he did not give consent for cataract surgery.

Injection of illicit drugs can cause many local and systemic infections. Cutaneous infections and endocarditis are the most common complications [2]. Intravenous drug addiction often results in searching for new sites of

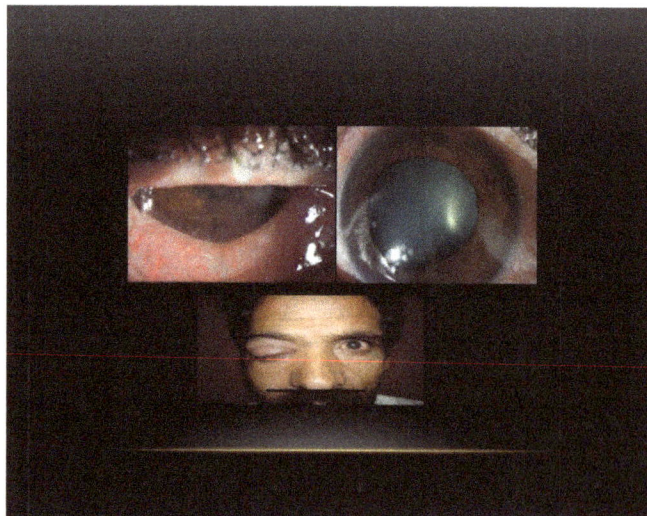

Figure 1. Right eye slit photograph shows multiple injection scars inferior of the cornea (left upper picture), left eye slit photograph shows sealed scarred corneal lacerations (Left upper picture); patient's face (lower picture).

injection. When most of the peripheral veins have been used up, the addict patient approaches the skin (subcutaneous injection) and other unusual sites that can cause unusual complications such as abscesses and tissue necrosis [3]. There are many reported cases of unusual injection sites. For example, White *et al.* have reported a case of penile ulceration caused by drug injection [4], Alvi *et al.* and Holt *et al.* have reported cases of breast ulceration following drug abuse [5] [6] and Hawkins *et al.* have reported a case of Horner's syndrome due to sympathetic damage after injection into neck area [7].

In addition to the systemic consequences, common ocular manifestations of drug abuse include corneal ulcers, endogenous endophthalmitis and talc retinopathy [2]. However, several uncommon cases have been reported showing drug abuse directly affecting the eye. For example, a case of cocaine instillation into conjunctival fornix has been reported to lead to bilateral corneal ulcer [8]. Ghosheh *et al.* have reported a case of orbital cellulitis and superior ophthalmic vein thrombosis due to injecting heroin directly into the orbit [2]. Blackmon *et al.* have reported a case of periorbital injection of drugs that caused bacillus endophthalmitis and lens subluxation [9].

Endophthalmitis is the inflammation of the interior ocular tissue and is typically classified as postoperative, posttraumatic, or endogenous [10]. Although hematogenous spreading of pathogens resulted from drug injection is a known uncommon cause of endophthalmitis [10], direct exogenous traumatic endophthalmitis is rarely considered among drug abusers. Exogenous endophthalmitis is resulted from penetration into the eye such as in postoperative endophthalmitis. Exogenous endophthalmitis was resulted from direct traumatic injection into the eye in our case. Endophthalmitis can have a rapid progression and prognosis is related to prompt diagnosis and treatment. Unreliable history among drug abusers and their tendency not to reveal drug abuse can lead to delayed diagnosis and poor outcomes, so a high degree of suspicion is required for correct diagnosis.

This report illustrates that the orbit can be a potential site of drug injection and endophthalmitis should be considered in individuals who abuse drugs. To our knowledge there is not any previous report of bilateral eye injection among drug abusers, causing traumatic endophthalmitis, in the English literature and our report helps ophthalmologists to think about rare sources of endophthalmitis.

Conflicts of Interest

None.

References

[1]   Mathews, A.S., Pillai, G.S., Natasha, R. and Shetty, M. (2011) Endogenous Endophthalmitis—A Review. *Kerala Journal of Ophthalmology*, **23**, 25-31.

[2]   Ghosheh, F.R. and Kathuria, S.S. (2006) Intraorbital Heroin Injection Resulting in Orbital Cellulitis and Superior Ophthalmic Vein Thrombosis. *Ophthalmic Plastic & Reconstructive Surgery*, **22**, 473-475. http://dx.doi.org/10.1097/01.iop.0000248991.71690.eb

[3]   Del Giudice, P. (2004) Cutaneous Complications of Intravenous Drug Abuse. *British Journal of Dermatology*, **150**, 1-10. http://dx.doi.org/10.1111/j.1365-2133.2004.05607.x

[4]   White, W.B. and Barrett, S. (1982) Penile Ulcer in Heroin Abuse: A Case Report. *Cutis*, **29**, 62-63, 69.

[5]   Alvi, A. and Ravichandran, D. (2006) An Unusual Case of Breast Ulceration. *Breast*, **15**, 115-116. http://dx.doi.org/10.1016/j.breast.2004.11.004

[6]   Holt, R.W. and Miller, D.L. (1988) Cocaine Abuse and Unusual Injection Sites. *Annals of Emergency Medicine*, **17**, 186-187. http://dx.doi.org/10.1016/S0196-0644(88)80332-9

[7]   Hawkins, K.A., Bruckstein, A.H. and Guthrie, T.C. (1977) Percutaneous Heroin Injection Causing Horner Syndrome. *JAMA*, **237**, 1963-1964. http://dx.doi.org/10.1001/jama.1977.03270450053022

[8]   Ravin, J.G. and Ravin, L.C. (1979) Blindness Due to Illicit Use of Topical Cocaine. *Annals of Ophthalmology*, **11**, 863-864.

[9]   Blackmon, D.M., Calvert, H.M., Henry, P.M. and Westfall, C.T. (2000) Bacillus Cereus Endophthalmitis Secondary to Self-Inflicted Periocular Injection. *Arch Ophthalmol*, **118**, 1585-1586. http://dx.doi.org/10.1001/archopht.118.11.1585

[10] Kim, R.W., Juzych, M.S. and Eliott, D. (2002) Ocular Manifestations of Injection Drug Use. *Infectious Disease Clinics of North America*, **16**, 607-622. http://dx.doi.org/10.1016/S0891-5520(02)00013-2

26

Suicide after Excimer Laser Refractive Surgery: On the Importance of Matching Expectations

Gysbert van Setten

St Eriks Eye Hospital, Karolinska Institutet, Stockholm, Sweden
Email: gysbert-botho.vansetten@sankterik.se

Abstract

Background: Refractive surgery may change the individual life to the better largely eliminating the need for spectacles. However, expectations may vary and postoperative reality may come as a surprise. Aim: To emphasize the need for thorough alignment of expectations and options between surgeon and patient. Methods: A case is presented in which a successful refractive laser operation is a part of a trigger mechanism for a depressive episode leading to suicide. It emphasizes the crucial importance of constructive alignment of expectations between patient and treating physician prior to surgery. Results: The case presented outlines that ophthalmic surgery at the edge of high-tec with all its tempting features is also very attractive to individuals with very well defined and less flexible expectations. The possible irreversibility of some of the refractive surgery may force the patient postoperatively into a psychological corner, immobilizing him/her and restricting his/her options. Conclusions: High-tec operations dealing with one of the most elementary senses we have, vision, demand a thorough estimation of the patients profile prior to any surgery. Only matching expectations between the possible and desired outcome and reconfirmation of the match may reduce the risk of postoperative crisis which may carry a risk the patient's life.

Keywords

Suicide, Excimer Laser Surgery, Ophthalmology, Refractive Surgery

1. Introduction

It is known that some ocular diseases such as glaucoma, chronic inflammation and decreased visual acuity may lead to depression [1]-[5]. Depression is known to possibly lead to suicide attempts. However, suicide attempts following ophthalmic surgery are the exception as no such case has (to the best knowledge of the author) this far been reported. Excimer surgery has been accepted very well by suitable patients and the success rate is very high [6]. However, the persons undergoing excimer laser surgery have often high expectations and the demand for a successful outcome is imminent. Hence, the current draw backs of excimer laser surgery such as halos, glares etc. often cause more discomfort that the bare clinical picture would allow to expect. As commonly known, such side effects are mostly temporary. However, an extremely rare but very severe incident after excimer laser surgery has been observed which has not been reported earlier.

2. The Case

A young patient, age 33 (altered in order to protect the identity of the individual), was operated on both eyes for the existing myopia with excimer laser. There was a history of a period with psychological instability many years ago and the patient had received psychiatric consultancy that successfully solved the crisis. A few weeks after an uneventful excimer laser surgery the patient appeared at the emergency ward of an ophthalmological clinic. The patient was deeply depressive due to the result of the operation which resulted in emmetropia. Having missed the myopic condition the patient wanted the same to be reinstalled. This was attempted to be achieved by buying hyperopic contact lenses via internet, without achieving the desired result. The patient had in the meantime also consulted a psychiatrist who tried to help him accept the new conditions of sight. The ophthalmological examination showed a visual acuity of 16/20 on the right and 20/20 on the left eye without correction. The cornea showed only minor traces of the recently performed operation which clinically has led to the desired outcome. The patient complained of dryness and irritation and was prescribed lubricating drops and ointments. Such complaint has been increasingly reported after excimer laser surgery but is still considered to be transient. Dry eye complaints and effects themselves are known to have a negative effect on the quality of life [7].

However, a few weeks passed until the patient presented himself again at the eye clinic again at night in an acute stage of depression due to the refractive condition achieved complaining that the current situation as interfering with working capacity and capability. The visual acuity was the same and reading at distance was achieved with an addition of +1.75 dpt. It was considered that a possible overcorrection towards hyperopia has been the cause of the patients complaint but the refraction in cycloplegia showed a nearly perfect condition close to emmetropic condition with an astigmatism not exceeding −0.75 dpt. After a long discussion the patient relaxed and could be convinced that the problem could be solved by fitting suitable spectacles after an appointment with an ophthalmologist or an optician. The patient left the clinic in a condition that was considered psychologically stabilized. However, the patient appeared again a few weeks later, again during midnight hours, and again in a depressive state and after having consumed alcohol. There was not yet any further arrangement for an appointment with the ophthalmologist but the patient promised to return to arrange this at working hours to make this visit happen. Concerned about the psychological state, psychological consultancy was offered to the patient. This offer was declined by the patient saying that such a visit happened just the day before. The patient left the clinic with the promise to come back next morning to get the specialist consultancy performed.

The patient never came back. Instead, the author was informed some weeks later that the patient had committed suicide.

3. Discussion

Although depression has been considered the main cause of this suicide, it can not be excluded that desperation about the clinical outcome of the refractive surgery might have been one element in the decision process.

Although an event like this is extremely rare, the impact to the social environment and the importance for the ophthalmological surgeons is so high that I feel urged to convey this event to the ophthalmologic and medical community in order to emphasize the extremely important role of the preoperative evaluation of motivation and indication for refractive surgery. A number of factors and variables that do not usually come together like they did in this case could have certainly played a role the case presented. The decision behind a suicide seldom based on one event only although this does depends on the impact the event has or the impact value as it is perceived by the patient. However, it is strongly suggested that any patient with the history of psychological treatment or consultation in the past, no matter how long before this might have been, should receive a psychological evaluation before any refractive surgery is performed. After all are amongst the predictors of suicide male gender, mental illness, and ongoing or previous psychiatric treatment [8] (Nordentoft 2007). As this tragic case shows, our psychological understanding and training as ophthalmologists is probably not always sufficient enough to judge if this type of surgery is suitable for this special category of patients. Hence, if there is any indicator of mental illness, further tests currently available [9] (Terluin *et al.* 2009), should be applied by professionals prior to any treatment.

4. Conclusion

If there is any suspicion that the expectations of surgical outcome and the definition of success of both patient and surgeon do not completely match, no surgery should be performed. Extensive counselling and inculcating realistic expectations prior to excimer surgery have been recommended earlier [10]. The nature of refractive surgery as a voluntary procedure does emphasize the need for sufficient and thorough information on all known and the individual aspects of the procedure. For any individual with high demands and having a history of psychological weakness, any outcome worse than expected can be devastating. The importance of the occupation in the gap between expectations and perceptions has been reported [11]. It is strongly recommended to alter the selection of patients for excimer surgery giving higher value to the psychological background and considering any history of psychological abnormality as a relative contraindication for excimer laser treatment. Although extremely rare, this case shows what surgery might lead to, when the patient's expectations are not fully understood.

Commercial Interests

Commercial Interests: None.

Acknowledgements

The author is very thankful to Aviation-Ophthalmology, Danderyd, Sweden for the support allowing the publication of this manuscript.

References

[1]   Mabuchi, F., Yoshimura, K., Kashiwagi, K., Shioe, K., Yamagata, Z., Kanba, S., Iijima, H. and Tsukahara, S. (2008) High Prevalence of Anxiety and Depression in Patients with Primary Open-Angle Glaucoma. *Journal of Glaucoma*, **17**, 552-557. http://dx.doi.org/10.1097/IJG.0b013e31816299d4

[2]   Popescu, M.L., Boisjoly, H., Schmaltz, H., Kergoat, M.J., Rousseau, J., Moghadaszadeh, S., Djafari, F. and Freeman, E.E. (2012) Explaining the Relationship between Three Eye Diseases and Depressive Symptoms in Older Adults. *Investigative Ophthalmology & Visual Science*, **53**, 2308-2313. http://dx.doi.org/10.1167/iovs.11-9330

[3]   Wang, S.Y., Singh, K. and Lin, S.C. (2012) Prevalence and Predictors of Depression among Participants with Glaucoma in a Nationally Representative Population Sample. *American Journal of Ophthalmology*, **154**, 436-444. http://dx.doi.org/10.1016/j.ajo.2012.03.039

[4]   Maca, S.M., Wagner, J., Weingessel, B. and Vécsei-Marlovits, P.V. (2013) Acute Anterior Uveitis Is Associated with Depression and Reduction of General Health. *British Journal of Ophthalmology*, **97**, 333-337. http://dx.doi.org/10.1136/bjophthalmol-2012-302304

[5]   Li, M., Gong, L., Sun, X. and Chapin, W.J. (2011) Anxiety and Depression in Patients with Dry Eye Syndrome. *Current Eye Research*, **36**, 1-7. http://dx.doi.org/10.3109/02713683.2010.519850

[6]   McAlinden, C., Skiadaresi, E. and Moore, J.E. (2011) Visual and Refractive Outcomes Following Myopic Laser-Assisted Subepithelial Keratectomy with a Flying-Spot Excimer Laser. *Journal of Cataract & Refractive Surgery*, **37**, 901-906. http://dx.doi.org/10.1016/j.jcrs.2011.01.013

[7]   Li, M., Gong, L., Chapin, W.J. and Zhu, M. (2012) Assessment of Vision-Related Quality of Life in Dry Eye Patients. *Investigative Ophthalmology & Visual Science*, **53**, 5722-5727. http://dx.doi.org/10.1167/iovs.11-9094

[8]   Nordentoft, M. (2007) Prevention of Suicide and Attempted Suicide in Denmark. Epidemiological Studies of Suicide and Intervention Studies in Selected Risk Groups. *Danish Medical Bulletin*, **54**, 306-369.

[9]   Terluin, B., Brouwers, E.P., van Marwijk, H.W., Verhaak, P. and van der Horst, H.E. (2009) Detecting Depressive and Anxiety Disorders in Distressed Patients in Primary Care; Comparative Diagnostic Accuracy of the Four-Dimensional Symptom Questionnaire (4DSQ) and the Hospital Anxiety and Depression Scale (HADS). *BMC Family Practice*, **10**, 58. http://dx.doi.org/10.1186/1471-2296-10-58

[10] Shah, S., Perera, S. and Chatterjee, A (1998) Satisfaction after Photorefractive Keratectomy. *Journal of Refractive Surgery*, **14**, S226-S227.

[11] Lin, D.J., Sheu, I.C., Pai, J.Y., Bair, A., Hung, C.Y., Yeh, Y.H. and Chou, M.J. (2009) Measuring Patient's Expectation and the Perception of Quality in LASIK Services. *Health and Quality of Life Outcomes*, **7**, 63.
http://dx.doi.org/10.1186/1477-7525-7-63

27

Periorbital Necrotizing Fasciitis Caused by Streptococcus Viridians

Belinda Pustina, Naser Salihu

Department of Ophthalmology, University Clinical Center of Kosovo, Prishtina, Kosovo
Email: belindapustina@gmail.com

Abstract

Necrotizing fasciitis (NF) is a life threatening soft tissue infection characterized by necrosis of fascia and subcutaneous tissue. If this disease is misdiagnosed and mistreated, because of the fast spreading, it can lead to death. Prompt treatment with antibiotics and surgical debridement is necessary and lifesaving in this disease. In uncomplicated cases and early stages of the disease it can be treated only with intravenous antibiotics. This study presents a 70-year-old female, farmer who approached in our clinic with edema of periorbital region and a minor trauma in her lower eyelid. First skin anthrax of eyelids was considered in differential diagnosis, because the patient was in contact with animals. Culture taken from the wound resulted positive for *Streptococcus viridians* α hemolytic Streptococcus: the viridians group. Treatment with Ceftriaxone + Penicillin was initiated immediately. Patient responded to intravenous antibiotics and after 2 days the edema began to regress. After 2 weeks patient was discharged from the hospital and the clinical outcome was satisfactory. Based on this case early diagnosed necrotizing fasciitis may be treated only with antibiotics.

Keywords

Periorbital Necrotizing Fasciitis, Streptococcus Viridians, Minor Trauma

1. Introduction

Periorbital NF caused by Streptococcus viridians is a severe and uncommon bacterial infection primary involving superficial fascia and subcutaneous tissue. Minor trauma may be the way for bacteria to enter subcutaneous tissue.

Treatment of necrotizing fasciitis involves intravenous antibiotics and surgical debridement. Delayed treatment is associated with increased morbidity and mortality [1]. Streptococcus produces toxins in the blood which causes Systemic Inflammatory Response (SIRS) that may lead to septic shock [2] and death [3] [4].

Even though aggressive surgical debridement should be started as soon as possible, there are some case reports supporting the evidence that in selected uncomplicated cases there is no need for aggressive surgical debridement in necrotizing fasciitis. They can be treated only with antibiotics [5]-[7].

In this study we represent a case of periorbital NF after minor trauma that was successfully treated only with systemic antibiotics, because it was diagnosed in early stages.

2. Case Presentation

A 70-year-old female farmer with diabetes was presented in our clinic with edema of the eyelids and right periorbital region. She came to our clinic in a febrile and lethargic condition. Diffuse eyelid swelling was noticed. Although she had skin anesthesia she was complaining for the pain. The skin was pink to purple color. On clinical examination she had edema and discharge in her upper eyelid and lower eyelid. In the lower eyelid there was a minor wound that looked like an insect bite (**Figure 1**). It was ulcerated with the crust and had raised margins. Crusts and necrosis was noticed also (**Figure 2**). Since she was at contact with animals, and farmers are at great risk of exposure to infected materials of animals, skin anthrax was considered.

Culture was taken from the wound and resulted positive for Streptococcus Viridians. Intravenous Ceftriaxone 2 g q12 h and Penicilin G 4 milion q4h units IV in three divided doses was applied immediately. The clinical signs regressed only with antibiotic therapy. After two days the edema started to regress and the clinical condition started to improve (**Figure 3**). Eyes were also examined and there were no pathological findings in her right eye. The visual acuity and intraocular tension were normal.

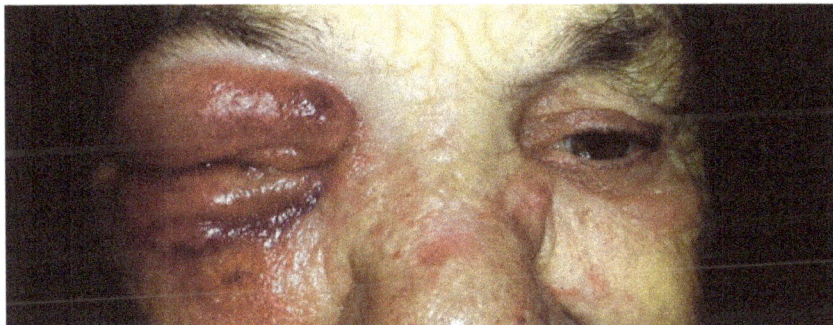

Figure 1. Periorbital edema with tissue necrosis, violet discoloration and fluid filled bullae.

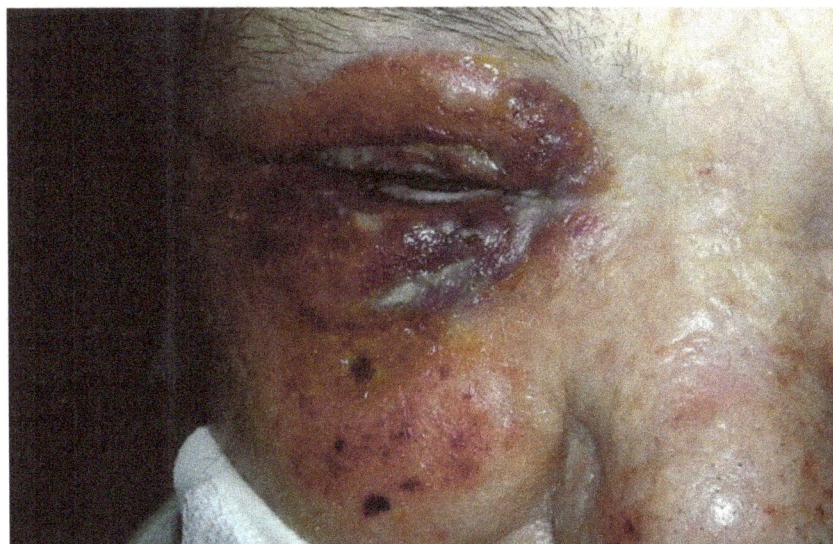

Figure 2. Crusts and necrosis of eyelids.

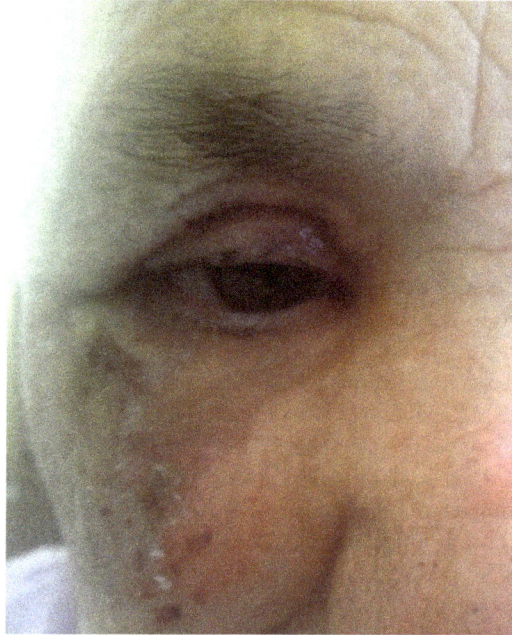

Figure 3. Regression of edema and necrosis of eyelids.

3. Discussion

Based on the involved layer infections of periorbital soft tissue with necrosis can be classified as cellulitis, fasciitis or myositis [8]. NF is a rare, rapidly progressive infection of soft tissue. Periorbital NF is uncommon because of the excellent blood supply to that area [9].

There are some types of the NF. Type I infections are polymicrobial, they are more often and tend to occur in patients with significant co-morbidities such as diabetes or cancer in which host defenses are compromised favoring the development of these infections.

Type II infections are caused by group A Streptococcus and are most common in otherwise healthy individuals with a history of trauma, intravenous drug abuse or surgery [10].

Rarity of the disease leads to misdiagnosis and mistreatment. Necrotizing fasciitis should not be misdiagnosed with preseptal cellulitis and orbital cellulitis. The differences between them are presence of cyanosis (violet discoloration) and serous fluid filled bullae [11].

Antibiotics may not be enough, because of the possibility of thrombosis in blood vessels in that region, that's why debridement is needed in complicated cases. To avoid ectropion and keratitis during debridement underlying muscles and eyelids must be protected [12] [13].

Based on a BOSU study in UK an incidence of 0.24 per 1.000.000 NF per annum was identified over a 2-year period. β hemolytic Streptococcus A was identified in 76% and systemic complications in 66.66% with sepsis and death occurred in 10% [14].

It is reported mainly in adults with a female predominance 54% were about one half previously healthy. Following blunt trauma were reported 17%, penetrating injury 22% and 11% after face surgery. In 28% no cause was identify [15].

Even though periorbital NF is a rare disease it should be considered after minor trauma in patients with weaken immune system as in this case with diabetes.

It is difficult to differentiate it from other common soft tissue infections. One of the infections that should be considered is skin anthrax. It is important to have suspicions especially in cases with history of contact with animals or animal products. Although the history is very important in putting the right diagnosis gram staining and culture confirm the diagnosis [16].

Periorbital redness and edema leading to a formation of large bullae and skin color progressing from rose to blue gray are characteristics of periorbital NF. Also one of the signs that can lead to diagnosis of NF is complaint of pain and anesthesia over the affected area and swelling around the lesion. One of the signs that can increase the suspicion of the skin anthrax is black eschar, not seen in NF [17] [18].

In conclusion periorbital NF is a rare disease and if it's not diagnosed in early stages it can cause serious and life threatening problems. The viridians group of α hemolytic Streptococcus should be considered in etiology of periorbital necrotizing fasciitis after minor trauma in patients with co-morbidities. Warning signs that can lead us to right diagnosis are violet skin discoloration and skin anesthesia. Early treatment may prevent functional and esthetic side effects.

4. Conclusion

Necrotizing fasciitis in early and uncomplicated stages may be treated successfully only with conservative treatment.

Disclosure

The authors declare that there is no conflict of interests regarding the publication of this paper.

References

[1] Lazzeri, D., Lazzeri, S., Figus, M., et al. (2010) Periorbital Necrotising Fasciitis. British Journal of Ophthalmology, 94, 1577-1585. http://dx.doi.org/10.1136/bjo.2009.167486

[2] Bustos, B.R., Soto, G.G., Hickmann, O.L. and Torres, B.C. (2009) Necrotizing Fasciitis of the Eyelids and Toxic Shock Syndrome Due to Streptococcus pyogenes. Revista Chilena de Infectología, 26, 152-155.

[3] Stevens, D.L. (2000) Streptococcal Toxic Shock Syndrome Associated with Necrotizing Fasciitis. Annual Review of Medicine, 51, 271-288. http://dx.doi.org/10.1146/annurev.med.51.1.271

[4] Sartelli, M. (2010) A Focus on Intra-Abdominal Infections. World Journal of Emergency Surgery, 5, 9. http://dx.doi.org/10.1186/1749-7922-5-9

[5] Majeski, J.A. and Alexander, J.W. (1983) Early Diagnosis, Nutritional Support and Immediate Extensive Debridement Improve Survival in Necrotizingfasciitis. American Journal of Surgery, 145, 784-787. http://dx.doi.org/10.1016/0002-9610(83)90140-X

[6] Lee Hooi, L., Hou, B.A. and Lay Leng, S. (2012) Group A Streptococcus Necrotizing Fasciitis of the Eyelid: A Case Report of Good Outcome with Medical Management. Ophthalmic Plastic Reconstructive Surgery, 28, e13-e15. http://dx.doi.org/10.1097/IOP.0b013e31821282ee

[7] Pessa, M.E. and Howard, R.J. (1985) Necrotizing Fasciitis. Surgery, Gynecology Obstetrics, 161, 357-361.

[8] McHenrv, C.R. and Malangoni, M.A. (1995) Necrotizing Soft Tissue Infections. In: Fry, D.E., Ed., Surgical Infections, Little, Brown and Co., Boston, 161-168.

[9] Kihiczak, G.G., Schwartz, R.A. and Kapila, R. (2006) Necrotizing Fasciitis: A Deadly Infection. Journal of the European Academy of Dermatology and Venereology, 20, 365-369. http://dx.doi.org/10.1111/j.1468-3083.2006.01487.x

[10] Kronish, J.W. and McLeish, W.M. (1991) Eyelid Necrosis and Periorbital Necrotizing Fasciitis. Report of a Case and Review of the Literature. Ophthalmology, 98, 92-98. http://dx.doi.org/10.1016/S0161-6420(91)32334-0

[11] Lazzeri, D., Lazzeri, S., Figus, M., et al. (2010) Periorbital Necrotizing Fasciitis. British Journal of Ophthalmology, 94, 1577-1585. http://dx.doi.org/10.1136/bjo.2009.167486

[12] Saldana, M., Gupta, D., Khandwala, M., Weir, R. and Beigi, B. (2010) Periorbital Necrotizing Fasciitis: Outcomes Using a CT-Guided Surgical Debridement Approach. European Journal of Ophthalmology, 20, 209-214.

[13] Stone, H.H. and Martin, J.D. (1972) Synergistic Necrotizing Cellulitis. Annals of Surgery, 175, 702-711. http://dx.doi.org/10.1097/00000658-197205000-00010

[14] Flavahan, P.W., Cauchi, P., Gregory, M.E., Foot, B. and Drummond, S.R. (2014) Incidence of Periorbital Necrotising Fasciitis in the UK Population: A BOSU Study. British Journal of Ophthalmology, 98, 1177-1180. http://dx.doi.org/10.1136/bjophthalmol-2013-304735

[15] Lazzeri, D., Lazzeri, S., Figus, M., Tascini, C., Bocci, G., Colizzi, L., Giannotti, G., Lorenzetti, F., Gandini, D., Danesi, R., Menichetti, F., Del Tacca, M., Nardi, M. and Pantaloni, M. (2010) Periorbital Necrotising Fasciitis. British Journal of Ophthalmology, 94, 1577-1585. http://dx.doi.org/10.1136/bjo.2009.167486

[16] Karahocagil, M.K., Akdeniz, N., Akdeniz, H., Calka, O., Karsen, H., Bilici, A., Bilgili, S.G. and Evirgen, O. (2008) Cutaneous Anthrax in Eastern Turkey: A Review of 85 Cases. Clinical and Experimental Dermatology, 33, 406-411. http://dx.doi.org/10.1111/j.1365-2230.2008.02742.x

[17] Kanski, J.J. (2003) Clinical Ophthalmology, a Systematic Approach. 5th Edition, Butterworth Heinemann, Elsevier Science Limited, Edinburgh, 9.

[18] American Academy of Ophthalmology (2004) Basic and Clinical Science Course. Orbit, Eyelids, and Lacrimal System: Section 7, 2004-2005. American Academy of Ophthalmology, San Francisco, 44.

28

The Missing Piece in Glaucoma?

Syed S. Hasnain

General Ophthalmology, Porterville, CA, USA
Email: hasnain40@sbcglobal.net

Abstract

Glaucoma is defined as an optic disc neuropathy meaning the nerve fibers are being atrophied similar to the fate occurring in non-glaucomatous optic atrophies. Furthermore, the nerve fibers are always being destroyed randomly in all the non-glaucomatous optic atrophies. In contrast, the nerve fibers in glaucoma are invariably destroyed in an orderly tandem fashion, from peripheral to central, never randomly. Is glaucoma really an optic disc neuropathy in light of orderly destruction of nerve fibers in glaucoma? The current prevailing theories in glaucoma such as posterior bowing of the lamina cribrosa or cupping can't explain the orderly destruction of nerve fibers occurring in glaucoma. In fact, there is no biological mechanism acting directly on the nerve fibers or their RGCs which could lead to their orderly destruction. Therefore, there should be some mechanical way, which could result in the orderly destruction of nerve fibers even though this mechanical scenario may have resulted from the direct biological effect of raised IOP on some important component of the optic disc. It is proposed that the border tissue of Elschnig (BT) atrophies due to chronic ischemia caused by raised IOP, and as a result, the lamina cribrosa (LC) begins sinking in the scleral canal—a mechanical problem. Due to sinking of the LC, the nerve fibers get stretched and broken starting with the most peripheral nerve fibers being closest to the edge of the scleral opening and ending with the most central nerve fibers in an orderly tandem fashion. Therefore, in view of the orderly destruction of nerve fibers, glaucoma may not be an optic disc neuropathy but an optic disc axotomy.

Keywords

Glaucoma, Normal Tension Glaucoma, Severance, Arcuate Field Defects, Disc Notching, Disc Hemorrhage, Sinking Disc, Cupping Disc, Excavated Disc, RNFL

1. Introduction

Chronic glaucoma has been a mystery ever since it was given a separate entity 160 years ago [1]. Ophthalmologists of the time found the optic discs of chronic glaucoma subjects being cupped, instead of being normally flat. It is presumed that the disc becomes cupped due to the force of raised intraocular pressure (IOP) resulting in atrophy and shrinkage of the nerve fibers. Until now, cupping of the disc and atrophy of the nerve fibers are still considered the salient features of the glaucomatous disc and thus glaucoma is defined as an optic disc neuropathy.

However, the concept of cupping disc and atrophy of the nerve fibers has failed to answer many pathognomonic features of glaucoma including predictable visual field defects. I believe the concept of cupping was given mistakenly in the 1850s, which has put us on the wrong path in glaucoma. One hundred years later, the term cup/disc ratio was introduced which gave further credence to the cupping concept but at the same time created conundrum in glaucoma diagnosis since ironically we started using the same parameter of "cupping" in describing both physiological as well as glaucomatous cupping of the disc.

It is imperative to mention the arrangement of nerve fibers in this discussion. There are three main aspects in which the nerve fibers are arranged in the retina and in the optic disc. First, the nerve fibers in the retina are arranged in layers superficial to deep. Second, the most central vision fibers originate closest to the disc, like most superficial (closest to vitreous) and exit from the most central part of the disc. In contrast, the most peripheral nerve fibers originate from the most distant retina or farthest from the optic disc, lie deepest (closest to sclera) and exit closest to the edge of the scleral opening, **Figure 1**. Third, the nerve fibers originating from the nasal retina proceed directly to the nasal part of the optic disc. However, the situation is different in the temporal retina because of the presence of the macular fibers. The nerve fibers originating from the nasal aspect of the macular area proceed directly to the central temporal part of the disc. The fibers originating from the temporal macular and peripheral retina have to arch above and below the macular fibers to reach the superior and inferior poles of the optic disc respectively and hence are known as the arcuate fibers.

We may differ on many aspects in glaucoma but on one issue we all have consensus: that the million or so nerve fibers densely packed in a disc are always invariably being destroyed, one by one, from peripheral to central in an orderly tandem fashion, and never randomly. If the nerve fibers are not destroyed in a predictable orderly sequence, the role of visual field tests in glaucoma would be meaningless.

The cupping disc/atrophy of the nerve fibers paradigm has failed to explain the orderly destruction of nerve fibers [2], which is hallmark of glaucoma. For any glaucoma theory to prevail, it must explain the orderly destruction of nerve fibers otherwise it will not be valid. In light of the orderly destruction of nerve fibers all the prevailing glaucoma theories such as the direct role of raised IOP, apoptosis, neurodegeneration [3], increased sensitivity of the disc to IOP, posterior bowing of the lamina cribrosa or cupping become wrong as none of them can explain the orderly destruction of nerve fibers occurring in glaucoma. If the nerve fibers are being destroyed

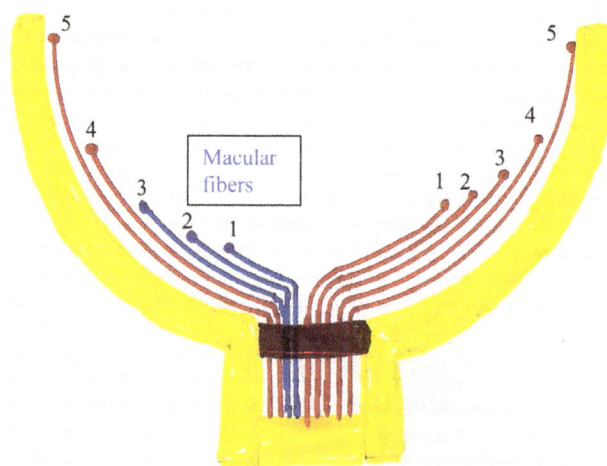

Figure 1. Arrangement of nerve fibers in the retina and optic disc. Most peripheral fiber (5) originates farthest from the disc, lies closest to the sclera and exit closest to the scleral edge. Most central fiber (1) originates closest to the disc, lies closest to vitreous and exits from the most central part of scleral opening.

in an orderly tandem fashion in glaucoma, then we should expect the mechanism for their destruction to be orderly as well.

In fact, there is no biological mechanism which acting directly on the nerve fibers or their RGCs could result in their orderly destruction. Therefore, for the orderly destruction of nerve fibers to occur in glaucoma, there must be some mechanical way even though that mechanical scenario may have resulted from the direct biological effect of raised IOP on some very important component of the optic disc.

2. What May Be the Mechanical Scenario?

The border tissue of Elschnig (BT) keeps the LC firmly in place in the scleral opening. The LC is sinking due to atrophy of the border tissue which is solely supplied by ciliary circulation. Systemic circulatory pressure supplying the BT and IOP are opposing forces. Normally, the circulatory pressure supplying the BT should be higher than the IOP for the proper perfusion and healthy maintenance of the BT, **Figure 2**.

However, if this delicate situation is reversed, either due to raised IOP or if pressure supplying the BT becomes lower than the IOP due to systemic problems such as chronic hypotension, then even normal range IOP can take the upper hand. Thus, even the normal range IOP will begin compressing the circulation of the BT thereby inducing chronic ischemia and its atrophy and NTG will ensue. Therefore, it is the IOP becoming higher than the circulatory pressure of the BT resulting in both HTG and NTG.

The eyeball is supplied by dual circulation, the central retinal artery (CRA)—a high pressure system and ciliary circulation—a comparatively lower pressure system. In acute glaucoma, when IOP exceeds pressure of the CRA, it compresses circulation of the retina resulting in immediate death of neuronal tissue and optic atrophy. Furthermore, the optic atrophy resulting from acute glaucoma is a flat disc (non-excavated) as there is no sinking of the LC and thus no severance of nerve fibers taking place.

In contrast, chronic glaucoma develops when IOP becomes higher than the ciliary pressure supplying the BT. Since the ciliary pressure is a lower pressure system, even a moderate elevation of IOP can become higher than ciliary pressure and chronically compress circulation of the BT, resulting in its atrophy. As the BT beocmes atrophied, the LC begins sinking and the nerve fibers get stretched and severed at the scleral edge. In summary,

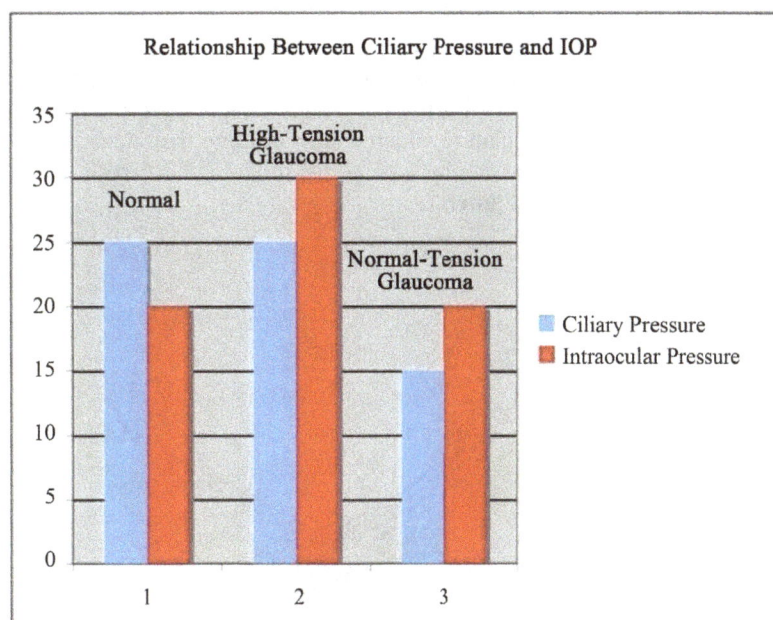

Figure 2. Relationship between ciliary pressure and IOP. Normally, ciliary circulatory pressure supplying the border tissue should be higher than IOP for healthy perfusion as in column (1). In column (2), the IOP is increased to 30 whereas the ciliary pressure remains the same at 25, this will result in high-tension glaucoma. In column (3) the ciliary pressure is decreased to 15 mm but the IOP is same, normal at 20, resulting in normal-tension glaucoma.

the nerve fibers are being atrophied in a non-orderly fashion in acute glaucoma whereas, the nerve fibers are being severed in an orderly fashion in chronic glaucoma.

Due to atrophy of the BT, the LC starts sinking [4] [5] resulting in stretching and ultimately breakage of the prelaminar nerve fibers since one end is attached to the soma of the RGC and the other end anchored in the pores of the LC. Only the prelaminar nerve fibers can be destroyed in an orderly tandem fashion since they are still loose and have not yet fastened in bundles in the pores of the LC. Once the nerve fibers are anchored in the pores of the LC, they can't be separated individually and thus their orderly tandem severance is not possible. Therefore, the LC may not be the site of injury in glaucoma as commonly believed.

3. Why Are the Nerve Fibers Being Destroyed in an Orderly Fashion?

The sinking of the LC and severance of the nerve fibers can explain their orderly destruction in glaucoma. As the LC sinks, the peripheral nerve fibers closest to the scleral edge are stretched and broken first, **Figure 3**. As a result, the next central fiber will move towards the periphery to occupy the space vacated by the preceding severed fiber and thus also get stretched and severed at the scleral edge.

In addition to the border tissue, the 360 degrees of nerve fibers also anchor the LC as roots anchor a tree. Thus, the severance of nerve fibers leads to further disc sinking. The cascade of severance of the nerve fibers and sinking disc would become self-propagated and will continue until all the nerve fibers have moved in an orderly tandem fashion to the scleral edge and get severed. This may explain the unstoppable nature of glaucoma despite maximum lowering of IOP. The severed segments undergo phagocytosis and thus will create empty spaces or excavation that we may be interpreting as cupping of the disc.

4. Do We Have Evidence of Severance of Nerve Fibers?

Progressive thinning of the RNFL in glaucoma can only be explained due to severance of nerve fibers as it is not occurring in non-glaucomatous optic atrophies. The arcuate retinal empty spaces [6] in glaucoma are due to severance and depletion of arcuate nerve fibers and notching due to their depletion at the site of their entry in the disc. All of the 360 degrees of nerve fibers are being severed simultaneously, however the arcuate fibers being fewer in number are depleted earlier, thus producing the arcuate field defects, **Figure 4** and **Figure 5**. Notching at the poles of the disc is the initial excavation in the disc and a confirmatory sign of glaucoma. At this stage, the pathognomonic arcuate field defects will appear on perimetry.

The histology of the end-stage glaucomatous disc is not 100% cupped LC, but an empty crater left over after the phagocytosis of severed nerve fibers, **Figure 6**. Splinter hemorrhages and characteristic whitish pallor of the disc are due to severance of the vasculature which is also meeting the fate of nerve fibers. In contrast, the histology of the non-glaucomatous optic atrophy such as due to multiple sclerosis, reveals the presence of nerve fibers though atrophied and shrunken, **Figure 7**.

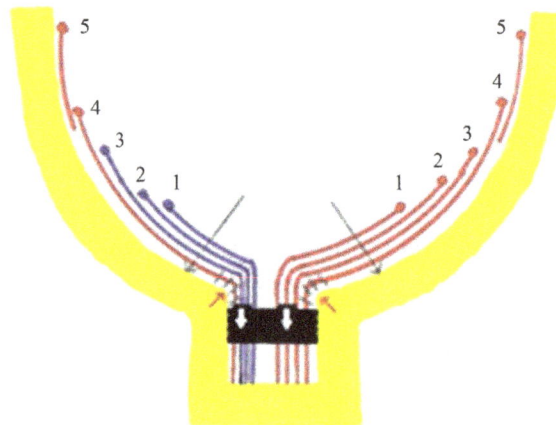

Figure 3. Note the sinking of the disc resulting in stretching and severing of the peripheral fibers. Most Peripheral fiber (5) has been severed and disappeared and this process will continue until central most fiber (1) has been severed. There will be movement of the central fibers to the periphery to occupy the space created by severance of the peripheral fibers.

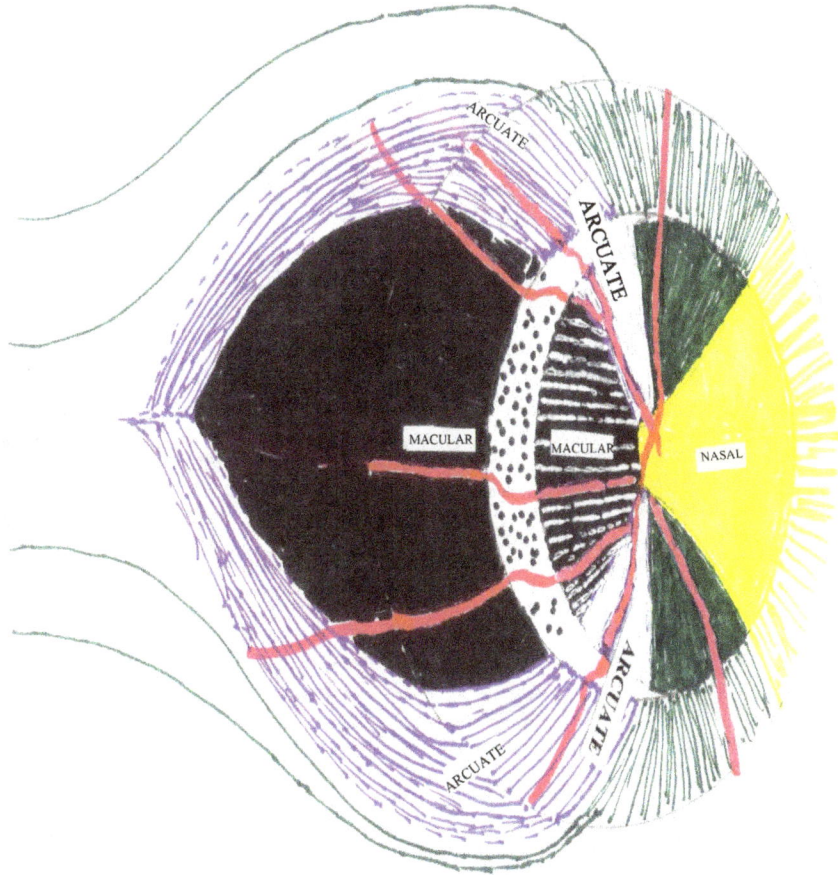

Figure 4. Due to temporal sinking all the temporal fibers (Macular, superior and inferior arcuate) are being axotomized. However, the arcuate fibers being fewer in number will be depleted earlier resulting in arcuate field defects as in **Figure 5**.

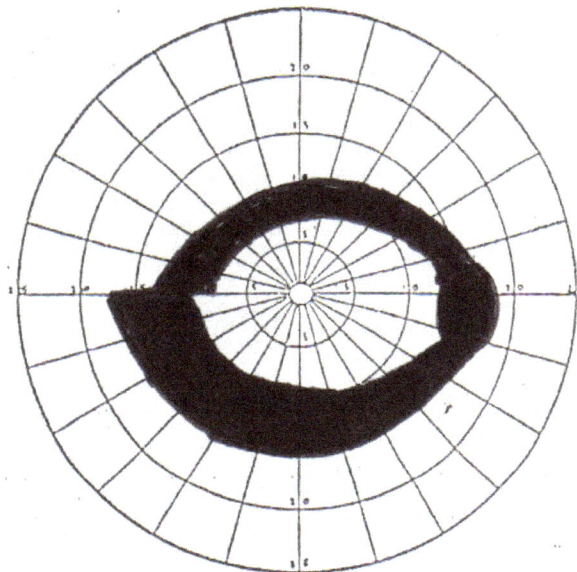

Figure 5. Right eye: Double arcuate/ring scotoma after arcuate fibers have been severed. Arcuate fibers being fewer in number compared to macular fibers, will be depleted earlier resulting in arcuate field defects.

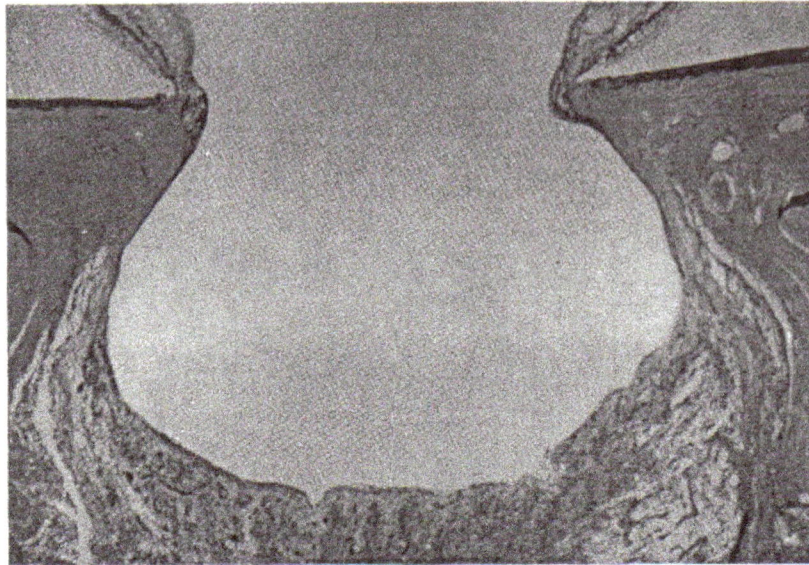

Figure 6. End-stage glaucomatous disc. Bean-pot excavation is not a deeply cupped disc/lamina but a left over crater which once housed the disc. The lamina is probably lying at the bottom of the crater after being emptied of all the nerve fibers after their severance. Kolker AE, Hetherington Jr J. Becker-Shaffer's diagnosis and therapy of the glaucoma, Mosby, 1976, p 146.

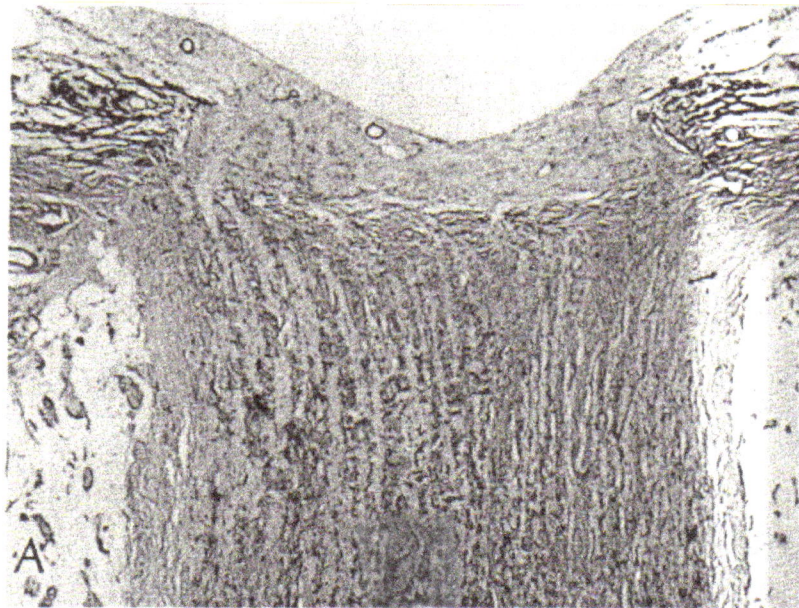

Figure 7. Flat disc atrophy due to multiple sclerosis. Note the nerve fibers though atrophied and shrunken are still present in contrast to glaucomatous disc. There is no excavation of the disc since there is no sinking and thus no severance of nerve fibers is occurring in flat disc atrophy. Copy from Yanoff, Ocular Pathology 1975.

5. Conclusion

The severance of the nerve fibers appears to be the missing piece in glaucoma mystery. The sinking disc and severance of nerve fibers is able to corroborate with their orderly destruction, a hallmark of glaucoma. In essence, the nerve fibers along with vasculature are being severed in glaucoma. Therefore, glaucoma may not be an optic disc neuropathy but an optic disc axotomy.

References

[1] Duke-Elder, S. and Barrie, J. (1969) Diseases of the Lens and Vitreous, Glaucoma and Hypotony. *System of Ophthalmology*, Vol. X1, Henry Kimpton, London, 385.

[2] Hasnain, S.S. (2006) Scleral Edge, Not Optic Disc or Retina Is the Primary Site of Injury in Chronic Glaucoma. *Medical Hypothesis*, **67**, 1320-1325. http://dx.doi.org/10.1016/j.mehy.2006.05.030

[3] Hasnain, S.S. (2012) Can Glaucoma Be a Neurodegenerative Disease? Highlights of Ophthalmology. *Panama*, **40**.

[4] Hasnain, S.S. (2010) Optic Disc May Be Sinking in Chronic Glaucoma. *Ophthalmology Update*, **8**, 22-28.

[5] Yang, H. (2010) Optic Nerve Head (ONH) Lamina Cribrosa Insertion Migration and Pialization in Early Non-Human Primate Experimental Glaucoma. *Poster Presentation ARVO Meeting*, 3 May 2010.

[6] Hasnain, S.S. (2013) Arcuate Field Defects in Glaucoma Ophthalmology Update.

29

Novel Mechanistic Interplay between Products of Oxidative Stress and Components of the Complement System in AMD Pathogenesis

Hongjun Du[1,2], Xu Xiao[3], Travis Stiles[2], Christopher Douglas[2], Daisy Ho[2], Peter X. Shaw[2*]

[1]Department of Ophthalmology, Xijing Hospital, Xi'an, China
[2]Department of Ophthalmology and Shiley Eye Institute, University of California San Diego, San Diego, USA
[3]Sichuan Provincial People's Hospital, Chengdu, China
Email: *pshaw@ucsd.edu

Abstract

Age-related macular degeneration (AMD) is a leading cause of vision loss affecting tens of millions of elderly worldwide. Early AMD includes soft drusen and pigmentary changes in the retinal pigment epithelium (RPE). As people age, such soft confluent drusen can progress into two forms of advanced AMD, geographic atrophy (GA, or dry AMD) or choroidal neovascularization (CNV, or wet AMD) and result in the loss of central vision. The exact mechanism for developing early AMD and progressing to advanced stage of disease is still largely unknown. However, significant evidence exists demonstrating a complex interplay of genetic and environmental factors as the cause of AMD progression. Together, complement factor H (CFH) and HTRA1/ARMS polymorphisms contribute to more than 50% of the genetic risk for AMD. Environmentally, oxidative stress from activities such as smoking has also demonstrated a powerful contribution to AMD progression. To extend our previous finding that genetic polymorphisms in CFH results in OxPLs and the risk-form of CFH (CFH Y402H) has reduced affinity for oxidized phospholipids, and subsequent diminished capacity which subsequently diminishes the capability to attenuate the inflammatory effects of these molecules, we compared the binding properties of CFH and CFH related protein 1 (CFHR1), which is also associated with disease risk, to OxPLs and their effects on modulating inflammation and lipids uptake. As both CFH-402H and CFHR1 are associated with increased risk to AMD, we hypothesized that like CFH-402H, CFHR1 contribution to AMD risk may also be due to its diminished affinity for OxPLs. Interestingly, we found that association of CFHR1 with OxPLs was not statistically different than CFH. However, binding of CFHR1 did not elicit the same protective ben-

---

*Corresponding author.

efits as CFH in that both inflammation and lipid uptake are unaffected by CFHR1 association with OxPLs. These findings demonstrate a novel and interesting complexity to the potential interplay between the complement system and oxidative stress byproducts, such as OxPLs, in the mechanistic contribution to AMD. Future work will aim to identify the molecular distinctions between CFH and CFHR1 which confer protection by the former, but not latter molecules. Understanding the molecular domains necessary for protection could provide interventional insights in the generation of novel therapeutics for AMD and other diseases associated with oxidative stress.

Keywords

Age-Related Macular Degeneration, Oxidative Stress, Complement Factor H, Inflammation

1. Introduction

It is established that AMD is a disease of aging and chronic inflammation. The hallmark of early AMD is lipid accumulation leading to the presence of drusen. Drusen are pockets of lipid and other extracellular material that aggregate between the Bruch's membrane and the retinal pigment epithelium (RPE) of the eye [1]. Typically, sparse "hard" drusens are benign artifacts of aging but as the number and size (often leading to a "soft" designation) of drusen increase, so does the risk of progression to both forms of advanced AMD. The two forms of advanced AMD are: 1) geographic atrophy (GA) of the retinal pigment epithelium (RPE) and overlying photoreceptors (also called advanced "dry" AMD) and 2) choroidal neovascularization (CNV, also called "wet" AMD). GA AMD is characterized by confluent areas of photoreceptor and RPE cell death, and GA without CNV is responsible for over 10% of the legal blindness from advanced AMD [2]. Interestingly, just over half of GA AMD presents bilaterally, further demonstrating an environmental component of disease [3]. Currently, approximately 900,000 persons in the United States are affected by GA AMD [4]. However, despite the high correlation demonstrated between various genetic and environmental contributors the etiology remains largely unknown and there exists no approved treatment [5].

There is substantial evidence suggesting that contributing mechanisms to GA AMD require a combination of insults such as photo-oxidative stress, complement activation, cellular senescence, and microbial assault. This paradigm is supported by earlier work which demonstrated that loci at the complement factor H (CFH), C2 and C3 are associated with all phenotypic variants of AMD, including early AMD and GA [6]. Genes involved in lipid metabolism, such as ApoE and LIPC are also significantly associated with dry AMD [7] [8]. Central to many of these proposed factors, oxidative stress can have multifactorial influences amongst a number of the proposed pathways and is known to play a critical role in many aging diseases including cardiovascular disease and AMD [9]. Oxidative stress in the eye is of particular importance as the burden of purposeful sunlight exposure in combination with high metabolic demand and oxygen content creates a disproportionate burden of oxidative stress that requires tight homeostatic regulation to maintain function. A major product of this increased oxidative burden of the eye is a relatively large amount of OxPLs shed by photoreceptors [10]-[13]. These OxPLs are inherently inflammatory in systemic context, but the inflammatory burden is tightly controlled in the eye by largely unappreciated mechanisms. We hypothesize that, at least in part, functional abnormalities of the innate immune system incurred via high risk genotypes contribute to the pathogenesis of AMD by altering the tight homeostatic control of the OxPLs contribution to inflammation. This disruption leads to a state of chronic inflammation and pathologic progression.

The documented contribution of oxidative stress, inflammation, and genetic variations in complement factors indicates a strong probability that genetic risk modifies the aspects of the complement system in a manner which leads to perturbation and exacerbation of the cycle of oxidation, inflammation and pathogenic progression of this disease. We have shown that risk genotypes associated with CFH proteins interact with less affinity with OxPLs, and the decreased association leads to an increased inflammatory burden by these molecules [12]. The purpose of this study is to examine the potential mechanism underlying the increased risk of AMD progression that results from expression of CFHR1, and whether the contribution to the disease is reminiscent of phenomenon observed in the decreased interaction of CFH Y402H with OxPLs.

2. Material and Methods

2.1. Preparation of Native and Oxidized Phospholipid

Since phospholipids have low aqueous solubility, in plasma they typically co-exist with proteins in the form of lipoproteins, such as ApoB in low density lipoprotein (LDL). We thus chose LDL as a carrier for native or oxidized phospholipids moiety in this study. We first isolated LDL from plasma of normolipidemic donors (normal lipid level) by sequentialultracentrifugation [14]. OxLDL was generated by incubating LDL (1 mg/mL) with an oxidation agent (10 μM CuSO$_4$) for 18 hours at 37˚C where native phospholipids on the surface of LDL were oxidized into OxPLs [15]. Malondialdehyde-modified LDL (MDA-LDL), another form of oxidatively modified LDL, is made as described previously [16]. Native (non-oxidized) phospholipids moiety on native LDL were used as a control.

2.2. Preparation of Recombinant CFH and CFHR1

The gene encoding human CFH and CFHR1 was sub-cloned into a mammalian expression vector pRK5 [12]. The same amount of constructs was then transfected into HEK293 cells using Fugene 6 kit following the manufacturer's instruction (Roche, Indianapolis, IN). The medium containing rCFH or rCFHR1 protein was harvested and concentrated using Amicon Ultra (Millipore, Billerica, MA). All recombinant proteins are assayed for endotoxin contamination using Gen Script ToxinSensor™ Chromogenic-LAL Endotoxin Assay Kit to ensure the free of LPS and avoid the bias of the stimulation.

2.3. Chemiluminescent ELISA

For ELISA studies, lipoprotein antigens (in PBS, 2 μg/ml of protein concentration) were coated on microtiter plates at 4˚C overnight. A 1:100 dilution of conditioned medium with the indicated construct was added to the plate, followed by biotinylated anti-CFH antibody (ab112197, abcam, Cambridge, MA, USA) or anti-CFHR1 antibody (ABIN1405357, antibodies-online, Atlanta, GA, USA). The amount of bound CFH or CFHR1 was detected with neutral avidin-alkaline phosphatase (AP) followed by light emission substrate Lumiphos 530. The chemiluminescence was measured and expressed as RLU/100 ms.

2.4. Culturing of RPE Cells and Stimulation

Human ARPE-19 cells were grown for 14 days in DMEM/F12 (1:1) plus 10% FCS to allow for forming of a truly differentiated epithelial layer. After serum starvation, cells were stimulated with oxidatively modified LDL or a control of non-modified LDL at 50 μg/ml for 18 hours (under our culture condition, most of inflammatory cytokine's transcripts are exponentially expressed within 6 hours and most of gene transcripts peaked at 18 hours). To study the effect of binding of CFH or CFHR1 protein to OxLDL on stimulation of pro-inflammatory cytokines, we pre-incubated 50 μg/ml of OxLDL with concentrated conditioned media containing rCFH or rCFHR1 protein (50 μg/ml protein concentration by Thermo Scientific BCA assay).The OxPLs/CFH or CFHR1 complex was added to ARPE-19 cells for 18 hours incubation for gene expression or 48 hours for lipids accumulation.

2.5. Gene Expression Assays

After stimulation, RNA was purified using RNeasy Mini Kit (Qiagen) and used for cDNA synthesis using Superscript III (Invitrogen, Carlsbad, CA, USA). The expression of inflammatory cytokines/chemokines known to associated with AMD pathology was then assessed by quantitative PCR with SYBR Green Real-Time PCR Master Mixes (Thermo Fisher Scientific, Waltham, MA USA) using athermocycler (Bio-Rad Labs, Irvine, CA, USA). Sample sizes of 6 were used to reach the 80% of power when 0.25 fold change was expected, sigma = 0.25 and $\alpha = 0.05$.

2.6. Western Blot

Cell extractions for protein assessment studies were performed as previously described [12]. Briefly, cells were lysed with Cell Lysis Buffer (#9803, Cell Signaling Technology, Boston, MA, USA) containing 0.5 mM of phenylmethanesulfonyl fluoride (PMSF) (Sigma-Aldrich, St. Louis, MO, USA). Protein concentration was standardized by BCA protein assay (Thermo Fisher Scientific, Grand Island, NY, USA). Samples (25 μg) were separated by SDS-PAGE in 4% - 20% gradient Tris-glycine precast gels (Invitrogen, Carlsbad, CA, USA) and transferred to a polyvinylidene difluoride (PVDF) membrane (Millipore, Billerica, MA, USA). The membrane was incubated for 1 hour in blocking solution containing 5% non-fat milk powder and 0.1% Tween-20, pH 7.6. This was followed by overnight incubation at 4°C in the blocking buffer containing rabbit primary antibodies against CD36 (Abcam, ab133625, 1:500). Subsequently, the labeled proteins were visualized by incubation with a horseradish peroxidase (HRP)-conjugated anti-goat or rabbit IgG (1:2000; Santa Cruz Biotechnology) followed by development with a chemiluminescence substrate for HRP (Thermo Fisher Scientific). The images of western blots were captured by GE imageQuant imager. Relative band intensities were analyzed using Image J software and normalized to GAPDH.

2.7. Oil-Red O Staining

Lipid accumulation in ARPE-19 cells was assessed *in vitro* as previously described [17]. Briefly, ARPE-19 cells were resuspended into 0.5 ml of DMEM containing 20% FCS and seeded to each well of a 12-well culture plate laid with a round cover slip. The following day, 25 μg/ml of native or OxLDL (50 μg/ml of OxLDL is toxic to cells during an extended incubation) as OxPLs/rCFH or rCFHR1 was added to the medium and extended the incubation for another 48 hours. After 48 hour of incubation, the cells were used to assess lipids uptake. The cells were washed with PBS and fixed with formaldehyde/sucrose solution and then stained with heated Oil red O/propylene glycol solution and mounted. The number of lipid droplets/cell of a total of 100 cells was counted using a microscope with a visual grid.

3. Results

3.1. Complement Factor H Related Protein 1 Has the Similar Binding Property to OxPLs as the Protective Form of CFH

We previously showed that CFH derived from the risk (C) and protective (T) alleles bind differentially to OxPLs. Plasma containing CFH (rs1061170) homozygous CC (402H, risk genotype) vs. homozygous TT (402Y, protective genotype) in our experiment can be respectively exemplified with recombinant CFH402Y and CFH402H proteins, and as a result it can be shown that the protective form of CFH402Y binds to OxPLs stronger than risk form of CFH402H [12]. In this report, we also show that under the same assay conditions, both recombinant CFH and CFHR1 bind significantly stronger to OxPLs than to native LDL. However, there is no difference in binding to either native or OxLDL between CFH402Y and CFHR1 (**Figure 1**).

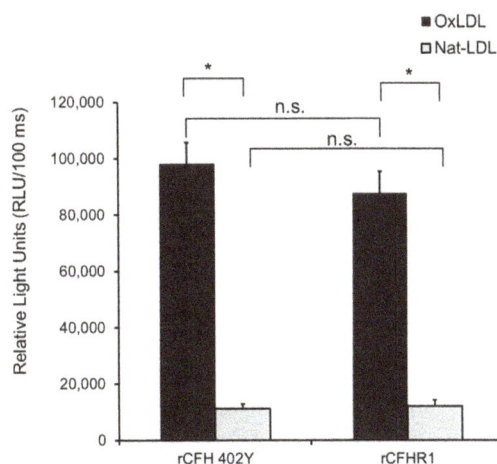

Figure 1. Relative binding property of CFH variants to oxidized phospholipids. The binding of recombinant protein rCFH 402Y (protective) and rCFHR1 to native or oxidized LDL antigens was measured using relative light units (RLUs) of chemiluminescence. Data are expressed in RLU and as mean ± SEM. N = 6 for each sample point, n.s., not significant, *P < 0.05.

3.2. Oxidized Phospholipids Stimulate the Elevated Expression of Inflammatory Cytokines in Cultured RPE Cells

RPE plays an important role in maintaining the health of the retina through outer segment lipid turnover [18]. Like macrophages, they engulf the released outer segment vesicles from photoreceptors. When extensive oxidative stress occurs, such as smoking and sunlight exposure, the RPE vesicles accumulate oxidative modified products like OxPLs, which in turn stimulate inflammation and the expression of cell-surface receptors, including CD36. CD36 is a scavenger receptor that will mediate uptake of OxLDL in an unregulated fashion [19]. These processes can lead to intracellular accumulation of debris and lipofuscin and further induction of cytokines critical for activation of pro-inflammatory cascades. We investigated gene-expression profiles in cultured ARPE-19 cells upon exposure to oxidative modified lipoproteins including OxLDL and MDA-LDL. Our results showed that comparing to native LDL control, the OxLDL and MDA-LDL significantly up-regulated the expression of scavenger receptor CD36, pro-inflammatory cytokine IL-6 and pro-angiogenic protein VEGF (**Figure 2**).

3.3. CFH and CFHR1 Protein Modulate CD36 Expression and Inflammatory Cytokine IL-6 Expression Stimulated OxPLs

To investigate whether the binding of CFH or CFHR1 would attenuate the scavenger receptor expression on ARPE-19 cells stimulated by OxPLs, we pre-incubated OxPLs with rCFH or rCFHR1. As expected, the interaction of rCFH with OxPLs significantly reduced the level of CD36 protein. Conversely, rCFHR1 failed to modulate the CD36 levels (**Figure 3(A)**) indicating an inability to recapitulate the protective benefits of CFH. The absence of protective capacity was further observed in assessing the IL-6 inflammatory response of ARPE-19 cells to OxPLs stimulation, which was significantly reduced by pre-incubation with rCFH but not with rCFHR1 (**Figure 3(B)**). These data indicated that even with the similar binding property to OxPLs, these two related proteins displayed different function in attenuating pro-inflammatory events *in vitro*.

3.4. Incubation of OxLDL Results in Lipids Accumulation in RPE Cells *in Vitro*

As lipid-mediated inflammatory changes are closely linked to lipid accumulation and drusen formation in AMD, we extended the inflammatory characterization and investigated the lipids accumulation in cultured RPE cells following the *in vitro* incubation with native or OxLDL. To accomplish this, low-density seeded ARPE-19 (as shown in **Figure 4(A)**) were treated with 25 µg/ml concentration of native or OxLDL for 48 hours and assessed for lipid accumulation as visualized by Oil Red-O staining. As anticipated, the lipid vesicles were greatly increased in OxLDL treated RPE cells (**Figure 4(C)**) relative to native LDL treated cells (**Figure 4(B)**). Interestingly, addition of excess (50 µg/ml) of rCFH into the OxLDL containing medium led to significant reduction in the accumulation of lipids (**Figure 4(D)**), while the addition of rCFHR1 showed no significant effect on lipid

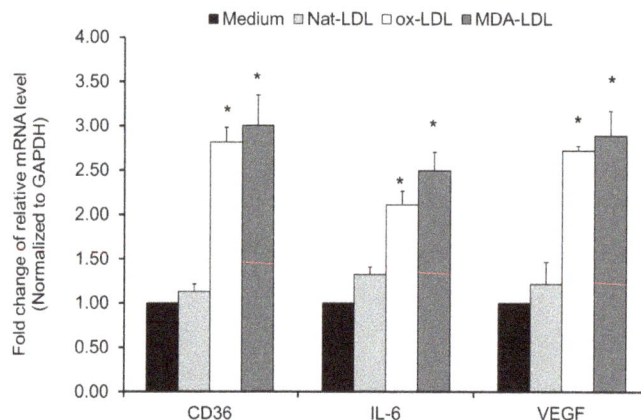

Figure 2. Gene expression as assayed by quantitative PCR on mRNA from ARPE-19 cells treated with 50 µg/mL of native LDL, OxLDL or MDA-LDL for 18 hour. Relative mRNA levels of indicated genes were calculated by normalizing results with GAPDH and are expressed relative to untreated samples. Data are shown as mean ± SEM. N = 6, $^{*}P < 0.05$.

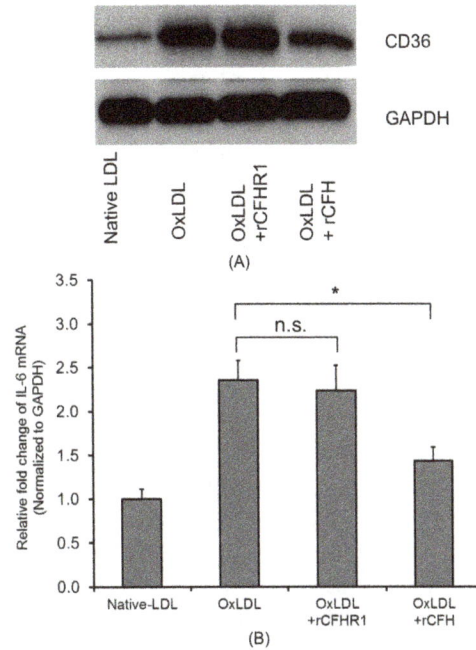

Figure 3. (A) CD36 protein level increased following treatment with OxLDL. ARPE-19 cells were treated with 50 μg/mL of native LDL, OxLDL or OxLDL and pre-incubated with the equal amount (50 μg/mL) of recombined rCFHR1 or rCFH as indicated, for 18 hours. The protein levels were assessed via SDS-PAGE and western blot using anti CD36 antibody. (B) CFH, but not CFHR1, inhibited expression of IL-6 stimulated by OxLDL. Gene expression was assayed by quantitative PCR on mRNA from ARPE19 cells treated with 50 μg/mL of native LDL, OxLDL or OxLDL pre-incubated with the equal amount (50 μg/mL) of recombined rCFHR1 or rCFH for 18 hours. Relative mRNA levels of indicated genes were calculated by normalizing results with GAPDH and are expressed relative to untreated samples. Results are shown as mean ± SEM. N = 6, $^*P < 0.05$.

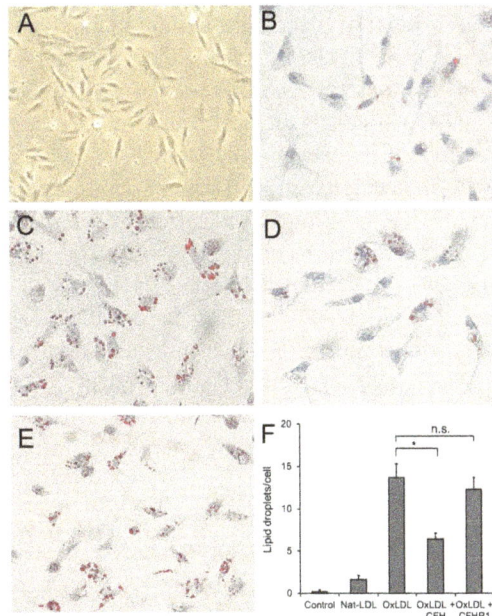

Figure 4. OxLDL3. Oxidized LDL enhances the uptake of lipids in cultured RPE cells. ARPE-19 cells were seeded and incubated for 48 hours with 25 μg/ml native-LDL (B), or 25 μg/ml OxLDL (C) alone, or OxLDL plus 25 μg/ml of rCFH (D), or OxLDL plus 25 μg/ml of rCFH (E). At the end of incubation, the cells were fixed and stained with Oil Red O. (A) is a picture of untreated ARPE-19 cells. (F), The lipid droplets were qualified for positive Oil Red O staining. Results are shown as stained lipid droplets/cell (mean ± SEM, $^*P < 0.05$).

accumulation (**Figure 4(E)**). **Figure 4(F)** shows the quantitative analysis of lipid droplets among untreated cells or cells treated with indicated agents. These data suggest that the scavenger receptor mediated uptake of OxLDL can be interfered by the binding of CFH to the OxPLs on the surface of OxLDL presumably by restricting the interaction between OxPLs and scavenger receptors. However, the interaction of CFHR1, which has the similar binding property as CFH, does not affect the OxLDL internalization.

4. Discussion

While we have uncovered increasingly more details concerning the speculative contributors to AMD progression, the mechanisms underlying how these factors intertwine to lead to advanced disease has largely remained elusive. Our previous work characterized a novel interaction of CFH with OxPLs, as well as mechanistic insight into how CFH proteins might restrict the inflammatory effects of these molecules. Additionally, we found that CFH variants associated with increased risk of AMD demonstrated a decreased affinity of the CFH protein for OxPLs, which led to a greater inflammatory burden [12]. The diminished protective capacity of these risk-associated variants in our studies represent a key mechanistic insight into the potential interplay between genetic risk factors and environmental stressors that cumulatively contribute to AMD progression. As a largely homologous protein to CFH, the fact that CFHR1 expression leads to increased AMD disease risk as opposed to protection has persisted as a somewhat enigmatic proposition. For example, while CFHR1 expression confers risk for AMD, it is protective against atypical hemolytic uremic syndrome [20]. As risk variants of CFH conferred disease risk via diminished association with OxPLs, we hypothesized that CFHR1 conferred risk by having similarly reduced OxPLs affinity, thereby enabling OxPLs to freely interact with inflammation-promoting factors. While CFHR1 is known to not be protective, we showed statistically identical association of CFHR1 and CFH with OxPLs. Indeed, the work represented herein demonstrates that OxPL/CFHR1 complexes offer no ability to attenuate the inflammatory effects of OxPLs. In addition to its ability to restrict inflammation in RPE cells, we had previously shown that the protective benefits of CFH extended to a diminished intake and accumulation of undesirable OxPL molecules, which logically would extend into a reduction in drusen formation. Despite its similar affinity and homology to CFH, CFHR1 does not impede the intake and accumulation of OxPLs into RPE cells, further shining light on its lack of protective capacity.

While the initial hypothesis of diminished OxPL association did not prove accurate, the work herein clearly demonstrates an intricate mechanism by which differential components of the CFH family contribute to AMD progression. What we conclude from this work is that simple association of CFH family members with OxPLs is not sufficient for blocking interactions between these molecules and RPE receptors which internalize these oxidized lipids. As this was a closed system with no other cellular contributors, the likely explanation for the observed phenomenon is that steric differences in the larger CFH protein somehow restrict, likely in a steric fashion, interaction of the OxPL molecules with RPE receptors that typically trigger internalization and inflammation. This paper indicates one of the most important aspects of complement regulators such as CFH and CFHR1. In addition to their protective function for complement activation triggered by external pathogens, CFH also blocks the inflammation triggered by OxLDL while CFHR1, loses such ability. Future work will focus on the molecular dissection of the CFH protein to elucidate the domains responsible for this restricted interaction in hopes of identifying the minimal essential components needed for the restriction of inflammation and lipid accumulation. By better understanding these mechanisms, we can provide valuable insight into both AMD pathology, and other conditions associated with oxidative stress. This will provide specific intervention points by which we can theorize and design future therapeutic approaches to improving outcomes of patients with these conditions.

Acknowledgements

The work was supported by the National Natural Science Foundation of China (No. 30973253, 81470654 to HJD and National Eye Institute grants (R01-EY-025693 to PXS and P30EY022589).

References

[1]   Jager, R.D., Mieler, W.F. and Miller, J.W. (2008) Age-Related Macular Degeneration. *New England Journal of Medicine*, **358**, 2606-2617. http://dx.doi.org/10.1056/NEJMra0801537

[2]   Sunness, J.S. (1999) The Natural History of Geographic Atrophy, the Advanced Atrophic Form of Age-Related Macular Degeneration. *Molecular Vision*, **5**, 25.

[3]   Fleckenstein, M., Adrion, C., Schmitz-Valckenberg, S., Gobel, A.P., Bindewald-Wittich, A., Scholl, H.P., *et al.* (2010) Concordance of Disease Progression in Bilateral Geographic Atrophy Due to AMD. *Investigative Ophthalmology & Visual Science*, **51**, 637-642. http://dx.doi.org/10.1167/iovs.09-3547

[4]   Friedman, D.S., O'Colmain, B.J., Munoz, B., Tomany, S.C., McCarty, C., de Jong, P.T., *et al.* (2004) Prevalence of Age-Related Macular Degeneration in the United States. *Archives of Ophthalmology*, **122**, 564-572. http://dx.doi.org/10.1001/archopht.122.4.564

[5]   Wei, C.X., Sun, A., Yu, Y., Liu, Q., Tan, Y.Q., Tachibana, I., *et al.* (2016) Challenges in the Development of Therapy for Dry Age-Related Macular Degeneration. *Advances in Experimental Medicine and Biology*, **854**, 103-109. http://dx.doi.org/10.1007/978-3-319-17121-0_15

[6]   Cameron, D.J., Yang, Z., Gibbs, D., Chen, H., Kaminoh, Y., Jorgensen, A., *et al.* (2007) HTRA1 Variant Confers Similar Risks to Geographic Atrophy and Neovascular Age-Related Macular Degeneration. *Cell Cycle*, **6**, 1122-1125. http://dx.doi.org/10.4161/cc.6.9.4157

[7]   Yu, Y., Reynolds, R., Fagerness, J., Rosner, B., Daly, M.J. and Seddon, J.M. (2011) Association of Variants in the LIPC and ABCA1 Genes with Intermediate and Large Drusenand Advanced Age-Related Macular Degeneration. *Investigative Ophthalmology &Visual Science*, **52**, 4663-4670. http://dx.doi.org/10.1167/iovs.10-7070

[8]   Toops, K.A., Tan, L.X. and Lakkaraju, A. (2016) Apolipoprotein E Isoforms and AMD. *Advances in Experimental Medicine and Biology*, **854**, 3-9. http://dx.doi.org/10.1007/978-3-319-17121-0_1

[9]   Jarrett, S.G. and Boulton, M.E. (2012) Consequences of Oxidative Stress in Age-Related Macular Degeneration. *Molecular Aspects of Medicine*, **33**, 399-417. http://dx.doi.org/10.1016/j.mam.2012.03.009

[10] Beatty, S., Koh, H., Phil, M., Henson, D. and Boulton, M. (2000) The Role of Oxidative Stress in the Pathogenesis of Age-Related Macular Degeneration. *Survey of Ophthalmology*, **45**, 115-134. http://dx.doi.org/10.1016/S0039-6257(00)00140-5

[11] Suzuki, M., Kamei, M., Itabe, H., Yoneda, K., Bando, H., Kume, N., *et al.* (2007) Oxidized Phospholipids in the Macula Increase with Age and in Eyes with Age-Related Macular Degeneration. *Molecular Vision*, **13**, 772-778.

[12] Shaw, P.X., Zhang, L., Zhang, M., Du, H., Zhao, L., Lee, C., *et al.* (2012) Complement Factor H Genotypes Impact Risk of Age-Related Macular Degeneration by Interaction with Oxidized Phospholipids. *Proceedings of the National Academy of Sciences of the United States of America*, **109**, 13757-13762. http://dx.doi.org/10.1073/pnas.1121309109

[13] Salomon, R.G., Hong, L. and Hollyfield, J.G. (2011) Discovery of Carboxyethylpyrroles (CEPs): Critical Insights into AMD, Autism, Cancer, and Wound Healing from Basic Research on the Chemistry of Oxidized Phospholipids. *Chemical Research in Toxicology*, **24**, 1803-1816. http://dx.doi.org/10.1021/tx200206v

[14] Havel, R.J., Eder, H.A. and Bragdon, J.H. (1955) The Distribution and Chemical Composition of Ultracentrifugally Separated Lipoproteins in Human Serum. *Journal of Clinical Investigation*, **34**, 1345-1353. http://dx.doi.org/10.1172/JCI103182

[15] Palinski, W., Yla-Herttuala, S., Rosenfeld, M.E., Butler, S.W., Socher, S.A., Parthasarathy, S., *et al.* (1990) Antisera and Monoclonal Antibodies Specific for Epitopes Generated during Oxidative Modification of Low Density Lipoprotein. *Arteriosclerosis*, **10**, 325-335.http://dx.doi.org/10.1161/01.ATV.10.3.325

[16] Shaw, P.X., Horkko, S., Tsimikas, S., Chang, M.K., Palinski, W., Silverman, G.J., *et al.* (2001) Human-Derived Anti-Oxidized LDL Autoantibody Blocks Uptake of Oxidized LDL by Macrophages and Localizes to Atherosclerotic Lesions *in Vivo. Arteriosclerosis, Thrombosis, and Vascular Biology*, **21**, 1333-1339. http://dx.doi.org/10.1161/hq0801.093587

[17] Tsimikas, S., Miyanohara, A., Hartvigsen, K., Merki, E., Shaw, P.X., Chou, M.Y., *et al.* (2011) Human Oxidation-Specific Antibodies Reduce Foam Cell Formation and Atherosclerosis Progression. *Journal of the American College of Cardiology*, **58**, 1715-1727. http://dx.doi.org/10.1016/j.jacc.2011.07.017

[18] Kevany, B.M. and Palczewski, K. (2010) Phagocytosis of Retinal Rod and Cone Photoreceptors. *Physiology*, **25**, 8-15. http://dx.doi.org/10.1152/physiol.00038.2009

[19] Boullier, A., Bird, D.A., Chang, M.K., Dennis, E.A., Friedman, P., Gillotre-Taylor, K., *et al.* (2001) Scavenger Receptors, Oxidized LDL, and Atherosclerosis. *Annals of the New York Academy of Sciences*, **947**, 214-222; Discussion 222-213.

[20] Hofer, J., Janecke, A.R., Zimmerhackl, L.B., Riedl, M., Rosales, A., Giner, T., *et al.* (2013) Complement Factor H-Related Protein 1 Deficiency and Factor H Antibodies in Pediatric Patients with Atypical Hemolytic Uremic Syndrome. *Clinical Journal of the American Society of Nephrology*: *CJASN*, **8**, 407-415. http://dx.doi.org/10.2215/CJN.01260212

30

Oculo Orbital Complications of Sinusitis

Nada Otmani[1]*, Serheir Zineb[2], Housbane Sami[2], Oudidi Abdellatif[1], Bennani Othmani Mohamed[2]

[1]Hassan II Hospital, Fez, Morocco
[2]Faculty of Medicine, Casablanca, Morocco
Email: *nada.oudidi@gmail.com, abdellatif.oudidi@usmba.ac.ma, nada.otmani@usmba.ac.ma, pr.oudidi@gmail.com, alanine@gmail.com

Abstract

The ocular-orbital complications of sinusitis constitute a diagnostic and therapeutic urgency that requires a correct multidisciplinary assumption. Objectives: The description of clinical and therapeutic data of the orbital complications of acute sinusitis. Methods: Our work is based on a retrospective study of 86 cases of ocular-orbital complications of sinusitis hospitalized at the ENT-department of Hassan II Hospital in Fes (Morocco), between the years of 2006 and 2014. Results: It is about 56 men and 30 women. The average age was 24 years, with the extremes of 3 years and 65 years. The average time of consultation was 13 dates. The achievement was frontal-ethmoido in 26 cases, and it is about a pan sinusitis in 24 cases. About 13% and 7% of cases were classified respectively in the stage III and the stage IV of chandler. The surgery was done for 24 cases. Bacteriological sample was performed among 24 patients and allowed to isolate a streptococcus (3.5%), and a staphylococcus (5.8%), and a poly microbial flora for 15.1% of patients. A death in sepsis panel was noted for a patient who presented a thrombosis of cavernous sinus. And we have noted a persistent left exophthalmia without the diminution of visual acuity for another patient. Conclusion: The orbital complications of sinusitis require a multi-disciplinary medical approach associated to ear specialist, ophthalmologist, and neuro-radiology. A precocious diagnosis, an appropriate anti-biotic therapy, and sometimes an associated surgical treatment, can significantly diminish the mortality and the morbidity related to this pathology.

Keywords

Oculo Orbital, Sinusitis, Complication, CT Scan, Endoscopic Surgery

---

*Corresponding author.

1. Introduction

The ophthalmologic complications of chronic and acute sinusitis are more frequent than the cranial and endo-cranial complications [1] [2]. The severity of complications attached to the sinus infections resides in the risk of blindness by damage of the optic nerve. The vital prognosis can be included in the forms reaching the orbital apex, by the spread of infection towards the cavernous sinus and the cerebro-meningeal structures [3] [4].

Current thinking supports that the pathogenesis of these complications is predominantly a multifactorial in-flammatory disease [1] [3]. The role of bacteria in the pathogenesis of these complications; is currently being reassessed. Repeated and persistent sinus infections can develop in persons with severe acquired or congenital immunodeficiency states or with a disruption of the intrinsic mucociliary transport system [5] [6].

Despite the fact that the incidence and the severity of these complications have been gradually diminished in recent years in the western countries, they continue to have a serious medico-surgical challenge in our society [1] [5]. Therefore, the objective of our study was to describe the clinic, bacteriologic and therapeutic characteristics of these lesions and their evolution.

2. Patients and Method

We bring a number of cases of the ocular-orbital complications of sinusitis, treated in the ENT department of Hassan II Hospital in Fes (Morocco) during a period of 10 years from January 2006 to September 2014.

The informations were collected from patients' records. The variables collected were about the demographic data, the front door, the time delay before consultation, the ocular-orbital complications observed, the result of bacteriological examination when it is performed, the performed treatment and long-term development. We used the classification of chandler to determine the different anatomic-clinical stages of orbital attacks. This classifi-cation is based on the extension inflammation in relation to the anatomic-physiological boundaries which are the septum and the periosteum by order of increasing severity. The different characteristics have been described as percentage except for age and the time delay before consultation for which the average and the extremes are re-lated. The statistical analysis has been realized using the software Epi Info 3.5.1.

3. Results

During the period of study, 86 cases of ocular-orbital complications have been noted for the patients suffering from sinusitis. The average age of patients was 24 years, with the extremes from 3 years to 65 years with a male predominance (sex ratio of 3/1).

Concerning the antecedents, nine patients were diabetic (10.5%), 27 had a chronic rhinitis and one patient had an antecedent of the old maxilla-facial trauma. Eight cases had chronic smocking.

The search of the sinus gateway, though hard to find at admission, helped us to note a rhinogenic cause in 34 cases (39.5%), dental in three cases (3.4%) and secondary to maxillofacial trauma in one case (1.1%).

The consultation period has been précised for all patients and ranged from three days to 60 days with the me-dian of 13 days.

3.1. Clinical Features and Review

Two thirds of patients (69%) presented the first signs of sinus damage between September and February, which is the period of nasopharyngitis.

The eyelid edema and the periorbital pain were constant symptoms that lead the patients to consult (**Figure 1**). The ENT examination includes systematically a nasal endoscopy which helped to retain the sinus origin in front of mucosal inflammation, festering rhinorrhea and the nasal obstruction.

One of the patients was presented with a bilateral eyelid edema associated to the consciousness troubles. His neurological examination found a state of gradual mental clouding, and imagery found a thrombosis of cavern-ous sinus.

The contribution of ophthalmologists was very successful (**Figure 2**). Their clinic examination allowed to note an eyelid edema and a periorbital pain for all the patients associated with:

- An exophthalmia in 19 cases (22%),
- A conjunctival redness in 11 cases (12.8%),
- Chemosis in 11 cases (12.8%),
- A mydriasis in one case (1.1%),

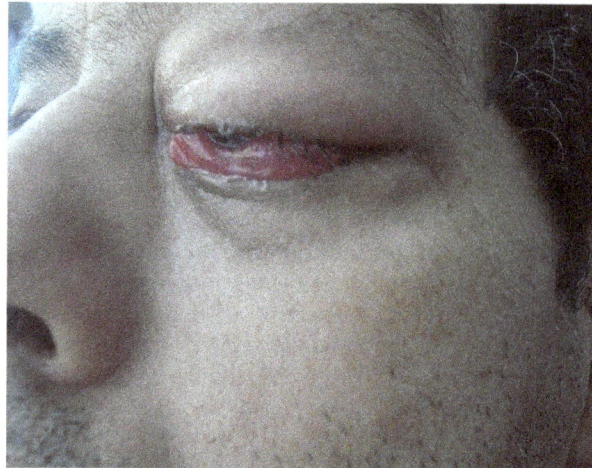

Figure 1. Orbital abscess secondary to a left frontal sinusitis.

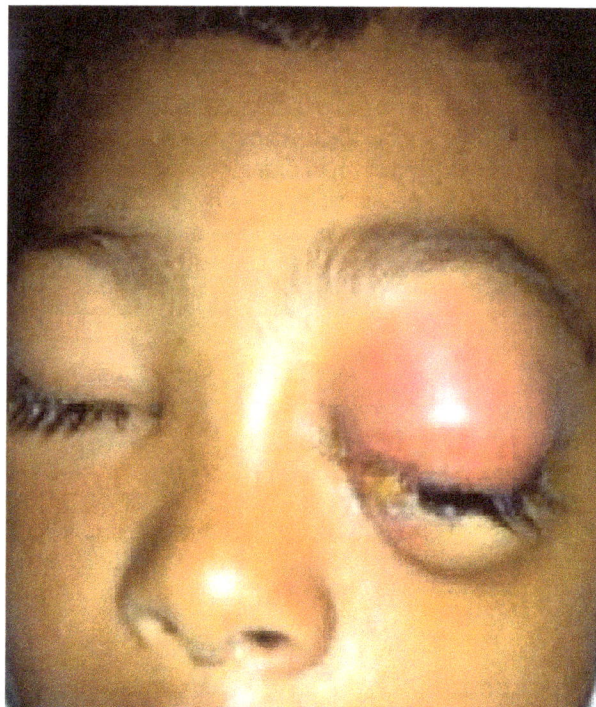

Figure 2. Orbital abscess secondary to a ethmoiditis.

- A squint in 1 case (1.1%),
- Ocular Motility Disorders in five cases (5.8%).

A decrease of visual acuity in 5 cases (5.8%), two cases of blindness: one unilateral (a very pale ischemic papilla in a patient having a pan sinusitis), and the other in a patient with diabetic retinopathy.

3.2. Imagery Results

The ocular echography was done for 12 patients and returned normal in 7 cases and showed an orbital abscess collection in other cases.

The orbital-frontal brain and nasal sinus CT helped appreciating the siege and the extent of sinus damage and assessing the degree of orbital and intracranial complications (**Figure 3**). The frontal ethmoido sinusitis was the most frequent (30.2%) followed by the pansinusitis (27.9%) (**Figure 4**).

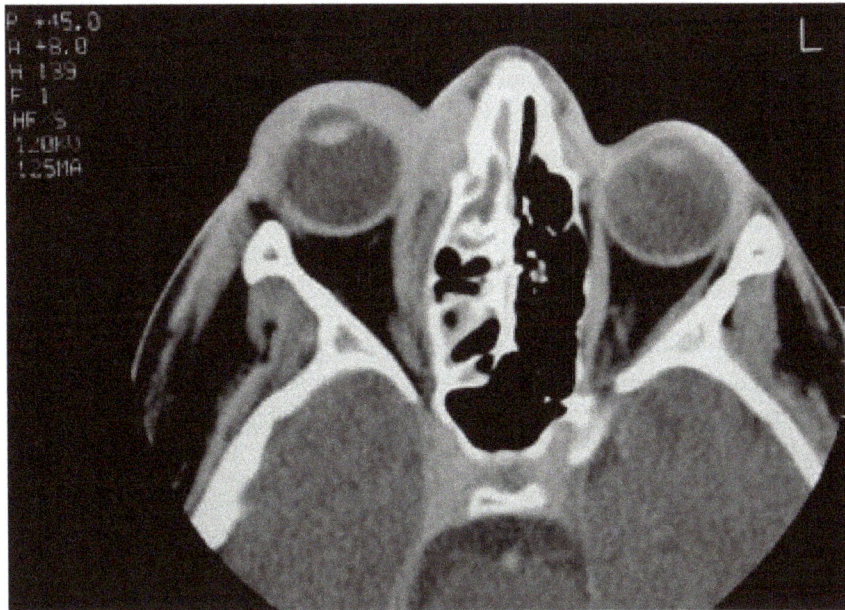

Figure 3. CT image in axial section showing a filling right ethmoid extended to the ipsilateral orbit with subperiosteal abscess and exophthalmia.

Different localizations of sinusitis

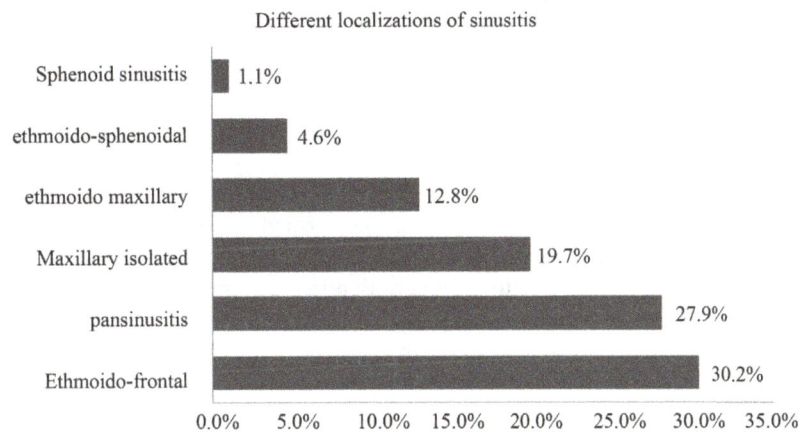

Sphenoid sinusitis 1.1%
ethmoido-sphenoidal 4.6%
ethmoido maxillary 12.8%
Maxillary isolated 19.7%
pansinusitis 27.9%
Ethmoido-frontal 30.2%

Figure 4. Landforms sinusitis.

Distribution of patients according to the classification of Chandler

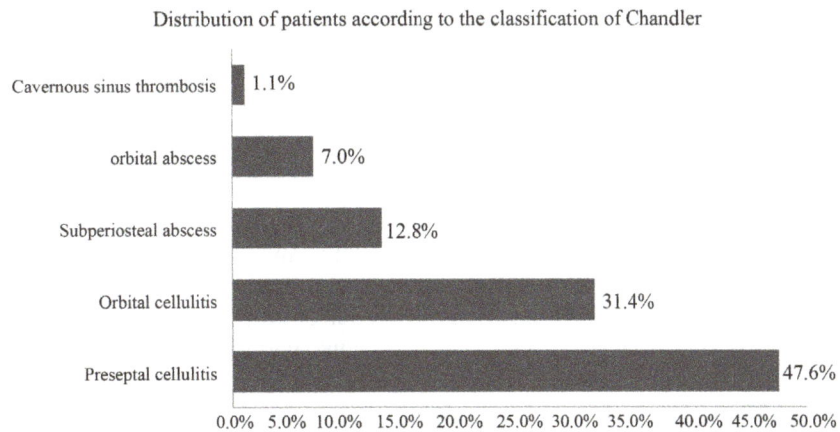

Cavernous sinus thrombosis 1.1%
orbital abscess 7.0%
Subperiosteal abscess 12.8%
Orbital cellulitis 31.4%
Preseptal cellulitis 47.6%

Figure 5. Distribution of patients according to the Chandler's classification.

According to the Chandler's classification, the patients were divided into five stages: 47.6% had a preseptal cellulite, and 31.4% had an orbital cellulite (**Figure 5**).

One single patient had an orbital fistula in addition to the preseptal cellulite. A diabetic patient unbalanced and having the chronic pan-sinusitis neglected, presented a hearth of intracranial suppuration.

3.3. Biological Examination

The biological assessment confirmed inflammatory nature showing a hyper-leucocytosis to neutrophil for 66 patients (76.7%) with a very accelerated sedimentation rate for 59.3% of patients and an elevated CRP for 52% of patients. no blood culture was performed.

The HIV serology was requested for three patients whose clinical condition was very noisy, and it came negative.

The bacteriological examination to find the germ was performed for 24 patients (27.9%). The sample was taken in consultation for a patient with left upper eyelid fistula, and to the operating block during orbital or sinus drainage for 23 cases. The result was in favor of a polymicrobial flora for 13 patients (15.1%); no germ was found for 9 patients (10.4%). The most frequent germs were staphylococcus aureus (5.8%), streptococcus (3.5%), Haemophilus (2.4%) and Bacteroides (1.1%).

3.4. Support and Evolution

During hospitalization, a medical treatment was administered for all patients, based on probabilistic broad-spectrum antibiotic therapy by the parental route sometimes adjusted according to the antibiogram data when available. The length of antibiotic therapy was from 5 to 6 days for the orally injectable route relayed for two weeks. This treatment was associated with:

- A nasal local treatment (washing and trimming of the nasal cavity), in 27 patients or 31.4%.
- An antibiotic collyrium in 19 cases, 20% of patients.
- An oral corticosteroid therapy of short length for 8 patients, 9.3%.

Anticoagulant treatment was prescribed for curative dose in the case of cavernous sinus thrombosis.

The surgery was up every time which conveyed a compressive abscessed collection and before the medical treatment failure. It was performed for 21 patients (24.4%). The surgical gesture consisted of:

- Drainage of orbital abscess in 6 cases, of which one is by endoscopic route and five by external route.
- Drainage of a subperiosteal abscess in one case, performed by endoscopic route.
- A decompressive orbitotomy in one case of orbital cellulite with the aggravation of ocular function.
- An average meatotomy associated to the anterior ethmoidectomy by endoscopic route for seven patients.
- Drainage of an abscess collection of soft parts in two cases.
- A biopsy (after drainage of orbital abscess) in one case.
- A dissection of the fistula in one case, with the curettage of the mucosa of correspondent sinus.

The surveillance under treatment was based on clinical signs (ophthalmologic, rhinologic, and neurologic) and the radiologic signs (the control scanner done in 3 cases). Regular monitoring was conducted for a year. Additionally, the patients consulted in need.

The decline of patients ranged from 14 months to 5 years with an average of 41 months. While monitoring, the patient who presented a carvenous sinus thrombosis passed away in a septicemia table. The persistence of left exophthalmia during eight months without diminution of visual acuity was noted for one patient of 52 years, who has refused the surgery for an abscess under periosteum.

Most of patients were male, with a median age of 24 years and about 11% were diabetic. The frontal-ethmoido damage was the most frequent (30.2%) followed by pan-sinusitis (27.9%). Almost (47.6%) of patients presented a stage I of Chandler (preseptal cellulite) of the orbital complications of sinusitis, while about one third (31.4%) of them had orbital cellulite (stage II). The bacteriological evaluation was generally in favor of polymicrobial flora. Staphylococcus aureus was the most germ found.

All patients have benefited from the antibiotic treatment associated to local treatment. The surgical treatment was performed for 24, 4% of cases, before an abscess collection or treatment failure. The evolution was favorable for all patients, except for the patient having presented a carvenous sinus thrombosis, who died in a septicemia table.

4. Discussion

The ocular-orbital complications are the most frequent (80%) of acute sinusitis complications [1] [3]. In fact 60 to 75% of inflammatory damages of orbit are consecutive for sinusitis [3] [5]. The predominance of ophthalmological complications for children and young people is usually reported in the majority of the literature series [3] [5]-[7]. In the series of Lui the proportion was lower (38.7%) [8].

The male predominance of the orbital complications of acute sinusitis was pointed out by most of the authors [1] [9] [10]. However, in the series reported by Ben Ammor [5], the female predominance was remarked. The immunosuppression is a favorable ground for complicated acute sinusitis [11]. Diabetes is considered as the most classic factor of immunosuppression and the most predisposing for carvenous sinus thrombosis [12]. The infection to VIH [11], medullary aplasia post chemotherapy, treatment by radiotherapy [3] [5] [10], the troubles of local nasal immunity and hypogammaglobulinaemia are also the causes of immunosuppression.

The bilateralization of ophthalmological signs is a factor of poor prognosis, and the visual function can be compromised. The cavernous sinus thrombosis generally includes vital prognosis [12] [13], but it can also appear by an isolated paralysis of VI and simply chemosis and/or ptosis [11] [13].

In most studies, the preseptal cellulites were the most frequently encountered complications [8] [10]. A study conducted in Tunisia [14] proved that about half of the patients presented subperiosteal abscesses.

The ophthalmological complications of acute sinusitis are most often secondary to ethmoiditis [4] [15] [16]. The orbital sonography is effective for the study of the lesions located in front of the orbit and is less efficient in the regions of apex and the back of eyeball. This examination maintains its interest in monitoring under medical treatment abscesses [3] [5] [16] [17]. Furthermore, cerebral CT performed with and without the injection of the contrast material allows searching for possible signs in favor of cavernous sinus damage, or the indirect orbital signs. The RMN is essentially requested before a suspected intracranial spread of infection [6] [18] [19]. It is less available in urgency, and it has not totally replaced the scanner for the initial diagnosis of sinusitis complications, but becomes the choice of examination for monitoring. It is more efficient than scanner in the diagnosis of venous thrombosis, its evolution, and of possible associated parenchymal lesions.

The germs involved are mainly aerobic bacteria. The anaerobic germs will be found in association in 43% of cases, most frequently isolated for adults [5] [10]; they are probably under-estimated infrequency and require an appropriate research in order to adapt the treatment [2] [20] [21]. Some germs seem to present a significant aggressiveness as evidenced by the rapid evolution towards complications. However, the increasing resistances to antibiotic treatment in the first intention must be evoked primarily [3] [14] [15]. For certain authors, the staphylococcus aureus, the streptococcus, anaerobes are most often responsible for orbital complications [21] [22]. For most authors, the common causative organism of carvenous sinus thrombosis is staphylococcus aureus [12] [22]. And the progression towards irreversible blindness is possible in case of methi-resistent staphylococcus aureus [22]. The poly-microbial damage is frequent; especially for adults. The aspergillosis of maxillary sinus on a foreign body of dental origin is the most classical picture of fungal sinusitis [5] [21].

According to Klosselk [4], the patients in the stage I of Chandler can be outpatients. The hospitalizations with an ophtalmological examination, a bacteriological levy, an antibiotic treatment by venous lane are recommended for the stages II, III, IV, and V [4] [23] [24].

The frequency of these complications has been decreased significantly with the advent of new antibiotic molecules [1] [6]. The therapeutic management of sinusitis complications is an urgency, which still relies on a probabilistic broad-spectrum antibiotic therapy, active against the main usual bacteria (aerobic and anaerobic) in the foreground [24]-[26], associated or not to a surgical treatment [1] [17] [25], and undertaken as soon as the samples are done [6] [24]-[26]. This treatment must be adapted secondly in terms of bacteriological results [3] [6] [25] [26]. The duration of intravenous antibiotic therapy is from 5 to 10 days with oral relay soon as apyrexia is durable, and after the disappearance of local inflammatory signs, and it must last between 10 and 15 days [15] [24] [26].

The local treatments are important to facilitate airing and the sinus drainage. This treatment is always necessary. The use of corticoids is very controversial. Some authors advocate corticoids before a suspicion of the optic nerve infringement with the decrease of visual acuity [5]. It has a short duration that ranges from 5 to 6 days [27].

In case of thrombophlebitis; heparin therapy is recommended by some authors [8] [12] and discussed by some others [24] [27]. A randomized clinical attempt confirmed without ambiguity, the benefit of aspirin on the vital and the functional prognosis of the patient. Even in case of the presence of cerebral hemorrhagic lesions [15].

The surgical orbital drainage, using a bacteriological examination, is indicated before tomodensitometric examination of an orbital collection or before the clinical aggravation under treatment [6] [15]. It must be performed in urgency, in order to avoid having serious complications, such as optic nerve compression or of the cavernous sinus thrombosis [12] [28].

The sinus drainage is also systematic. It often helps ameliorating drainage and ventilation of the cells of anterior ethmoid, eliminating the inflammatory pathology which causes the obstruction of drainage tract [5] [15]. The surgical drainage allows having, in good conditions, often difficult bacteriological samples, or impossible to perform in consultation, to open the sinuses widely, and to wash, and to drain. However, since the advent of endoscopic equipments, the endoscopy is becoming increasingly widespread and sets two objectives [23] [28] [29]; the creation of a wide communication between sinuses and nasal pits, and the maximum preservation of anatomy and respiratory mucosa. However, the endoscopic route is not recommended for the pediatric patients, view of the ethmoid size. Thus, the increased risk of the post-operatory complications.

The Endonasal endoscopic surgery allows for a functional gesture of sinonasal cavities while preserving the physiological properties of the lining and providing nasal and sinus ventilation. It allows to limit complications and disfigurement external routes. Its development required the creation of an appropriate instrumentation. Thus the videosurgery, took his booming, making possible the operating comfort, better control gestures and unparalleled quality of teaching [23] [29].

It is noteworthy that even an earlier and aggressive surgical treatment does not ensure the prevention of ocular sequela. Harris [30] reported a sequelar blindness incidence of 14% and Spires an incidence of 33% [31]. Hence, the preventive treatment of complicated acute sinusitis must go through the management of viral rhinopharyngitis since they constitute the front door of sinusitis in most cases, and therefore that of complications. No study to date has investigated the role of vaccines through the general route in preventing the acute rhino-sinus infection of the child [32]. It is likely that the Hib conjugated vaccines (1992) and Heptavalent conjugated pneumococcus are induced by reducing the nasopharyngeal carriage of vaccine serotypes and their transmission, an individual but also collective protection [31] [33].

The pre-septal cellulites, the orbitals, and the sub-periosteal abscesses often have a favorable development without sequella under medical treatment [5] [24]. Yet we can sometimes remark a clinical aggravation (the decrease of visual acuity) in case of sub-periostal abscess. The indication of drainage is formal at this stage [9] [21] [30].

The visual prognosis is strongly undermined despite the urgent establishment of a surgical and medical treatment of intra-orbital abscess. The evolution may do so towards a carvenous sinus thrombosis or a cerebral abscess, bringing into play the vital prognosis [12] [21] [31].

The cavernous sinus thrombosis was a frequent pathology whose mortality is 100% [3] [6]. With the antibiotic treatment, this rate is actually reduced to attain the percentage between 23% and 50% with the neurologic and the ophthalmologic sequela in over half of the cases [3] [6] [9]. The recurrences of ophthalmologic complications must seek an endonasal anomaly; detect a mucoviscidosis or an allergic terrain [31].

The prevention of these complications passes through proper treatment planning. This should include a thorough clinical examination, detailed history taking, and appropriate imaging. In addition to a proper medical history, it is appropriate to take a history of sinus disease, predisposition to colds and sinusitis, as well as a history of any operations that might have been carried out. The immunotherapy reduces the reaction of body against allergens and treats the infection [6] [21].

5. Conclusions

The ocular-orbital complications are rare but severe. Their diagnosis must be urgent and adaptable due to the serious consequences.

Clinical signs help us to determine the type of complications and to evaluate the degree of severity. Imagery confirms diagnosis.

Management is based on a parenteral antibiotic therapy which is mostly directed against the key germs presumed in these conditions. The cooperation of ENT specialists, ophthalmology and radiology is often helpful.

The surgical treatment can be associated in case of an abscessed collection. The radiological and clinical surveillance is unavailable.

Acknowledgements

The accomplishment of this manuscript benefits of the help and direction from my dear supervisor-Prof. A Oudidi. Prof. Oudidi is always happy and willing to help me solve the confusions and direct me approach to the final result of the study. Without his encouragement, I would not finish this final work. Furthermore, I would like to show my grateful feeling to Prof. Bennani, with whose supervision I accomplish my study in time. He is always patient to help me out with questions in terms of administration and rules.

Competing Interests

The authors declare that they have no competing interests.

Authors' Contributions

1) NO: contributions to conception and design, and acquisition of data.
2) AO and SH: analysis and interpretation of data.
3) ZS: participate in drafting the article and revising it critically for important intellectual content.
4) BOM: give final approval of the version to be submitted and any revised version.

References

[1]   Chahed, H., Bachraoui, R., Kedous, S., Ghorbel, H., Houcine, A., Mediouni, A., Marrakchi, J., *et al.* (2014) Management of Ocular and Orbital Complications in Acute Sinusitis. *Journal Français d'Ophtalmologie*, **37**, 702-706. http://dx.doi.org/10.1016/j.jfo.2014.02.010

[2]   Souldi, H., Bouchareb, N., Khassime, S., Abada, R., Rouadi, S., Mahtar, M., *et al.* (2013) Complications Oculo-Orbitaires des sinusites aiguës. *Ann Fr Oto-Rhino-Laryngol Pathol Cervico-Faciale*, **130**, A124.

[3]   Belhoucha, B., Hssaine, K., Rochdi, Y., Nouri, H., Aderdour, L. and Raji, A. (2014) Les complications oculo-orbitaires des sinusites : Etude prospective à propos de 20 cas. *Ann Fr Oto-Rhino-Laryngol Pathol Cervico-Faciale*, **131**, A158-A159. http://dx.doi.org/10.1016/j.aforl.2014.07.370

[4]   Klossek, J.-M., Quinet, B., Bingen, E., François, M., Gaudelus, J., Larnaudie, S., *et al.* (2007) État actuel de la prise en charge des infections rhinosinusiennes aiguës de l'enfant en France. *Médecine et Maladies Infectieuses*, **37**, 127-152. http://dx.doi.org/10.1016/j.medmal.2006.11.008

[5]   Ben Amor, M., Khalifa, Z., Romdhane, N., Zribi, S., Ben Gamra, O., Mbarek, C., *et al.* (2013) Les complications orbitaires des sinusites. *Journal Français d'Ophtalmologie*, **36**, 488-493. http://dx.doi.org/10.1016/j.jfo.2012.06.027

[6]   Sova, J. and Raczyńska, K. (2004) Ocular and Orbital Complications of Paranasal Sinusitis. *Klin Oczna*, **106**, 525-527.

[7]   Nwaorgu, O.G.B., Awobem, F.J., Onakoya, P.A. and Awobem, A.A. (2004) Orbital Cellulitis Complicating Sinusitis: A 15-Year Review. *Nigerian Journal of Surgical Research*, **6**, 14-16.

[8]   Liu, I.-T., Kao, S.-C., Wang, A.-G., Tsai, C.-C., Liang, C.-K. and Hsu, W.-M. (2006) Preseptal and Orbital Cellulitis: A 10-Year Review of Hospitalized Patients. *Journal of the Chinese Medical Association*, **69**, 415-422. http://dx.doi.org/10.1016/S1726-4901(09)70284-9

[9]   Oxford, L.E. and McClay, J. (2006) Medical and Surgical Management of Subperiosteal Orbital Abscess Secondary to Acute Sinusitis in Children. *International Journal of Pediatric Otorhinolaryngology*, **70**, 1853-1861. http://dx.doi.org/10.1016/j.ijporl.2006.05.012

[10]   Ryan, J.T., Sumit, B. and Preciado, D.A. (2008) Orbital Cellulitis in 465 Children: A Review of 465 Cases. *Otolaryngology—Head and Neck Surgery*, **139**, P162. http://dx.doi.org/10.1016/j.otohns.2008.05.436

[11]   Del Borgo, C., Del Forno, A., Ottaviani, F. and Fantoni, M. (1997) Sinusitis in HIV-Infected Patients. *Journal of Chemotherapy*, **9**, 83-88. http://dx.doi.org/10.1179/joc.1997.9.2.83

[12]   Nagi, C.K. (2008) Thrombose de la loge caverneuse secondaire à une sinusite: Cavernous sinus thrombosis secondary to sinusitis. *Journal of Radiology*, **89**, 803-805. http://dx.doi.org/10.1016/S0221-0363(08)73787-9

[13]   Chandler, J.R., Langenbrunner, D.J. and Stevens, E.R. (1970) The Pathogenesis of Orbital Complications in Acute Sinusitis. *The Laryngoscope*, **80**, 1414-1428. http://dx.doi.org/10.1288/00005537-197009000-00007

[14]   Chahed, H., Bachraoui, R., Kedous, S., Ghorbel, H., Houcine, A., Mediouni, A., *et al.* (2014) Prise en charge des complications oculo-orbitaires des sinusites aiguës. *Journal Français d'Ophtalmologie*, **37**, 702-706. http://dx.doi.org/10.1016/j.jfo.2014.02.010

[15]   Ozkurt, F.E., Ozkurt, Z.G., Gul, A., Akdag, M., Sengul, E., Yilmaz, B., *et al.* (2014) Managment of Orbital Complications of Sinusitis. *Arquivos Brasileiros de Oftalmologia*, **77**, 293-296. http://dx.doi.org/10.5935/0004-2749.20140074

[16]   Khaled, H., El korbi, A., Belhadj Rhouma, S., Chouchène, H., Kolsi, N. and Koubaa, J. (2014) Complications orbitaires des sinusites: Diagnostic et prise en charge thérapeutique. *Annales Françaises d'Oto-Rhino-Laryngologie et*

de Pathologie Cervico-Faciale, **131**, A155. http://dx.doi.org/10.1016/j.aforl.2014.07.360

[17] Dessi, P., Champsaur, P., Paris, J. and Moulin, G. (1999) Imaging of the Adult Sinusitis: Indications for Using Conventional Techniques, CT Scan and MRI. *Revue de Laryngologie Otologie Rhinologie*, **120**, 173-176.

[18] Grimbert, P., Vabres, B., Orignac, I., Lebranchu, P., Clairand, R., Gayet, M., *et al.* (2013) Intérêt diagnostique d'une réunion de concertation multidisciplinaire des pathologies orbitaires inflammatoires au CHU de Nantes. *Journal Français d'Ophtalmologie*, **36**, 809-814. http://dx.doi.org/10.1016/j.jfo.2013.02.009

[19] Idrissi, I.A., El Benna, N., Ouardi, F. and Abdelouafi, A. (2009) Imagerie des complications orbitaires de la pathologie naso-sinusienne. *Journal de Radiologie*, **90**, 1563-1564. http://dx.doi.org/10.1016/S0221-0363(09)76128-1

[20] Brook, I. (2009) Microbiology and Antimicrobial Treatment of Orbital and Intracranial Complications of Sinusitis in Children and Their Management. *International Journal of Pediatric Otorhinolaryngology*, **73**, 1183-1186. http://dx.doi.org/10.1016/j.ijporl.2009.01.020

[21] Kim, H.J. (2004) Clinical Analysis of Orbital Complications of Acute Sinusitis in Children and Adults. *Otolaryngology—Head and Neck Surgery*, **131**, P258. http://dx.doi.org/10.1016/j.otohns.2004.06.529

[22] Rutar, T., Zwick, O.M., Cockerham, K.P. and Horton, J.C. (2005) Bilateral Blindness from Orbital Cellulitis Caused by Community-Acquired Methicillin-Resistant *Staphylococcus aureus*. *American Journal of Ophthalmology*, **140**, 740-742. http://dx.doi.org/10.1016/j.ajo.2005.03.076

[23] Ikeda, K., Oshima, T., Suzuki, H., Kikuchi, T., Suzuki, M. and Kobayashi, T. (2003) Surgical Treatment of Subperiosteal Abscess of the Orbit: Sendai's Ten-Year Experience. *Auris Nasus Larynx*, **30**, 259-262. http://dx.doi.org/10.1016/S0385-8146(03)00060-9

[24] François, M., Mariani-Kurkdjian, P., Dupont, E. and Bingen, E. (2006) Ethmoïdites aiguës extériorisées de l'enfant: A propos d'une série de 125 cas. *Archives de Pédiatrie*, **13**, 6-10. http://dx.doi.org/10.1016/j.arcped.2005.09.032

[25] Société de pathologie infectieuse, Société française de pédiatrie, Société française d'ORL and Collège Francais d'ORL (1996) Les infections ORL. *Revue Médicale de l'Assurance Maladie*, **4**, 4-10.

[26] Chidiac, C. (2011) Antibiothérapie par voie générale dans les infections respiratoires basses de l'adulte. *Médecine et Maladies Infectieuses*, **41**, 221-228. http://dx.doi.org/10.1016/j.medmal.2010.10.001

[27] Wane, A.M., Ba, E.A., Ndoye-Roth, P.A., Kameni, A., Demedeiros, M.E., Dieng, M., Ndiaye, M.R., *et al.* (2005) Senegalese Experience of Orbital Cellulitis. *Journal Français d'Ophtalmologie*, **28**, 1089-1094. http://dx.doi.org/10.1016/S0181-5512(05)81143-X

[28] Teinzer, F., Stammberger, H. and Tomazic, P.V. (2015) Transnasal Endoscopic Treatment of Orbital Complications of Acute Sinusitis: The Graz Concept. *Annals of Otology, Rhinology & Laryngology*, **124**, 368-373.

[29] Facon, F. and Dessi, P. (2005) Chirurgie endonasale micro-invasive: Apport de l'endoscopie en chirurgie maxillo-faciale: Rapport pour le 41e Congrès français de Stomatologie et Chirurgie Maxillo-Faciale Marseille, 21-23 septembre 2005. *Revue de Stomatologie et de Chirurgie Maxillo-Faciale*, **106**, 230-242. http://dx.doi.org/10.1016/S0035-1768(05)85852-8

[30] Harris, G.J. (1994) Subperiosteal Abscess of the Orbit. Age as a Factor in the Bacteriology and Response to Treatment. *Ophthalmology*, **101**, 585-595. http://dx.doi.org/10.1016/S0161-6420(94)31297-8

[31] Spires, J.R. and Smith, R.J. (1986) Bacterial Infections of the Orbital and Periorbital Soft-Tissues in Children. *The Laryngoscope*, **96**, 763-767. http://dx.doi.org/10.1288/00005537-198607000-00012

[32] Capra, G., Liming, B., Boseley, M.E. and Brigger, M.T. (2015) Trends in Orbital Complications of Pediatric Rhinosinusitis in the United States. *JAMA Otolaryngology—Head & Neck Surgery*, **141**, 12-17. http://dx.doi.org/10.1001/jamaoto.2014.2626

[33] Lindstrand, A., Bennet, R., Galanis, I., Blennow, M., Ask, L.S., Dennison, S.H., *et al.* (2014) Sinusitis and Pneumonia Hospitalization after Introduction of Pneumococcal Conjugate Vaccine. *Pediatrics*, **134**, e1528-e1536.

List of Abbreviations

CT: Computed Tomography,

NMR: Nuclear Magnetic Resonance,

ENT: Ear, Nose and Throat.

31

Large Penetrating Keratoplasty in the Management of Keratoglobus: A Case Report

Lamprini Papaioannou, Miltiadis Papathanassiou

Cornea Clinic, 2nd Ophthalmology Department, Attikon University Hospital, Athens, Greece
Email: papathanassiou1@gmail.com

Abstract

Background: Keratoglobus is a rare noninflammatory corneal disorder characterized by diffuse corneal thinning and globular protrusion of the cornea. Surgical management of keratoglobus is challenging and the standard method has not yet been defined. Aim: To present the role of large penetrating keratoplasty (PK) in the management of keratoglobus. Case Presentation: A 29-year-old male patient with bilateral keratoglobus presented with acute corneal hydrops in his right eye following extensive Descemet's membrane rupture, with a visual acuity in this eye limited to hand movement. Peripheral cornea was extremely thin and blue sclera was present. Acute hydrops was managed conservatively at this stage and two months later large PK was performed in the right eye using 9.5 mm diameter graft over a 9 mm patient's cornea trephination. Minor aqueous leakage was seen on the first postoperative day, managed with 2 more interrupted 10.0 nylon sutures. No further complications were noticed and postoperative course was uneventful. Fifteen months postoperatively the graft was clear and best corrected visual acuity was 20/60. Conclusions: Large penetrating keratoplasty has an important role in the management of keratoglobus, in cases where peripheral tuck-in lamellar keratoplasty or epikeratoplasty present serious intraoperative difficulties in host lamellar dissection and in stabilizing the graft due to extensive peripheral corneal and scleral thinning.

Keywords

Keratoglobus, Large Penetrating Keratoplasty, Corneal Ectasia

1. Introduction

Keratoglobus is a rare noninflammatory corneal disorder characterized by diffuse corneal thinning from limbus to limbus, commonly maximal at the periphery and globular protrusion of the cornea [1]. Keratoglobus is primarily considered a congenital disorder, although acquired forms of keratoglobus have been reported. The congenital form of the disorder is always bilateral and it is assumed to be autosomal recessive but to our knowledge the inheritance pattern has not yet been defined [2]. It has also been associated with disorders of the connective tissue such as Ehlers-Danlos syndrome, Marfan syndrome, and Rubinstein-Taybi syndrome, with the former being the most common association. Other systemic associations include Leber's congenital amaurosis, Syphilis and Thyroid eye disease [1]. Aquired keratoglobus has been described in idiopathic orbital inflammation, possibly caused by anterior segment ischaemia and in vernal keratoconjuctivitis and chronic marginal blepharitis, possibly attributable to frequent eye rubbing. The most common ocular feature associated with keratoglobus is blue sclera caused by a thinned and more transparent sclera, maximally at the ciliary body. Patients with keratoglobus have clear corneas with normal diameter and the main cause of poor vision is high myopia with irregular astigmatism caused by excessive corneal thinning and protrusion. Corneal thinning and fragility can result in corneal perforations, either spontaneous or following minor trauma. Spontaneous tears in Descemet's membrane may also occur, resulting in acute hydrops [1] [3].

Surgical management of keratoglobus is challenging and the standard method has not yet been defined, considering the rarity and the special features of the condition, mainly including the corneal thinning from limbus to limbus. Several modifications of conventional penetrating and lamellar keratoplasty procedures have been reported, aiming to overcome the special difficulties and risk factors. We present the role of large penetrating keratoplasty (PK) in the management of the condition.

2. Case Presentation

A 29-year old male patient with known history of bilateral keratoglobus presented to the Cornea Clinic with pain, photophobia and blurred vision in his right eye of two days duration. Best corrected visual acuity was limited to hand movement in the right eye and 20/120 in left eye. The diagnosis of bilateral keratoglobus was established with corneal topography (Oculus Pentacam). Slit lamp examination revealed acute corneal hydrops caused by extensive Descemet's membrane rupture in his right eye (**Figure 1**), excessive thinning in the juxtalimbal periphery and coexisting blue sclera in both eyes (**Figure 2**). Intraocular pressure was 11 and 12 mmHg in the right and left eye respectively and further eye examination was unremarkable. No further systemic associations were present.

Acute hydrops was managed conservatively with topical hypertonic agents at this stage as the extent of the break made the use of intracameral gas for reattachment extremely difficult. Two months later, a large PK was performed in the right eye for visual rehabilitation. A 9.5 mm diameter graft was used over a 9 mm patient's cornea trephination. 22 interrupted 10.0 nylon sutures were placed and the procedure was uneventful.

Minor aqueous leak between 2nd and 3rd hour was noticed on the first postoperative day, managed with two additional interrupted 10.0 nylon sutures. No further complications were noticed. Fifteen months postoperatively the graft remained clear and best corrected visual acuity was 20/60 (**Figure 3**).

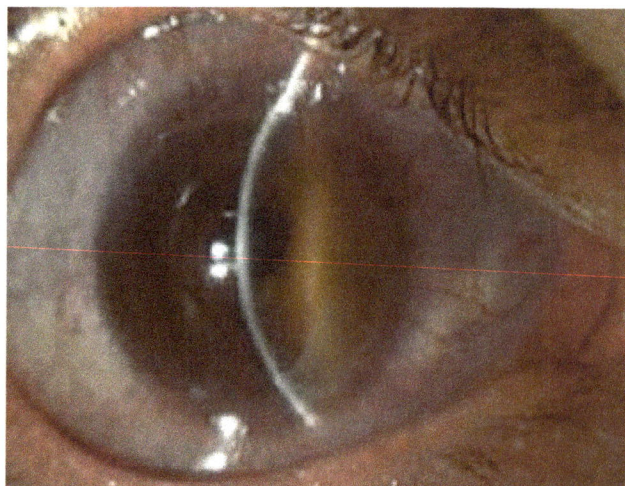

Figure 1. Extensive descemet's membrane rupture.

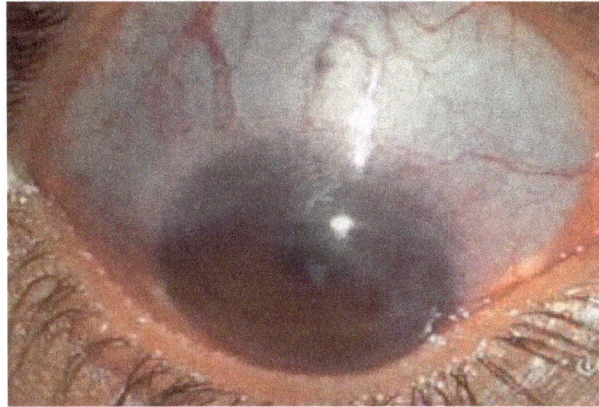

Figure 2. Co-existing blue sclera was present in our patient.

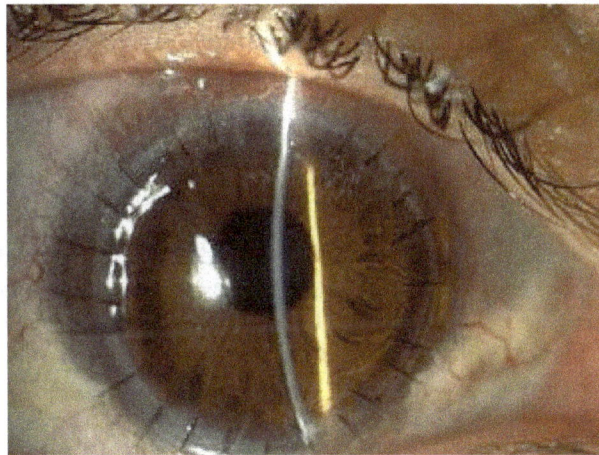

Figure 3. The 9.5 mm diameter graft remained clear 15 months postoperatively.

3. Discussion

The features of keratoglobus as discussed above, make the management of the condition challenging. Regarding the management of acute hydrops, it can be both conservative and invasive. Conventional treatment includes bandage contact lens, topical hypertonic saline and cycloplegics [3]. More invasive is the use of intracameral gas to tamponade the detached descemet's membrane to the posterior surface of the corneal stroma [4] [5]. Regarding the surgical management of keratoglobus, no golden standard has been defined. Conventional penetrating keratoplasty presents difficulties in wound closure, due to excessive mid-peripheral corneal thinning and graft to host thickness disparity. Therefore, an alternative option of penetrating keratoplasty has been described, using large limbus to limbus donor corneal grafts to avoid placement of the graft-host junction at the thinned mid-periphery [6]. Thereby, wound healing and tectonic stability are promoted, but the immunological privilege of corneal transplant is lost, while limbal stem cells are disrupted [7]. Several modifications of lamellar keratoplasty have also been described in the literature. Epikeratoplasty is such a technique that uses a donor graft, denuded from descemet's membrane, placed over the host cornea after posterior dissection of the conjunctiva [8]. The graft is sutured to the sclera and thus epikeratoplasty has the advantantage of avoiding suturing to the thin corneal periphery, but this advantage is limited in cases with coexisting scleral thinning. On the other hand, this technique disrupts limbal stem cells and could result in persistant epithelial defects. Promising were the results of a modified epikeratoplasty technique, described by Javadi *et al.*, aiming to avoid limbal stem cell damage, by creating a 360 degree peripheral lamellar intrastromal pocket in the host cornea for the insertion of the donor corneo-scleral button [9]. Epikeratoplasty followed by secondary penetrating keratoplasty for visual rehabilitation has also been reported [10]. An alternative technique is "Tuck-in" lamellar keratoplasty (TILK) that involves a central lamellar dissection along with a peripheral intrastromal pocket, where the peripheral donor flange is tucked in [11]. Further novel techniques have been reported, such as the use of an allograft corneoscleral ring around the limbus to support the mid-peripheral thinned cornea, described by Kanellopoulos and Pentacam-based big bubble deep anteriorlamellar keratoplasty, described by Riss *et al.* [12] [13] More recently, Karimian *et al.* described a limbal stem cell-sparing lamellar keratoplasty (LSCS-LKP) and Lockington *et al.* described a lamellar keratoplasty with a pleat creation to address the abnormal white-to-white diameter [14] [15].

In our case, excessive corneal thinning and scleral thinning were considered as high risk factors for serious intraoperative difficulties in host lamellar dissection and in stabilizing the graft in a tuck-in lamellar keratoplasty or epikeratoplasty. Additionally, the presence of an extensive descemet's membrane rupture would require a secondary PK for visual rehabilitation. Therefore large PK was felt a safer approach, as it allowed the replacement of the ruptured descemet's membrane, while the immune disadvantage of a limbus to limbus PK was limited due to the smaller size of the graft (9.5 mm). Furthermore, limbal stem cell and angle structure disruption was avoided. On the other hand, the graft suturing was still challenging and more sutures were placed compared to the standard PK technique. However, a minor aqueous leak was noticed on the first postoperative day, managed with two additional sutures. No further complications were noticed. To our knowledge, large PK has already been reported in a keratoglobus case by Kodjikian *et al.*, using a mid-sized graft of 9 mm diameter placed eccentrically [16]. However, since no standard method has yet been defined and no large series regarding the surgical management of keratoglobus are available in the literature, one additional report could contribute to this objective.

4. Conclusion

In conclusion, the rarity of the condition limits the ability of comparative studies or large case series. Therefore, reports of surgeons' experience, obtained even by single cases could be helpful in drawing conclusions for the options of keratoglobus surgical management. In this perspective, we believe that large penetrating keratoplasty has an important role in keratoglobus management, especially in cases with descemet's membrane rupture and co-existing blue sclera.

References

[1] Wallang, B.S. and Das, S. (2013) Keratoglobus. *Eye*, **27**, 1004-1012. http://dx.doi.org/10.1038/eye.2013.130

[2] Pouliquen, Y., Dhermy, P., Espinasse, M.A. and Savoldelli, M. (1985) Keratoglobus. *Journal Français d'Ophtalmologie*, **8**, 43-45.

[3] Grewal, S., Laibson, P.R., Cohen, E.J. and Rapuano, C.J. (1999) Acute Hydrops in the Corneal Ectasias: Associated Factors and Outcomes. *Transactions of the American Ophthalmological Society*, **97**, 187-198.

[4] Panda, A., Aggarwal, A., Madhavi, P., Wagh, V.B., Dada, T., Kumar, A., *et al.* (2007) Management of Acute Corneal Hydrops Secondary to Keratoconus with Intracameral Injection of Sulfur Hexafluoride (SF6). *Cornea*, **26**, 1067-1069. http://dx.doi.org/10.1097/ICO.0b013e31805444ba

[5] Shah, S.G., Sridhar, M.S. and Sangwan, V.S. (2005) Acute Corneal Hydrops Treated by Intracameral Injection of Perfluoropropane (C3F8) Gas. *American Journal of Ophthalmology*, **139**, 368-370. http://dx.doi.org/10.1016/j.ajo.2004.07.059

[6] Cowden, J.W., Copeland, R.A. and Schneider, M.S. (1989) Large Diameter Therapeutic Penetrating Keratoplasties. *Refractive & Corneal Surgery*, **5**, 244-248.

[7] Khodadoust, A.A. and Silverstein, A.M. (1972) Studies on the Nature of the Privilege Enjoyed by Corneal Allografts. *Investigative Ophthalmology*, **11**, 137-148.

[8] Cameron, J.A., Cotler, J.B., Risco, J.M. and Alvarez, H. (1991) Epikeratoplasty for Keratoglobus Associated with Blue Sclera. *Ophthalmology*, **98**, 446-452. http://dx.doi.org/10.1016/S0161-6420(91)32271-1

[9] Javadi, M.A., Kanavi, M.R., Ahmadi, M. and Yazdani, S. (2007) Outcomes of Epikeratoplasty for Advanced Keratoglobus. *Cornea*, **26**, 154-157. http://dx.doi.org/10.1097/01.ico.0000244878.38621.fc

[10] Jones, D.H. and Kirkness, C.M. (2001) A New Surgical Technique for Keratoglobus-Tectonic Lamellar Keratoplasty Followed by Secondary Penetrating Keratoplasty. *Cornea*, **20**, 885-887. http://dx.doi.org/10.1097/00003226-200111000-00022

[11] Kaushal, S., Jhanji, V., Sharma, N., Tandon, R., Titiyal, J.S. and Vajpayee, R.B. (2008) "Tuck-In" Lamellar Keratop-

lasty (TILK) for Corneal Ectasias Involving Corneal Periphery. *British Journal of Ophthalmology*, **92**, 286-290.
http://dx.doi.org/10.1136/bjo.2007.124628

[12] Kanellopoulos, A.J. and Pe, L.H. (2005) An Alternative Surgical Procedure for the Management of Keratoglobus. *Cornea*, **24**, 1024-1026. http://dx.doi.org/10.1097/01.ico.0000157411.31566.a7

[13] Riss, S., Heindl, L.M., Bachmann, B.O., Kruse, F.E. and Curseifen, C. (2012) Pentacam-Based Big Bubble Deep Anterior Lamellar Keratoplasty in Patients with Keratoconus. *Cornea*, **31**, 627-632.
http://dx.doi.org/10.1097/ICO.0b013e31823f8c85

[14] Karimian, F., Baradaran-Rafii, A., Faramarzi, A. and Akbari, M. (2014) Limbal Stem Cell-Sparing Lamellar Keratoplasty for the Management of Advanced Keratoglobus. *Cornea*, **33**, 105-108.
http://dx.doi.org/10.1097/ICO.0b013e3182a9b1ac

[15] Lockington, D. and Ramaesh, K. (2015) Use of a Novel Lamellar Keratoplasty with Pleat Technique to Address the Abnormal White-to-White Diameter in Keratoglobus. *Cornea*, **34**, 239-242.
http://dx.doi.org/10.1097/ICO.0000000000000315

[16] Kodjikian, L., Baillif, S., Burillon, C., Grange, J.D. and Garweg, J.G. (2004) Keratoglobus Surgery: Penetrating Keratoplasty Redux. *Acta Ophthalmologica Scandinavica*, **82**, 625-627.
http://dx.doi.org/10.1111/j.1600-0420.2004.00271.x

32

Effects of Cyclopentolate on Form Deprivation Myopia in Guinea Pigs

Tao Li[1], Xiaodong Zhou[1*], Zhi Chen[2], Xingtao Zhou[2]

[1]Department of Ophthalmology, Jinshan Hospital of Fudan University, Shanghai, China
[2]Department of Ophthalmology, Eye and ENT Hospital of Fudan University, Shanghai, China
Email: *xdzhou2013@126.com

Abstract

Purpose: To investigate the effects of intravitreal injection of cyclopentolate on form deprivation myopia in guinea pigs. Methods: Thirty-five guinea pigs at age of 3 weeks were randomly divided into 5 groups (n = 7 for each group): deprived, deprived plus saline, deprived plus cyclopentolate, normal control, and cyclopentolate group. Form deprivation was only performed in right eyes with translucent membranes for 4 weeks. Physiological saline and cyclopentolate were intravitreally injected into deprived eyes at four-day intervals. All the left eyes remained untreated as group control. Refraction was measured by retinoscopy after cycloplegia. The axial dimensions were measured by A-scan ultrasound. Subsequently, retinal histology was observed by light microscopy. Results: After 4 weeks of treatment, intravitreal injection of cyclopentolate significantly reduced the degree of myopia in the deprived eyes (from −3.92 D to −0.86 D, $P < 0.001$), and retarded the increase of vitreous chamber depth (from 3.83 ± 0.06 mm to 3.70 ± 0.05 mm, $P < 0.001$) and axial length (from 8.42 ± 0.04 mm to 8.30 ± 0.05 mm, $P < 0.001$) in the deprived eyes. Histological examination revealed no evidence of retinal damage of eyes injected with physiological saline or cyclopentolate compared with normal control eyes. Conclusions: Intravitreal administration of cyclopentolate reduces axial elongation of the deprived eyes in guinea pigs. Further investigations are required to identify the optimal dose.

Keywords

Cyclopentolate, Muscarinic Antagonist, Form Deprivation Myopia, Axial Length, Refraction

1. Introduction

Form deprivation myopia (FDM) in mammals has been linked to disruption of emmetropization due to poor

---

*Corresponding author.

image quality on the retina of deprived eye. A variety of ocular conditions that lead to varying degrees of visual deprivation in human eyes such as corneal opacity [1] and vitreous haemorrhage [2] are associated with myopia in humans. It has been demonstrated in a wide range of animal species including chicks [3], tree shrews [4], guinea pigs [5] [6], monkeys [7] [8], fish [9] and mice [10]. The experimental myopia of animal models shares similar characteristic features with human myopia, such as an increase in the axial length of the eye [11].

Muscarinic antagonists were reported to inhibit or decrease the development of FDM [12]-[16]. McBrien *et al.* [12] found that the non-selective muscarinic antagonist atropine inhibited experimentally induced myopia through chronic intravitreal injection. Tropicamide, another non-selective muscarinic antagonist, was also proved to be partially effective in inhibiting myopia in chicks [16]. The M1-selective antagonist pirenzepine was effective in reducing the axial elongation associated with experimental myopia in a dose-dependent manner [13] [14]. Cottriall *et al.* [15] revealed that the M4-selective antagonist himbacine was effective in preventing the development of myopia in chicks. Many other antagonists were tested in the deprived eyes of chicks as well [16].

Atropine is also the most widely investigated pharmacological agent for the prevention of children myopia progression. The higher the concentration of atropine is, the greater the control effect of myopia progression is, and the more the adverse effects are [17] [18]. The safety profile of atropine (*i.e.*, its effect on pupil size and accommodation) has always been of concern and prohibited many children from utilizing this medication. However, photophobia due to mydriasis and blurring of near vision from induced cycloplegia often disturb children and resulted in a high rate of noncompliance from children.

Cyclopentolate, a type of muscarinic antagonist, is widely used as a cycloplegic and mydriatic agent for eye examination in clinical practice. Yen and colleagues [19] found that the mean myopic progression of children with use of cyclopentolate 1% eye drops every night was statistically less than that with use of normal saline eye drops. Furthermore, topical administration of cyclopentolate dilated the pupil in all eyes of guinea pigs but did not change other ocular parameters (*i.e.*, refraction, vitreous chamber depth, axial length) [20]. However, the long-term effect of cyclopentolate on myopia control is not fully determined, and it has not yet been evaluated the effectiveness on FDM in animals.

The guinea pigs are a promising alternative to other mammals for experimental myopia, as they are born with a well-developed visual system [5] [6]. The purpose of this study was to investigate the effects of intravitreal injection of cyclopentolate on FDM in guinea pigs.

2. Materiors and Methods

2.1. Animals

Thirty-five pigmented guinea pigs at age of 3 weeks were obtained from the breeding room in Thai town, Fengxian District, Shanghai City, China. These animals were randomly divided into 5 groups (n = 7 in each group): deprived, deprived plus saline, deprived plus cyclopentolate, normal control, and cyclopentolate group. Guinea pigs were reared at 25°C with a 12-12 h light-dark cycle. The animal research was approved by the Animal Care and Ethics Committee at Jinshan Hospital of Fudan University, Shanghai, China. The treatment and care of the animals were conducted according to the ARVO Statement for the Use of Animals in Ophthalmic and Vision research.

2.2. Form Deprivation Myopia

The procedure of form deprivation has been detailed in a previous study [5]. Briefly, the right eyes of guinea pigs were occluded with self-made translucent membranes, which were held in place based on their rubber-band effect around the mouth and head of guinea pigs. The left eye, nose, mouth and ears were exposed. The guinea pigs cooperated well in the process of wearing the occluders, and anaesthesia was not necessary for this procedure. The diffusers did not compromise the cornea, and the right eyes could blink behind the occluders freely. The occluders made from milky white latex gloves were opaque, soft and elastic with the thickness less than 0.06 mm, and light transmission of 60%. The diffusers were examined once a day to ensure they were in place.

2.3. Treatment Protocols

Guinea pigs were intraperitoneally injected with 100 mg/kg ketamine HCL (Gutian Pharmaceutical Company,

Fujian, China). After anesthesia, the right eyes of the guinea pigs received intravitreal injections through the pars plana 1 mm from the limbus using a 26-gauge needle at four-day intervals for a total of 7 injections during 4-week treatment periods according to their treatment group. The deprived plus cyclopentolate group and cyclopentolate group received 10 µL of cyclopentolate (10 µg/µL; Alcon, US) at 9 a.m. To test for a possible vehicle effect, 10 µl of physiological saline were intravitreally injected in the right eyes in deprived plus saline group. The occluders were renewed after every injection. All the left eyes remained untreated as a control.

2.4. Refraction and Biometric Measurement

Each eye was measured before treatment and after 4 weeks of treatment. Cycloplegia and dilation of the pupil was induced by 4 drops of tropicamide 0.5%, and 30 minutes later ocular refraction was measured with a streak retinoscope. All refractive errors were measured in the horizontal and vertical meridians, which was described in Howlett *et al.* [6]. Refractions were reported as spherical equivalents (sphere plus half the cylinder). A refractive accuracy of 0.25 D has been determined previously by Zhou *et al.* [21].

The axial dimensions were measured by A-scan ultrasound (11 MHz; Hiscan A/B, Opticon, Italy) under corneal topical anesthesia (oxybuprocaine hydrochloride 0.4%, Santen, Japan), including axial length (a distance from the corneal apex to the vitreous-retinal interface, including cornea thickness), anterior chamber depth (a distance from the corneal apex to the front surface of the lens, including cornea thickness), lens thickness and vitreous chamber depth (a distance from the back of the crystalline lens to the vitreous-retinal interface). The ultrasound probe was directly in contact with the cornea during the axial measurement. A genuine measurement was confirmed when clear traces of various components of the eye with consistent waves and amplitudes were detected [22]. Peaks were selected for the front of the cornea, the front and back of the crystalline lens, and the vitreous-retinal interface. The average value was then used for analysis. All measurements were performed by the same examiner who was masked to the treatment group assignment.

2.5. Retinal Histology

Retinal tissue was acquired for retinal histology at the end of the treatment. Guinea pigs were administered a lethal dose of sodium pentobarbital (150 mg/kg). Right eyes of the animals were enucleated and fixed with paraformaldehyde 4% in 0.1 M phosphate buffer solution (PBS, pH 7.4) for 24 h at 4°C. The eyeballs were then hemisected equatorially with removal of the lens and vitreous body. The eyecups were immersed in fresh paraformaldehyde 4% solution, followed by a routine histological processing text. Sections of approximately 4-µm thickness (0.5 mm from the temporal margin of the optic disc) were cut on a microtome, mounted on slides, stained with hematoxylin and eosin. Slides were examined at ×200 magnification on an Olympus microscope fitted with a digital camera.

2.6. Statistical Analysis

Statistical Package for the Social Sciences software (version 16.0, SPSS, Inc.) was used for statistical analysis. Data were expressed as mean ± standard deviation (SD). Paired t tests were performed to compare intra-group differences. One-way analysis of variance (ANOVA) was used to compare inter-group differences. If ANOVA showed a significant difference, a Bonferroni post-hoc test was applied to determine whether there were significant differences between pairs of groups. $P < 0.05$ was considered statistically significant.

3. Results

3.1. Effect of Cyclopentolate on Refraction

The eyes of guinea pigs, at age of 3 weeks, initially showed mild hyperopia. No statistically significant difference in the refraction was observed between the right and left eyes. After the right eyes were occluded for 4 weeks, the deprived eyes became significantly myopic compared with the fellow eyes and normal control eyes ($P < 0.001$ and $P < 0.001$, respectively; **Table 1** and **Figure 1**).

Intravitreal injection of cyclopentolate (700 µg) significantly reduced the degree of myopia in the deprived eyes compared to deprived plus saline group (from -3.92 ± 0.64 D to -0.86 ± 0.69 D, $P < 0.001$; **Table 1**). However, FDM could still be induced in deprived eyes which had undergone cyclopentolate treatment, because

Table 1. Cycloplegic ocular refraction and biometric dimensions of the right and left eyes in guinea pigs at the end of 4-week treatment period.

Groups	Eye	Refraction (D)	Axial length (mm)	Anterior chamber depth (mm)	Lens thickness (mm)	Vireous chamber depth (mm)
Deprived	Right	−3.86 ± 0.65[c]	8.41 ± 0.06[c]	1.21 ± 0.04	3.39 ± 0.04	3.81 ± 0.05[c]
	Left	1.29 ± 0.31	8.24 ± 0.04	1.22 ± 0.03	3.39 ± 0.03	3.63 ± 0.04
Deprived + saline	Right	−3.92 ± 0.64[c]	8.42 ± 0.04[c]	1.21 ± 0.04	3.38 ± 0.04	3.83 ± 0.06[c]
	Left	1.18 ± 0.27	8.23 ± 0.03	1.21 ± 0.04	3.38 ± 0.04	3.64 ± 0.04
Deprived + cyclopentolate	Right	−0.86 ± 0.69[abc]	8.30 ± 0.05[abc]	1.21 ± 0.05	3.39 ± 0.04	3.70 ± 0.05[abc]
	Left	1.26 ± 0.28	8.23 ± 0.03	1.21 ± 0.04	3.38 ± 0.03	3.64 ± 0.04
Normal control	Right	1.27 ± 0.28	8.22 ± 0.04	1.21 ± 0.04	3.39 ± 0.04	3.62 ± 0.04
	Left	1.23 ± 0.27	8.22 ± 0.05	1.21 ± 0.03	3.38 ± 0.03	3.63 ± 0.05
Cyclopentolate	Right	1.26 ± 0.30	8.23 ± 0.04	1.20 ± 0.03	3.39 ± 0.03	3.64 ± 0.04
	Left	1.29 ± 0.24	8.24 ± 0.04	1.21 ± 0.03	3.39 ± 0.03	3.64 ± 0.05

Data were expressed in mean ± SD. [a]$P < 0.05$, compared with deprived group; [b]$P < 0.05$, compared with deprived plus saline group; [c]$P < 0.05$, compared with normal control group.

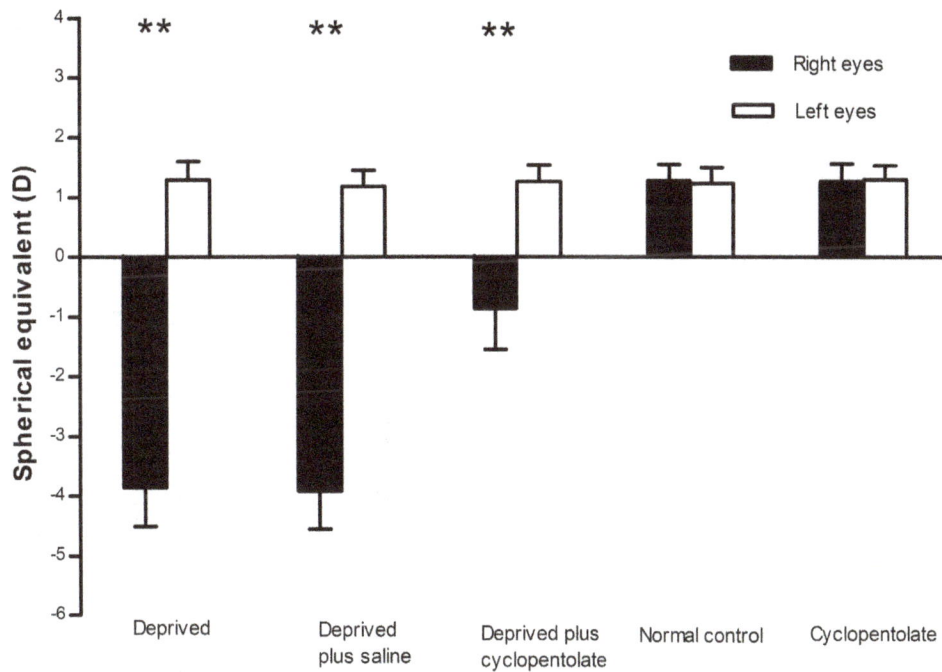

Figure 1. Average refraction (mean ± SD) of the right and left eyes at the end of 4-week treatment period in the different groups (n = 7 guinea pigs for each group). Asterisks refer to the difference between the right and left eyes in each group. [**]$P < 0.001$; [*]$P < 0.05$.

its refraction showed a statistically significant difference compared with fellow eyes ($P < 0.001$). In contrast, intravitreal injection of physiological saline caused no significant effect on the refraction of deprived eyes compared to the deprived eyes in the deprived group ($P = 1.00$). In non-deprived age-matched animals, there was no statistically significant difference in the ocular refraction of between cyclopentolate treatment and normal control. No statistically significant difference was observed in the refraction of fellow eyes in the different treatment groups (F = 0.475, $P = 0.75$).

3.2. Effects of Cyclopentolate on Ocular Biometric Dimensions

After 4 weeks of treatment, there were significant differences in vitreous chamber depth (VCD) and axial length (AL) between the deprived and fellow eyes in deprived plus cyclopentolate group ($P < 0.001$ and $P < 0.001$, respectively; **Figure 2**, **Figure 3**). Significant differences in VCD and AL were also observed between the deprived eyes in deprived plus cyclopentolate group and the deprived eyes in deprived plus saline group ($P < 0.001$ and $P < 0.001$, respectively; **Table 1**). Intravitreal injection of cyclopentolate (700 μg) significantly retarded the increase of VCD (from 3.83 ± 0.06 mm to 3.70 ± 0.05 mm, $P < 0.001$; **Table 1**) and AL (from 8.42 ± 0.04 mm to 8.30 ± 0.05 mm, $P < 0.001$; **Table 1**) in the deprived eyes compared to those of the deprived eyes in the deprived group and deprived plus saline group.

However, the increase of VCD and AL in the deprived eyes was not suppressed completely by cyclopentolate treatment, because its VCD and AL showed a statistically significant difference compared with fellow eyes. In contrast, intravitreal injection of physiological saline caused no significant effect on VCD and AL of deprived eyes compared to the deprived group. In non-deprived age-matched animals, there was no statistically significant difference in the VCD and AL of between cyclopentolate treatment and normal control.

As illustrated in **Table 1**, there were no statistically significant differences in anterior chamber depth, lens thickness, VCD, and AL between the right and left eyes in normal control group. There were no statistically significant differences in anterior chamber depth and lens thickness of deprived eyes in different treatment groups, as well as anterior chamber depth, lens thickness, VCD and AL of fellow eyes in different treatment groups.

3.3. Retinal Histology

As can be seen in **Figure 4**, guinea pigs showed a normal arrangement of ganglion cell layer (GCL), inner plexiform layer (IPL), inner nuclear layer (INL), outer plexiform layer (OPL), outer nuclear layer (ONL) and photoreceptor layer (PL). Histological examination revealed these layers were similar in retinal structure and integrity among all the 5 groups. There was no apparent evidence of retinal damage of eyes injected with physiological saline or cyclopentolate compared with normal control eyes.

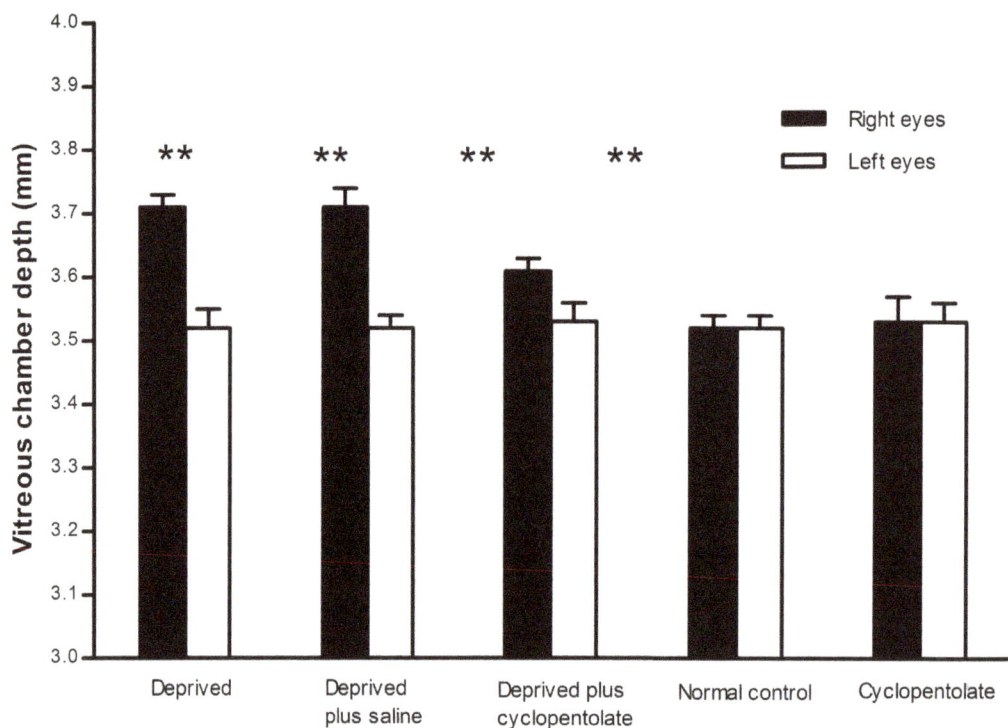

Figure 2. Average vitreous chamber depth (mean ± SD) of the right and left eyes at the end of 4-week treatment period in the different groups (n = 7 guinea pigs for each group). Asterisks refer to the difference between the right and left eyes in each group. $^{**}P < 0.001$; $^{*}P < 0.05$.

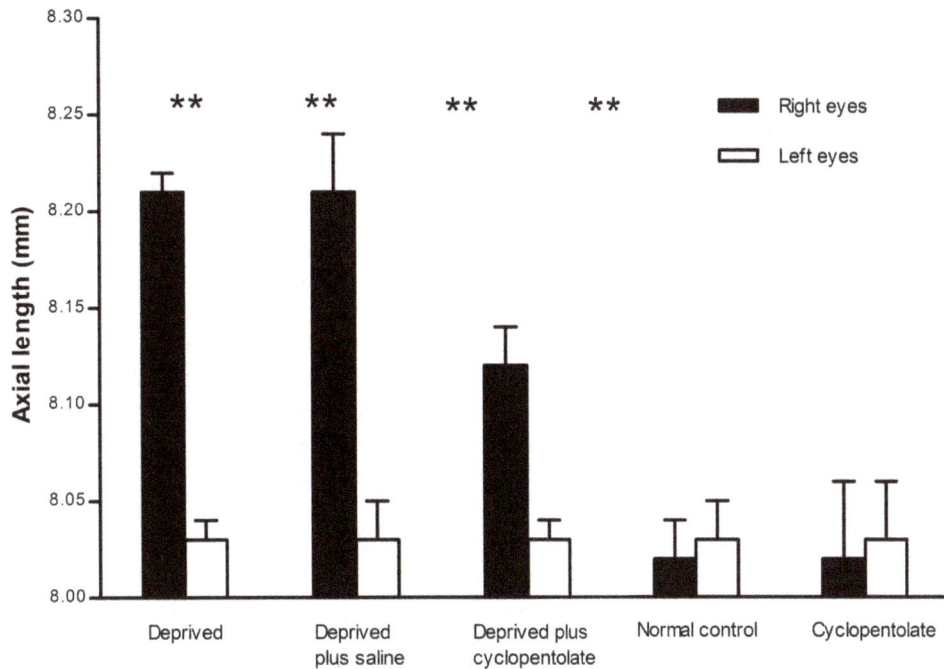

Figure 3. Average axial length (mean ± SD) of the right and left eyes at the end of 4-week treatment period in the different groups (n = 7 guinea pigs for each group). Asterisks refer to the difference between the right and left eyes in each group. [**]$P < 0.001$; [*]$P < 0.05$.

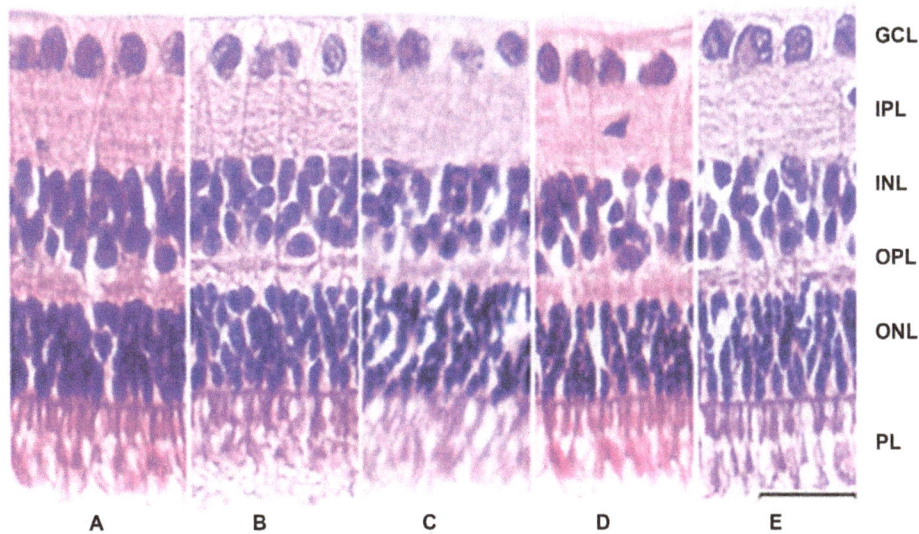

Figure 4. Light microscopy in right eyes of guinea pigs for the six groups. No abnormality was detected in any layers of the retinal tissue from posterior pole (0.5 mm away from optic disc). GCL: ganglion cell layer; IPL: inner plexiform layer; INL: inner nuclear layer; OPL: outer plexiform layer; ONL: outer nuclear layer; PL: photoreceptor layer; A: deprived group; B: deprived plus saline group; C: deprived plus cyclopentolate group; D: normal control group; E: cyclopentolate group; Bar: 50 μm.

4. Discussion

The present study demonstrated intravitreal administration of cyclopentolate could reduce the excessive axial elongation and the concomitant development of FDM in guinea pigs. Furthermore, our findings of similar results for anterior chamber depth and lens thickness across all the groups indicate that their development was unrelated to the different treatment modalites.

Cyclopentolate is a muscarinic receptor antagonist like atropine [23], which is widely used in clinical practice. Atropine has many ocular and systemic side effects (e.g., allergic conjunctivitis, glare, gastric pain) [18] compared to cyclopentolate, and hence it is not a popular choice of drug for myopia treatment. Although short-acting, minimal side effects of cyclopentolate make it a potential drug for anti-myopia therapy. Observing 96 children in Taiwan, Yen *et al.* [19] found that the mean myopic progression was −0.578 D/y in the cyclopentolate group and −0.219 D/y in the atropine group, both of which were statistically less than that in the control group. However, no further study reported the effect of cyclopentolate on myopia in children and animal models. To the best of our knowledge, this study is the first to evaluate the effectiveness of intravitreal injection of cyclopentolate on FDM in guinea pig eyes. In the current study, intravitreal injection of cyclopentolate showed a significant inhibitory effect on deprivation-induced myopia in guinea pigs, but there were still significant differences in refraction, VCD and AL between the deprived and fellow eyes. They could not completely inhibit the development of FDM, suggesting the doses of cyclopentolate (700 µg) or the frequency of its administration (intravitreal injections at four-day intervals) might be too low to induce a complete elimination of myopia. In addition, after intravitreal injection of cyclopentolate in the non-deprived animals, their refraction and ocular biometric dimensions showed no significant changes, indicating that local cyclopentolate had no effect on the normal refractive development in guinea pigs.

Topical administration of pirenzepine can prevent induced form-deprivation [24] and lens-induced [25] experimental myopia in guinea pigs by inhibiting axial elongation. Evaluating various concentrations of the muscarinic antagonists, Luft *et al.* [16] found that only atropine, pirenzepine, and oxyphenonium prevented FDM, whereas others including tropicamide, dexetimide, scopolamine, benztropine, dicyclomine, gallamine, mepenzolate, propantheline, procyclidine, 4-diphenylacetoxy-*N*-methylpiperidine, hexahydro-sila-difenidol, p-fluorohexahydro-sila-difenidol, methoctramine, AFDX-116, quinuclidinyl benzilate, were ineffective or partially effective. The action of cyclopentolate in the present study may be different from previous antagonists due to different types of antagonists or experimental species.

The deprived eyes whether injected or not showed a decrease in mean refraction, accompanied by an elongation of the VCD and AL. Previous studies revealed an increase in AL of the deprived eye was mainly due to elongation of the vitreous chamber [6] [26]. Compared with only deprivation, physiological saline injection had little effect on refraction and ocular biometric dimensions. Although the saline vehicle injection may disturb the intraocular balance [27], it had no significant influence on the natural development of eyes.

Histological evidence from the present study found no retinal damage at the effective dose of 700 µg cyclopentolate. Retinal structure and integrity in guinea pigs induced by intravitreal injection of cyclopentolate was consistent with the results of intravitreal administration of atropine, pirenzipine and tropicamide in chicks [16]. Le *et al.* [24] also found no obviously toxic effects on the eyes treated with topical administration of pirenzepine.

Muscarinic receptors are one of the important facts during the development of myopia. Although the ocular tissues of guinea pigs express muscarinic subtypes M1 to M5 [28], it remains unknown how the muscarinic antagonists affect ocular growth. The effect of atropine on myopia control is considered by a retinal based mechanism mediated via muscarinic receptor signaling and non-accommodative way [28]. Cyclopentolate is a nonspecific antagonist, and hence its interaction with different receptors is potentially complex. The mechanism for cyclopentolate treatment may be through molecular signals involved the local connection between the retina and sclera, which directly influence the sclera growth [29] or induce a series of signaling cascade from retinal pigment epithelial to sclera [30]. We don't know whether anti-myopia effects of cyclopentolate is also independent of accommodation (such as with atropine). In addition, further investigations are needed to confirm whether effects of cyclopentolate could be mediated by nonmuscarinic mechanism. It is well-known that muscarinic antagonist benztropine blocks dopamine transporter [31], thus cyclopentolate may also exert some similar activity through dopamine system.

5. Conclusion

In conclusion, intravitreal injections of cyclopentolate are effectively able to reduce the refraction, VCD and AL of deprived eyes in guinea pigs. Further investigations are required to identify the optimal dose of cyclopentolate treatment.

Conflict of Interests

The authors have no financial or proprietary interest in the subject matter of this paper.

Acknowledgements

This work was supported by Grant from Shanghai Municipality Health Bureau Youth Project (2013-121) and Grant from Shanghai Municipality Jinshan District Health Bureau Youth Project (JSKJ-KTQN-2013-02).

References

[1]   Gee, S.S. and Tabbara, K.F. (1988) Increase in Ocular AXIAL Length in Patients with Corneal Opacification. *Ophthalmology*, **95**, 1276-1278. http://dx.doi.org/10.1016/S0161-6420(88)33035-6

[2]   Miller-Meeks, M.J., Bennett, S.R., Keech, R.V. and Blodi, C.F. (1990) Myopia Induced by Vitreous Hemorrhage. *American Journal of Ophthalmology*, **109**, 199-203. http://dx.doi.org/10.1016/S0002-9394(14)75987-2

[3]   Wallman, J., Turkel, J. and Trachtman, J. (1978) Extreme Myopia Produced by Modest Change in Early Visual experience. *Science*, **201**, 1249-1251. http://dx.doi.org/10.1126/science.694514

[4]   Siegwart, J.J. and Norton, T.T. (1998) The Susceptible Period for Deprivation-Induced Myopia in Tree Shrew. *Vision Research*, **38**, 3505-3515. http://dx.doi.org/10.1016/S0042-6989(98)00053-4

[5]   Lu, F., Zhou, X., Zhao, H., Wang, R., Jia, D., Jiang, L., *et al.* (2006) Axial Myopia Induced by a Monocularly-Deprived Facemask in Guinea Pigs: A Non-Invasive and Effective Model. *Experimental Eye Research*, **82**, 628-636. http://dx.doi.org/10.1016/j.exer.2005.09.001

[6]   Howlett, M.H. and McFadden, S.A. (2006) Form-Deprivation Myopia in the Guinea Pig (*Cavia porcellus*). *Vision Research*, **46**, 267-283. http://dx.doi.org/10.1016/j.visres.2005.06.036

[7]   Smith, E.R., Huang, J., Hung, L.F., Blasdel, T.L., Humbird, T.L. and Bockhorst, K.H. (2009) Hemiretinal form Deprivation: Evidence for Local Control of Eye Growth and Refractive Development in Infant Monkeys. *Investigative Ophthalmology & Visual Science*, **50**, 5057-5069. http://dx.doi.org/10.1167/iovs.08-3232

[8]   Huang, J., Hung, L.F., Ramamirtham, R., Blasdel, T.L., Humbird, T.L., Bockhorst, K.H., *et al.* (2009) Effects of Form Deprivation on Peripheral Refractions and Ocular Shape in Infant Rhesus Monkeys (*Macaca mulatta*). *Investigative Ophthalmology & Visual Science*, **50**, 4033-4044. http://dx.doi.org/10.1167/iovs.08-3162

[9]   Shen, W., Vijayan, M. and Sivak, J.G. (2005) Inducing Form-Deprivation Myopia in fish. *Investigative Ophthalmology & Visual Science*, **46**, 1797-1803. http://dx.doi.org/10.1167/iovs.04-1318

[10] Tejedor, J. and de la Villa, P. (2003) Refractive Changes Induced by Form Deprivation in the Mouse Eye. *Investigative Ophthalmology & Visual Science*, **44**, 32-36. http://dx.doi.org/10.1167/iovs.01-1171

[11] Meng, W., Butterworth, J., Malecaze, F. and Calvas, P. (2011) Axial Length of Myopia: A Review of Current Research. *Ophthalmologica*, **225**, 127-134. http://dx.doi.org/10.1159/000317072

[12] McBrien, N.A., Moghaddam, H.O. and Reeder, A.P. (1993) Atropine Reduces Experimental Myopia and Eye Enlargement via a Nonaccommodative Mechanism. *Investigative Ophthalmology & Visual Science*, **34**, 205-215.

[13] Leech, E.M., Cottriall, C.L. and McBrien, N.A. (1995) Pirenzepine Prevents form Deprivation Myopia in a Dose Dependent Manner. *Ophthalmic and Physiological Optics*, **15**, 351-356. http://dx.doi.org/10.1016/0275-5408(95)00074-N

[14] Cottriall, C.L., McBrien, N.A., Annies, R. and Leech, E.M. (1999) Prevention of Form-Deprivation Myopia with Pirenzepine: A Study of Drug Delivery and Distribution. *Ophthalmic and Physiological Optics*, **19**, 327-335. http://dx.doi.org/10.1016/S0275-5408(98)00079-9

[15] Cottriall, C.L., Truong, H.T. and McBrien, N.A. (2001) Inhibition of Myopia Development in Chicks Using Himbacine: A Role for M4 Receptors? *Neuroreport*, **12**, 2453-2456. http://dx.doi.org/10.1097/00001756-200108080-00033

[16] Luft, W.A., Ming, Y. and Stell, W.K. (2003) Variable Effects of Previously Untested Muscarinic Receptor Antagonists on Experimental Myopia. *Investigative Ophthalmology & Visual Science*, **44**, 1330-1338. http://dx.doi.org/10.1167/iovs.02-0796

[17] Chua, W.H., Balakrishnan, V., Chan, Y.H., Tong, L., Ling, Y., Quah, B.L., *et al.* (2006) Atropine for the Treatment of Childhood Myopia. *Ophthalmology*, **113**, 2285-2291. http://dx.doi.org/10.1016/j.ophtha.2006.05.062

[18] Chia, A., Chua, W.H., Cheung, Y.B., Wong, W.L., Lingham, A., Fong, A., *et al.* (2012) Atropine for the Treatment of Childhood Myopia: Safety and Efficacy of 0.5%, 0.1%, and 0.01% Doses (Atropine for the Treatment of Myopia 2). *Ophthalmology*, **119**, 347-354. http://dx.doi.org/10.1016/j.ophtha.2011.07.031

[19] Yen, M.Y., Liu, J.H., Kao, S.C. and Shiao, C.H. (1989) Comparison of the Effect of Atropine and Cyclopentolate on Myopia. *Annals of Ophthalmology*, **21**, 180-182, 187.

[20] Fang, F., Huang, F., Xie, R., Li, C., Liu, Y., Zhu, Y., *et al.* (2015) Effects of Muscarinic Receptor Modulators on Ocular Biometry of Guinea Pigs. *Ophthalmic and Physiological Optics*, **35**, 60-69. http://dx.doi.org/10.1111/opo.12166

[21] Zhou, X., Lu, F., Xie, R., Jiang, L., Wen, J., Li, Y., *et al.* (2007) Recovery from Axial Myopia Induced by a Monocularly Deprived Facemask in Adolescent (7-Week-Old) Guinea Pigs. *Vision Research*, **47**, 1103-1111. http://dx.doi.org/10.1016/j.visres.2007.01.002

[22] Zhou, X., Qu, J., Xie, R., Wang, R., Jiang, L., Zhao, H., *et al.* (2006) Normal Development of Refractive State and Ocular Dimensions in Guinea Pigs. *Vision Research*, **46**, 2815-2823. http://dx.doi.org/10.1016/j.visres.2006.01.027

[23] Palamar, M., Egrilmez, S., Uretmen, O., Yagci, A. and Kose, S. (2011) Influences of Cyclopentolate Hydrochloride on Anterior Segment Parameters with Pentacam in Children. *Acta Ophthalmologica*, **89**, e461-e465. http://dx.doi.org/10.1111/j.1755-3768.2011.02122.x

[24] Le, Q.H., Cheng, N.N., Wu, W. and Chu, R.Y. (2005) Effect of Pirenzepine Ophthalmic Solution on Form-Deprivation Myopia in the Guinea Pigs. *Chinese Medical Journal*, **118**, 561-566.

[25] Ouyang, C.H., Chu, R.Y. and Hu, W.Z. (2003) Effects of Pirenzepine on Lens-Induced Myopia in the Guinea-Pig. *Chinese Journal of Ophthalmology*, **39**, 348-351.

[26] Mutti, D.O., Mitchell, G.L., Sinnott, L.T., Jones-Jordan, L.A., Moeschberger, M.L., Cotter, S.A., *et al.* (2012) Corneal and Crystalline Lens Dimensions before and after Myopia Onset. *Optometry and Vision Science*, **89**, 251-262.

[27] Gao, Q., Liu, Q., Ma, P., Zhong, X., Wu, J. and Ge, J. (2006) Effects of Direct Intravitreal Dopamine Injections on the Development of Lid-Suture Induced Myopia in Rabbits. *Graefe's Archive for Clinical and Experimental Ophthalmology*, **244**, 1329-1335. http://dx.doi.org/10.1007/s00417-006-0254-1

[28] McBrien, N.A., Stell, W.K. and Carr, B. (2013) How Does Atropine Exert Its Anti-Myopia Effects? *Ophthalmic and Physiological Optics*, **33**, 373-378. http://dx.doi.org/10.1111/opo.12052

[29] Liu, Q., Wu, J., Wang, X. and Zeng, J. (2007) Changes in Muscarinic Acetylcholine Receptor Expression in Form Deprivation Myopia in Guinea Pigs. *Molecular Vision*, **13**, 1234-1244.

[30] Bitzer, M., Kovacs, B., Feldkaemper, M. and Schaeffel, F. (2006) Effects of Muscarinic Antagonists on ZENK Expression in the Chicken Retina. *Experimental Eye Research*, **82**, 379-388. http://dx.doi.org/10.1016/j.exer.2005.07.010

[31] Coyle, J.T. and Snyder, S.H. (1969) Antiparkinsonian Drugs: Inhibition of Dopamine Uptake in the Corpus Striatum as a Possible Mechanism of Action. *Science*, **166**, 899-901. http://dx.doi.org/10.1126/science.166.3907.899

33

Vision-Related Quality of Life in Ocular Hypertension Patients: Effects of Treatment

Maria Kazaki[1], Ilias Georgalas[1], Alexandros Damanakis[1], Georgios Labiris[2], Sergios Taliantzis[1]*, Chryssanthi Koutsandrea[1], Dimitris Papaconstantinou[1]

[1]Department of Glaucoma, University of Athens, Athens, Greece
[2]Department of Ophthalmology, University of Alexandroupolis, Alexandroupolis, Greece
Email: *sergiotali@hotmail.com

Abstract

Purpose: To evaluate the quality of life related to vision (QoL) in patients with ocular hypertension under treatment. Methods: The study included two groups. The first one consisted of 60 ocular hypertension patients under topical hypotensive medications and the second one of 60 healthy persons. The Greek language version of the National Eye Institute Visual Function Questionnaire 25 (NEI VFQ-25) was completed by all patients. Results: The median scores of the total score and also for almost all the NEI VFQ-25 subscales were significantly decreased for the first group of ocular hypertension patients (OHT) under topical therapy. Females presented higher QoL than that of males. The patients who used one medication presented higher QoL than that of the patients who used more than one. The best corrected visual acuity (BCVA) and the intraocular pressure (IOP) were significantly correlated with QoL. The index of the visual fields, pattern standard deviation (PSD), was significantly related to the quality of life of OHT. The age, the cup to disk ratio and the central corneal thickness had also significant correlations with subscales of the QoL. Conclusions: The quality of life OHT patients under topical treatment is significantly decreased than healthy persons. Male sex and the number of medications affect QoL more. BCVA and IOP represent the clinical findings that best correlate with several subscales of QoL. PSD is a significant index that correlates well with the quality of life of OHT patients.

Keywords

Intraocular Pressure, Ocular Hypertension, Quality of Life, VFQ-25

---

*Corresponding author.

1. Introduction

Ocular hypertension (OHT) describes the condition in which the intraocular pressure lies above the 21 mmHg, with normal appearance of the optic nerve head and with visual fields with no signs of glaucomatous damage [1].

Since elevated IOP is the major risk factor for the development of glaucomatous visual loss, finding a "raised" intraocular pressure (IOP) indicates the need for further investigation. The decision to treat a patient with ocular hypertension should be made when the risk factor(s) are considered to outweigh the disadvantages of treatment [2]-[4].

Glaucoma and associated visual changes may negatively affect quality of life because of progressive visual field deterioration and lifetime treatment [5]. Multicenter studies such as the Ocular Hypertension Treatment Study (OHTS) and Collaborative Initial Glaucoma Treatment Study (CIGTS) have included questionnaires to evaluate quality of life related to vision (QoL) [6]-[8]. Intraocular pressure, visual field results and patient adherence cannot be used to assess the subjective experience of the quality of vision [9]. Furthermore, medication for treatment of glaucoma is negatively correlated with adherence and quality of life related to vision in patients with glaucoma [10].

Ocular hypertension patients represent a group with still mild glaucomatous type alterations but that may need treatment. The quality of life these patients has not been still evaluated nor the impact that topical medications have on them. To our knowledge a study of Wolfram and others included an ocular hypertension group but focused mainly on glaucomatous patients [11]. Instead this study examines QoL of OHT patients and its characteristics.

We hypothesized that the pharmacological treatment influences negatively QoL of OHT patients. The purpose of this study is to assess the quality of life related to vision of OHT patients under topical medications and the effect that those have on QoL.

2. Materials and Methods

2.1. Subjects

The study followed the guidelines of the Declaration of Helsinki and was approved by the ethics committee of G. Gennimatas Athens General Hospital. Informed consent was obtained from all subjects. For the purpose of our study, two groups meeting the inclusion criteria were considered. The first group included the first sixty patients with ocular hypertension that visited our department. Instead the second group included the first healthy sixty people with no ocular history.

Inclusion criteria for the first group were ocular hypertension under topical treatment with IOP up to 18 mmHg; abnormal appearance of optic nerve head; best corrected visual acuity (BCVA) 0.7 or better on Snellen chart test with spherical refractive error from −6.00 D to + 3.00 D. Inclusion criteria for the second group were individual with no history of ocular diseases nor use of medication for the eyes, BCVA 0.7 or better on Snellen chart test with spherical refractive error from −6.00 D to + 3.00 D, IOP up to 20 mmHg, vertical cup to disk ratio up to 0.4 and difference between the two eyes up to 0.2 with normal appearance of the optic disk and physiological visual fields. Abnormal appearance findings of optic nerve head include vertical cup-to-disc diameter ratio of >0.7 or asymmetry of cup/disc ratio (C/D) of >0.2, cup extension nasal to the rim vessels, kinking of the retinal vessels, baring of the circumlinear vessel and presence of splinter hemorrhages [12].

Exclusion criteria were glaucomatous or other findings on visual fields examination based on the Anderson-Patella criteria; IOP > 18 mmHg; ocular comorbidities such as diseases of the cornea, anterior chamber, lens, vitreous cavity, and retina that may reduce visual acuity; history of intraocular surgery; history of chronic systemic diseases that may affect general health; treatment duration of less than six months.

2.2. Evaluation

A specific examination protocol was applied to all patients, including general and ophthalmic history and complete ophthalmic examination that included determination of best corrected visual acuity, slit lamp examination, intraocular pressure measurement, fundus biomicroscopy, central corneal thickness measurement, C/D appreciation and visual fields examination.

The best corrected visual acuity was determined from Snellen chart testing. Slit lamp examination was performed to evaluate the anterior and posterior chambers. Fundus examination was performed with a (+78) D lens after dilation of the pupil with 1% tropicamide and 2.5% phenylephrine drops.

Intraocular pressure was determined with a Goldman applanation tonometer. All patients of the first group already used topical hypotensive therapy and underwent IOP measurement three times a day for three consecutive days. Topical treatment included prostaglandine analogs, β-blockers, carbonic any drase inhibitors, sympathomimetic and/or combination of the above. Central corneal thickness was measured with an ophthalmic ultrasonography system (Ocuscan RxP, Alcon Alcon Laboratories Inc, USA, city, state). Heidelberg Retina Tomograph was used to assess C/D (Heidelberg Engineering GmbH, Heidelberg, Germany). Visual field examination was performed with a white on white perimetry using the Swedish Interactive Threshold Algorithm standard 30-2 strategy (Humphrey Field Analyzer, Humphrey-Zeiss Systems, Dublin CA). A minimum 2 tests were performed to minimize the learning effect; if any 2 tests failed to satisfy the reliability criteria defined by the perimeter (false positive, false negative, and loss of fixation), the test was repeated. The Anderson-Patella criteria was used with 3 non edge points depressed to an extent of what is present in <5% of normal population with at least 1 point of these 3 depressed to an extent found in less than 1% of normal population, pattern standard deviation and corrected pattern standard deviation (PSD/CPSD) should be that found in <5% population and glaucoma hemifield test (GHT) should be "OUTSIDE NORMAL LIMITS" [13].

2.3. Questionnaire

The 25-item National Eye Institute Visual Function Questionnaire (NEI-VFQ 25) included questions about visual function of patients with chronic ophthalmic diseases. It had been developed for evaluation of patients with age-related cataracts, glaucoma, age-related macular degeneration, and diabetic retinopathy. The main purpose of the VFQ-25 was to assess the effect of ophthalmic diseases and related symptoms on the quality of life and social function of patients [14]. Several studies used this questionnaire to assess the quality of life of glaucoma patients [15]-[17]. The 25 questions had been grouped in 12 categories that were related to vision, and the total time requested to answer the entire questionnaire was 10 minutes [18]. The response to each question was converted in a 0 to 100 scale (lowest score, 0; highest score, 100). For each category, the mean score was calculated from the associated questions for the category. The total score for the entire questionnaire was calculated as the mean of the scores of the 12 subscales [19] [20]. The Greek language edition of NEI VFQ-25 was used [21].

2.4. Data Analysis

Data were analyzed using statistical software (SPSS for Windows 12.00, SPSS Inc., Chicago, IL). The Kolmogorov-Smirnov test was used to control the normality of the distribution. All the descriptive parameters were noted in the form of mean and standard deviation (SD) if the data were parametric or in the form of median with interquartile range if the data were nonparametric. Comparisons for normal distribution between the two groups were calculated using the Mann-Whitney U test for non parametric data and the independent sample t-test for parametric data. Correlations between quality of life and other variables were evaluated with the Spearman rank correlation. The multivariate linear regression analysis and the stepwise method, was used to calculate the significance that the clinical findings have on QoL. Statistical significance was defined by $P \leq 0.05$.

3. Results

One hundred and twenty persons were included in the study, in two separated groups. The first one included 60 OHT patients under topical treatment, thirty four women and twenty six men. The second group included 60 healthy people, thirty six women and twenty four men. **Table 1** presents the descriptive data and clinical characteristics of the two groups.

The main age of OHT group was higher than the healthy group (61 ± 6.23 and 57.31 ± 11.2 years of age respectively), with significantly worst BCVA ($P = 0.0001$), higher CD (0.6; $P = 0.0001$) and CCT of 525 μm, lower than the second group ($P = 0.001$). The global indices of the visual fields between the two groups were also significant different, with the mean MD and PSD of the first group to be -0.73 db ± 0.93 ($P = 0.0001$) and 1.87 db ± 0.52 respectively ($P = 0.0001$). The median number of medication of the first group was 2 with interquartile range from 1 to 2 and with interquartile range from 1 to 2 the median number of instillations to be 3 with interquartile range from 1 to 3. The median IOP of OHT under medication was 15 mmHg. The second group did not use treatment and had a median IOP of 13 mmHg.

Table 1. Descriptive data and Clinical Characteristics of the two groups.

Characteristic	First Group	Second Group	Probability Significance(S)
No. patients	60	60	-
Sex (female/male)	34/26	36/24	
Age (years)	61.18 ± 6.23	57.31 ± 11.2	S (0.001)
Best corrected visual acuity	10 (9 - 10)	10 (10 - 10)	S (0.0001)
Intraocular pressure (mmHg)	15 (14 - 16)	13 (12 - 15)	S (0.0001)
Daily number of medications	2 (1 - 2)	0	NA
Daily number of instillations	3 (1 - 3)	0	NA
Cup to disc ratio	0.6 (0.5 - 0.7)	0.2 (0.1 - 0.3)	S (0.0001)
Central corneal thickness (μm)	525 (514 - 541)	531(523 - 546)	S (0.001)
Mean deviation (db)	−0.73 ± 0.93	−0.06 ± 0.77	S (0.0001)
Pattern standard deviation (db)	1.87 ± 0.52	1. 84 ± 0.28	S (0.0001)

First Group of ocular hypertension patients under topical treatment. Second group of healthy individuals. Data reported as number of mean ± SD or median with interquartile range. Probability Mann-Whitney U test for nonparametric data. Independent sample t-test for parametric data. Significance $P \leq 0.05$. NA non applicable.

The median total score of QoL questionnaire of OHT group was 84.54 (interquartile range 77.45 - 91.14) while the total score of the healthy group was significantly higher with a median of 99.3 (interquartile range 97.91 - 100; $P = 0.0001$). **Table 2** presents the results of scores for all the subscales and the total score of NEI-VFQ questionnaire of the two groups. The median score for the general vision of OHT patients under topical medication was 75 with interquartile range between 50 and 75 lower than the healthy group ($P = 0.0001$). The median scores for almost all the subscales of the first group were significantly lower than those of the second one ($P = 0.0001$).

Males of the first group presented significantly lower median total score than the females of the same group (81.41 and 87.32 respectively, $P = 0.001$). **Table 3** presents the scores of NEI-VFQ 25 of OHT patients according to their gender. The subscales of general health, general vision, ocular pain near activities, role difficulty and peripheral vision were significantly worst for OHT men than for OHT women under topical treatment ($P < 0.05$).

Ocular hypertension patients of the first group that used one medication for treatment, presented a median total score of QoL questionnaire of 89.23 with interquartile range between 85.24 and 94.79, that is significantly higher from the median total score of the patients that used two medications (81.24, interquartile range between 77.45 and 85.32, $P = 0.0001$) or three medications (72.91 and with interquartile range between 70.39 and 77.16, $P = 0.0001$). The total score of OHT patients that used two medication were also significantly higher than the patients that used three drugs ($P = 0.004$). **Table 4** presents the scores of all the subscales of NEI-VFQ 25 for OHT patients that used one, two or three medications respectively. For all the categories the OHT patients with one topical medication, had significantly higher scores than the other patients ($P < 0.05$).

Best corrected visual acuity presents a significant correlation with the total score ($r = 0.237$, $P = 0.009$), the general health ($r = 0.327$, $P = 0.0001$) and the near activities ($r = 0.296$, $P = 0.001$) of QoL questionnaire of OHT patients. The intraocular correlates also significantly with most subscales of OHT patients. Instead daily number of medications does not present significant correlations with any of the subscales of NEI-VFQ 25 ($P > 0.05$). PSD is the global index of the visual fields that better correlates with the QoL of OHT patients. **Table 5** presents the correlations of the clinical characteristics of OHT patients' group with the subscales and the total score of the questionnaire.

Table 6 presents the results of the multivariate linear regression analysis for all the subscales of OHT patients. The clinical characteristic "daily number of medications" represents the index that influences almost all subscales and the total score (-7.775, $P = 0.0001$) of the questionnaire ($P < 0.05$). The near activities, role difficulty and total score are the subscales better explained by the clinical characteristics of OHT patients group ($R^2 = 0.279$, 0.539 and 0.383 respectively).

Table 2. Scores of the questionnaire (NEI-VFQ 25) for the two groups.

	1st Group (OHT under treatment)		2nd Group (Healthy Group)		Probability (Mann-Whitney U test)
	Median	(Interquartile range)	Median	(Interquartile range)	
1) General health	75	50 - 75	100	75 - 100	$P < 0.0001$
2) General vision	75	50 - 75	100	100 - 100	$P < 0.0001$
3) Ophthalmic pain	75	62.5 - 87.5	100	100 - 100	$P < 0.0001$
4) Near activities	87.5	66.6 - 100	100	100 - 100	$P < 0.0001$
5) Distance vision	91.63	77.08 - 100	100	100 - 100	$P < 0.0001$
6) Social activities	100	100 - 100	100	100 - 100	$P < 0.0001$
7) Mental health	75	62.75 - 85.93	100	93.75 - 100	$P < 0.0001$
8) Role Difficulty	100	75 - 100	100	100 - 100	$P < 0.0001$
9) Dependency	91.67	83.33 - 100	100	100 - 100	$P < 0.0001$
10) Driving	100	83.33 - 100	100	100 - 100	$P < 0.0001$
11) Color vision	100	100 - 100	100	100 - 100	$P < 0.0001$
12) Peripheral vision	100	100 - 100	100	100 - 100	$P < 0.0001$
Total score	84.54	77.45 - 91.14	99.3	97.91 - 100	$P < 0.0001$

Significance $P \leq 0.05$.

Table 3. Scores of the questionnaire (NEI-VFQ 25) of the ocular hypertension group according to their sex.

VFQ-25 category	Female	Male	Probability (Mann-Whitney U test)
1) General health	75 (50 - 75)	50 (25 - 75)	$P = 0.044$
2) General vision	75 (75 - 100)	75 (50 - 87.5)	$P = 0.001$
3) Ophthalmic pain	87.5 (62.5 - 100)	75 (50 - 87.5)	$P = 0.013$
4) Near activities	91.66 (83.33 - 100)	70.8 (58.33 - 83.33)	$P = 0.0001$
5) Distance vision	91.63 (83.33 - 100)	95.8 (75 - 100)	$P = 0.707$
6) Social activities	100 (100 - 100)	100 (100 - 100)	$P = 0.189$
7) Mental health	75 (62.75 - 81.25)	75 (50 - 87.5)	$P = 0.621$
8) Role difficulty	100 (75 - 100)	75 (62.5 - 100)	$P = 0.0001$
9) Dependency	91.66 (83.33 – 100)	91.66 (83.33 - 100)	$P = 0.271$
10) Driving	100 (83.33 - 100)	91.66 (83.33 - 100)	$P = 0.225$
11) Color vision	100 (100 - 100)	100 (100 - 100)	$P = 0.614$
12) Peripheral vision	100 (100 - 100)	100 (75 - 100)	$P = 0.009$
Total score	87.32 (82.07 - 93.09)	81.41 (72.39 - 85.59)	$P = 0.001$

Data reported as number of median (interquartile range). Mann Whitney U test; significance $P \leq 0.05$.

4. Discussion

Glaucoma decreases the quality of life for different reasons that include the diagnosis itself, the perimetric functional loss, the treatment itself, its side effects and costs [5]. Previous studies evaluated the relation between glaucoma, treatment, and health-related quality of life [22] including patients with established visual field defects [23]. Instead QoL of ocular hypertension patients under treatment has not been still estimated.

Table 4. Scores of the questionnaire (NEI-VFQ 25) of the ocular hypertension group according to the number of medication used.

VFQ-25 category	1 medication	2 medications	3 medications
1) General health	75 (50 - 81.25) (0.003) 1-2 (0.0001) 1-3	50 (25 - 75) (0.003) 1-2 (0.29) 2-3	50 (25 - 56.25) (0.0001) 1-3 (0.29) 2-3
2) General vision	75 (75 - 100) (0.0001) 1-2 (0.0001) 1-3	75 (50 - 75) (0.003) 1-2 (0.001) 2-3	50 (50 - 56.25) (0.0001) 1-3 (0.001) 2-3
3) Ophthalmic pain	87.5 (75 - 100) (0.001) 1-2 (0.004) 1-3	75 (62.5 - 87.5) (0.001) 1-2 (0.36) 2-3	62.5 (50 - 81.25) (0.004) 1-3 (0.36) 2-3
4) Near activities	91.66 (83.33 - 100) (0.017) 1-2 (0.0001) 1-3	83.33 (66.6 - 91.66) (0.017) 1-2 (0.001) 2-3	58.33 (58.33 - 75) (0.0001) 1-3 (0.001) 2-3
5) Distance vision	91.66 (81.24 - 100) (0.622) 1-2 (0.187) 1-3	91.66 (83.33 - 100) (0.622) 1-2 (0.046) 2-3	75 (75 - 100) (0.187) 1-3 (0.046) 2-3
6) Social activities	100 (100 - 100) (0.243) 1-2 (0.77) 1-3	100 (100 - 100) (0.243) 1-2 (0.297) 2-3	100 (100 - 100) (0.77) 1-3 (0.297) 2-3
7) Mental health	81.25 (75 - 87.5) (0.0001) 1-2 (0.042) 1-3	68.75 (62.5 - 81.25) (0.0001) 1-2 (0.66) 2-3	75 (50 - 75) (0.042) 1-3 (0.66) 2-3
8) Role difficulty	100 (100 - 100) (0.0001) 1-2 (0.0001) 1-3	75 (75 - 100) (0.0001) 1-2 (0.0001) 2-3	75 (62.5 - 75) (0.0001) 1-3 (0.0001) 2-3
9) Dependency	100 (89.57 - 100) (0.0001) 1-2 (0.001) 1-3	91.66 (66.66 - 91.66) (0.0001) 1-2 (0.367) 2-3	83.33 (58.33 - 93.74) (0.001) 1-3 (0.367) 2-3
10) Driving	100 (100 - 100) (0.001) 1-2 (0.0001) 1-3	83.33 (83.33 - 100) (0.001) 1-2 (0.041) 2-3	83.33 (75 - 87.49) (0.0001) 1-3 (0.041) 2-3
11) Color vision	100 (100 - 100) (0.0001) 1-2 (0.0001) 1-3	100 (75 - 100) (0.0001) 1-2 (0.682) 2-3	100 (93.75 - 100) (0.0001) 1-3 (0.682) 2-3
12) Peripheral vision	100 (100 - 100) (0.091) 1-2 (0.0001) 1-3	100 (75 - 100) (0.091) 1-2 (0.002) 2-3	75 (75 - 100) (0.0001) 1-3 (0.002) 2-3
Total score	89.23 (85.24 - 94.79) (0.0001) 1-2 (0.0001) 1-3	81.24 (77.45 - 85.32) (0.0001) 1-2 (0.004) 2-3	72.91 (70.39 - 77.16) (0.0001) 1-3 (0.004) 2-3

Data reported as number of median (interquartile range). Probability between patients that use 1 medication and 2 medications (1-2). Probability between patients that use 1 medication and 3 medications (1-3). Probability between patients that use 2 medication and 3 medications (2-3). Mann Whitney U test; significance $P \leq 0.05$.

The present study is focused on the quality of life related to vision of OHT patients that use topical medications with physiological achromatic visual fields and found a declined QoL when compared to that of healthy persons. For almost all of the qualitative subscales and the total score of QoL, OHT patients had worst results. This finding is in accordance with other studies assessing QoL of glaucomatous patients [24] [25]. Wolfram and other found that QoL impairment in glaucoma patients lies between OHT/early POAG versus moderate/severe POAG [11]. QoL in these two groups, OHT under treatment and glaucomatous patients, probably is in the same way compromised but further studies will probably explain better this relationship and clarify the impact that the different factors have on them.

Table 5. Spearman correlation between the Subscale Scores of the questionnaire NEI-VFQ 25 and the clinical Indices of the ocular hypertension patients under topical treatment.

VFQ-25 category	Age	Best corrected visual acuity	Intraocular pressure	Cup to disc ratio	Central corneal thickness	Mean deviation	Pattern standard deviation	Daily number of medications
1) General health (S)	−0.129 (0.16)	**0.327++** **(0.0001)**	**0.196+** **(0.032)**	−0.15 (0.102)	0.1 (0.277)	−0.089 (0.331)	−0.010 (0.913)	−0.089 (0.331)
2) General vision (S)	−0.012 (0.901)	0.162 (0.077)	**0.199+** **(0.029)**	−0.16 (0.081)	0.016 (0.861)	−0.04 (0.663)	**−0.224+** **(0.014)**	−0.040 (0.663)
3) Ophthalmic pain (S)	0.09 (0.328)	0.142 (0.122)	**−0.248)++** **(0.006)**	**−0.198+** **(0.03)**	0.068 (0.458)	−0.077 (0.403)	−0.017 (0.858)	−0.077 (0.403)
4) Near activities (S)	**−0.183⁺** **(0.045)**	**0.296++** **(0.001)**	**0.296++** **(0.001)**	**−0.210+** **(0.021)**	**0.278++** **(0.002)**	0.049 (0.593)	−0.107 (0.246)	0.049 (0.593)
5) Distance vision (S)	0.094 (0.309)	−0.029 (0.751)	0.130 (0.158)	−0.034 (0.712)	−0.149 (0.104)	−0.074 (0.421)	0.−124 (0.179)	−0.074 (0.421)
6) Social activities (S)	0.101 (0.272)	0.084 (0.359)	**−0.243++** **(0.008)**	−0.167 (0.068)	0.065 (0.483)	−0.047 (0.612)	−0.080 (0.383)	−0.04 (0.612)
7) Mental health (S)	0.055 (0.552)	0.117 (0.202)	0.078 (0.399)	0.036 (0.693)	0.08 (0.383)	−0.059 (0.521)	−0.085 (0.354)	−0.059 (0.521)
8) Role difficulty (S)	**0.386++** **(0.0001)**	−0.018 (0.841)	0.072 (0.437)	−0.114 (0.213)	0.066 (0.474)	−0.009 (0.920)	0.003 (0.976)	−0.009 (0.92)
9) Dependency (S)	0.038 (0.684)	0.159 (0.083)	**0.199+** **(0.029)**	0.073 (0.43)	−0.019 (0.841)	−0.163 (0.075)	−0.116 (−0.116)	−0.163 (0.075)
10) Driving (S)	−0.041 (0.653)	0.174 (0.157)	0.006 (0.947)	−0.054 (0.558)	0.077 (0.4)	−0.014 (0.879)	−0.169 (0.065)	−0.014 (0.879)
11) Color vision (S)	−0.057 (0.538)	0.179 (0.051)	−0.051 (0.584)	0.016 (0.866)	0.147 (0.110)	−0.028 (0.765)	**−0.258++** **(0.004)**	−0.028 (0.765)
12) Peripheral vision (S)	0.037 (0.689)	0.153 (0.095)	**0.231+** **(0.019)**	−0.162 (0.77)	0.109 (0.237)	−0.126 (0.172)	−0.095 (0.302)	−0.121 (0.172)
Total score (S)	0.133 (0.149)	**0.237++** **(0.009)**	0.151 (0.1)	−0.163 (0.076)	0.160 (0.081)	−0.046 (0.619)	−0.087 (0.345)	−0.046 (0.619)

Significance (S): ++ $P \leq 0.01$, + $P \leq 0.05$.

Males with preperimetric glaucoma under treatment presented worst QoL respect to women of the same group. This finding is in contrast with the study of Labiris and other [26] for pseudoexfoliative glaucoma patients. Tastan and other also found that depression and quality of life were decreased in women with glaucoma [27]. Instead in accordance to our study Odberg and collogues found that in patients with glaucoma, the women were in general more dissatisfied than the men [28].

Another finding of the study is that as the number of medications used by OHT patients increases their quality of life decreases. Skalicky and other also found that in patients with increasing glaucoma severity QoL is poorer as there is a higher probability of ocular surface disease because of benzalkonium chloride exposure [29]. The number of medications used by OHT patients is likely to be an important factor with negative impact on QoL ($P = 0.0001$) and according to the results of the regression analysis of the study is more sensitive than the other clinical characteristics. This finding is also in accordance with other studies focusing in glaucoma patients [26].

Best corrected visual acuity and intraocular pressure are both sensitive indices of QoL in OHT patients and possibly their impairment can explain the change of the qualitative subscales of the quality of life in preperimetric glaucoma group of patients. Previous studies in normal tension glaucoma patients also found the same impact of BCVA and IOP in QoL [25]. The age, CD ratio and CCT can affect different characteristics of QoL. PSD has been identified as the visual fields global index that correlates significantly with QoL. Nelson and other

Table 6. Multivariate linear regression analysis of the quality of life subscales' of ocular hypertension patients group.

VFQ-25 category	Adjusted R Square	B coef. Age (S)	B coef. BCVA (S)	B coef. IOP (S)	B coef. N.med (S)	B coef CD (S)	B coef. CCT (1)	B coef. MD (S)	B coef. PSD (S)
1) General health (S)	0.205	NS	14.163++ (0.002)	NS	−11.087++ (0.001)	NS	NS	NS	NS
2) General vision (S)	0.279	NS	NS	NS	−15.522++ (0.0001)	NS	−0.256+ (0.001)	NS	NS
3) Ophthalmic pain (S)	0.266	NS	NS	−5.684++ (0.0001)	−13.348++ (0.0001)	NS	NS	NS	NS
4) Near activities (S)	0.279	−0.851++ (0.001)	6.158+ (0.041)	2.423+ (0.043)	−6.038+ (0.015)	−30.179+ (0.039)	NS	NS	NS
5) Distance vision (S)	NA	NS	NS	NS	NS	NS	NS	NS	NS
6) Social activities (S)	0.07	NS	NS	−0.807++ (0.008)	NS	−8.542+ (0.027)	NS	NS	NS
7) Mental health (S)	0.92	NS	NS	NS	−6.441++ (0.001)	NS	NS	NS	NS
8) Role difficulty (S)	0.539	1.023++ (0.0001)	−4.64+ (0.019)	−2.260++ (0.001)	−16.491++ (0.0001)	NS	−0.114+ (0.034)	NS	NS
9) Dependency (S)	0.293	NS	NS	NS	−10.600++ (0.0001)	NS	−0.184++ (0.001)	NS	NS
10) Driving (S)	0.231	NS	NS	−1.496+ (0.017)	−6.774++ (0.0001)	NS	NS	NS	−3.39+ (0.03)
11) Color vision (S)	0.166	NS	NS	−1.248+ (0.026)	−4.319++ (0.0001)	NS	NS	NS	−4.112++ (0.004)
12) Peripheral vision (S)	0.162	NS	NS	NS	−6.915++ (0.0001)	NS	NS	NS	NS
Total score (S)	0.383	NS	NS	NS	−7.775++ (0.0001)	NS	NS	NS	NS

Significance (S): ++ $P \leq .01$, + $P \leq .05$. Abbreviations B coef.: B coefficient, BCVA: best corrected visual acuity, IOP: intraocular pressure, N med: number of medications, CD: cup to disk ratio, CCT: central corneal thickness, MD: mean deviation, PSD: pattern standard deviation. NS non significant. NA non applicable.

found that MD significantly related with QoL of glaucoma patients [30]. On the other hand Iester and colleagues found that QoL of glaucoma patients was significantly correlated with both MD and PSD [31]. Further studies need to be computed to clarify if the visual fields global indices, MD and PSD, have different impact on OHT and glaucoma patients.

A limitation of this study is the small number of OHT patients under treatment with different medications and/or different doses of medications. This will help to understand if a specific glaucoma medication is better correlated with QoL than another. Another limit is that a group of glaucoma patients was not included in the study and because of that no obvious comparisons can be computed between this group and a group of OHT patients. Further studies need to be done to clarify better these aspects.

5. Conclusion

In conclusion, the quality of life related to vision of OHT patients under topical treatment is significantly decreased than that of healthy persons. Male sex and the number of medications affect QoL more. The best corrected visual acuity and intraocular pressure represent the clinical findings that best correlate with several qualitative aspects of QoL. The pattern standard deviation is a significant index that correlates well with the quality of life of OHT patients.

Conflicts of Interest

None of the authors has conflict of interest with the submission.

Financial Support

No financial support was received for this submission.

Meeting Presentation

The paper has not been presented.

Informed Consent

The study was performed following all the guidelines for experimental investigations required by the Institutional Review Board or Ethics Committee of which all authors are affiliated. Informed consent was obtained from all subjects.

References

[1] Cowan Jr., C.L., Worthen, D.M., Mason, R.P. and Anduze, A.L. (1988) Glaucoma in Blacks. *Acta Ophthalmologica*, **106**, 738-739. http://dx.doi.org/10.1001/archopht.1988.01060130808027

[2] Cate, H., Bhattacharya, D., Clark, A., Holland, R. and Broadway, D.C. (2013) Patterns of Adherence Behaviour for Patients with Glaucoma. *Eye*, **27**, 545-553. http://dx.doi.org/10.1038/eye.2012.294

[3] Odberg, T. (1993) Visual Field Prognosis in Early Glaucoma. A Long-Term Clinical Follow-Up. *Acta Ophthalmologica*, **71**, 721-726. http://dx.doi.org/10.1111/j.1755-3768.1993.tb08590.x

[4] Schwartz, G.F. and Quigley, H.A. (2008) Adherence and Persistence with Glaucoma Therapy. *Survey of Ophthalmology*, **53**, S57-S68. http://dx.doi.org/10.1016/j.survophthal.2008.08.002

[5] Iester, M. and Zingirian, M. (2002) Quality of Life in Patients with Early, Moderate and Advanced Glaucoma. *Eye*, **16**, 44-49. http://dx.doi.org/10.1038/sj.eye.6700036

[6] Weinstein, J.M., Duckrow, R.B., Beard, D. and Brennan, R.W. (1983) Regional Optic Nerve Blood Flow and Its Autoregulation. *Investigative Ophthalmology & Visual Science*, **24**, 1559-1565.

[7] Mills, R.P., Janz, N.K., Wren, P.A. and Guire, K.E. (2001) Correlation of Visual Field with Quality-of-Life Measures at Diagnosis in the Collaborative Initial Glaucoma Treatment Study (CIGTS). *Journal of Glaucoma*, **10**, 192-198. http://dx.doi.org/10.1097/00061198-200106000-00008

[8] Nelson, P., Aspinall, P., Papasouliotis, O., Worton, B. and O'Brien, C. (2003) Quality of Life in Glaucoma and Its Relationship with Visual Function. *Journal of Glaucoma*, **12**, 139-150. http://dx.doi.org/10.1097/00061198-200304000-00009

[9] Watson, P.G. and Grierson, I. (1981) The Place of Trabeculectomy in the Treatment of Glaucoma. *Ophthalmology*, **88**, 175-196. http://dx.doi.org/10.1016/S0161-6420(81)35051-9

[10] Sleath, B., Robin, A.L., Covert, D., Byrd, J.E., Tudor, G. and Svarstad, B. (2006) Patient-Reported Behavior and Problems in Using Glaucoma Medications. *Ophthalmology*, **113**, 431-436. http://dx.doi.org/10.1016/j.ophtha.2005.10.034

[11] Wolfram, C., Lorenz, K., Breitscheidel, L., Verboven, Y. and Pfeiffer, N. (2013) Health- and Vision-Related Quality of Life in Patients with Ocular Hypertension or Primary Open-Angle Glaucoma. *Ophthalmologica*, **229**, 227-234. http://dx.doi.org/10.1159/000350553

[12] Shaffer, R. (1977) "Glaucoma Suspect" or "Ocular Hypertension". *Archives of Ophthalmology*, **95**, 588. http://dx.doi.org/10.1001/archopht.1977.04450040054004

[13] Asaoka, R., Iwase, A., Hirasawa, K., Murata, H. and Araie, M.I. (2014) Identifying "Preperimetric" Glaucoma in Standard Automated Perimetry Visual Fields. *Investigative Ophthalmology & Visual Science*, **55**, 7814-7820. http://dx.doi.org/10.1167/iovs.14-15120

[14] Mangione, C.M., Lee, P.P., Gutierrez, P.R., Spritzer, K., Berry, S. and Hays, R.D. (2001) Development of the 25-Item National Eye Institute Visual Function Questionnaire. *Archives of Ophthalmology*, **119**, 1050-1058. http://dx.doi.org/10.1001/archopht.119.7.1050

[15] Wren, P.A., Musch, D.C., Janz, N.K., Niziol, L.M., Guire, K.E. and Gillespie, B.W., CIGTS Study Group (2009) Contrasting the Use of 2 Vision-Specific Quality of Life Questionnaires in Subjects with Open-Angle Glaucoma. *Journal of Glaucoma*, **18**, 403-411. http://dx.doi.org/10.1097/IJG.0b013e3181879e63

[16] Lisboa, R., Chun, Y.S., Zangwill, L.M., Weinreb, R.N., Rosen, P.N., Liebmann, J.M., Girkin, C.A. and Medeiros, F.A. (2013) Association between Rates of Binocular Visual Field Loss and Vision-Related Quality of Life in Patients with Glaucoma. *JAMA Ophthalmology*, **131**, 486-494. http://dx.doi.org/10.1001/jamaophthalmol.2013.2602

[17] Sawada, H., Fukuchi, T. and Abe, H. (2011) Evaluation of the Relationship between Quality of Vision and the Visual Function Index in Japanese Glaucoma Patients. *Graefe's Archive for Clinical and Experimental Ophthalmology*, **249**, 1721-1727. http://dx.doi.org/10.1007/s00417-011-1779-5

[18] Mangione, C.M., Lee, P.P., Pitts, J., Gutierrez, P., Berry, S. and Hays, R.D. (1998) Psychometric Properties of the National Eye Institute Visual Function Questionnaire (NEI-VFQ). *Archives of Ophthalmology*, **116**, 1496-1504. http://dx.doi.org/10.1001/archopht.116.11.1496

[19] Mangione, C.M., Berry, S., Spritzer, K., Janz, N.K., Klein, R., Owsley, C. and Lee, P.P. (1998) Identifying the Content Area for the 51-Item National Eye Institute Vision Function Questionnaire: Results from Focus Groups with Visually Impaired Persons. *Archives of Ophthalmology*, **116**, 227-233. http://dx.doi.org/10.1001/archopht.116.2.227

[20] Cole, S.R., Beck, R.W., Moke, P.S., Gal, R.L. and Long, D.T. (2000) The National Eye Institute Visual Function Questionnaire: Experience of the ONTT. Optic Neuritis Treatment Trial. *Investigative Ophthalmology & Visual Science*, **41**, 1017-1021.

[21] Laboratory of Experimental Ophthalmology of Aristotle University (2000) Greek Language Translation of the National Eye Institute Visual Function Questionnaire. Aristotle University, Thessaloniki. Http://www.rand.org/content/dam/rand/www/external/health/surveys_tools/vfq/vfq25survey_greek.pdf

[22] Massof, R.W. and Fletcher, D.C. (2001) Evaluation of the NEI Visual Functioning Questionnaire as an Interval Measure of Visual Ability in Low Vision. *Vision Research*, **41**, 397-413. http://dx.doi.org/10.1016/S0042-6989(00)00249-2

[23] Yamagishio, K., Keiji, Y., Kimura, T., Yamabayashi, S. and Katsushima, H. (2009) Quality of Life Evaluation in Elderly Normal Tension Glaucoma Patients Using the Japanese Version of VFQ-25. *Nippon Ganka Gakkai Zasshi*, **113**, 964-971.

[24] Richman, J., Lorenzana, L.L., Lankaranian, D., Dugar, J., Mayer, J.R., Wizov, S.S. and Spaeth, G.L. (2010) Relationships in Glaucoma Patients between Standard Vision Tests, Quality of Life, and Ability to Perform Daily Activities. *Ophthalmic Epidemiology*, **17**, 144-151. http://dx.doi.org/10.3109/09286581003734878

[25] Hyman, L.G., Komaroff, E., Heijl, A., Bengtsson, B. and Leske, M.C., Early Manifest Glaucoma Trial Group (2005) Treatment and Vision-Related Quality of Life in the Early Manifest Glaucoma Trial. *Ophthalmology*, **112**, 1505-1513. http://dx.doi.org/10.1016/j.ophtha.2005.03.028

[26] Labiris, G., Katsanos, A., Fanariotis, M., Zacharaki, F., Chatzoulis, D. and Kozobolis, V.P. (2010) Vision-Specific Quality of Life in Greek Glaucoma Patients. *Journal of Glaucoma*, **19**, 39-43. http://dx.doi.org/10.1097/IJG.0b013e31819d5cf7

[27] Tastan, S., Iyigun, E., Bayer, A. and Acikel, C. (2010) Anxiety, Depression, and Quality of Life in Turkish Patients with Glaucoma. *Psychological Reports*, **106**, 343-357. http://dx.doi.org/10.2466/pr0.106.2.343-357

[28] Odberg, T., Jakobsen, J.E., Hultgren, S.J. and Halseide, R. (2001) The Impact of Glaucoma on the Quality of Life of Patients in Norway. I. Results from a Self-Administered Questionnaire. *Acta Ophthalmologica Scandinavica*, **79**, 116-120. http://dx.doi.org/10.1034/j.1600-0420.2001.079002116.x

[29] Skalicky, S.E., Goldberg, I. and McCluskey, P. (2012) Ocular Surface Disease and Quality of Life in Patients with Glaucoma. *American Journal of Ophthalmology*, **153**, 1003-1004.

[30] Nelson, P., Aspinall, P., Papasouliotis, O., Worton, B. and O'Brien, C. (2003) Quality of Life in Glaucoma and Its Relationship with Visual Function. *Journal of Glaucoma*, **12**, 139-150. http://dx.doi.org/10.1097/00061198-200304000-00009

[31] Iester, M. and Zingirian, M. (2002) Quality of Life in Patients with Early, Moderate and Advanced Glaucoma. *Eye*, **16**, 44-49. http://dx.doi.org/10.1038/sj.eye.6700036

34

Cycloplegic Refraction in Children: A Complete Audit Cycle

Suma Ganesh[1]*, Priyanka Arora[2], Sumita Sethi[3], Chandra Gurung[4]

[1]Department of Pediatric Ophthalmology and Strabismus, Dr Shroff's Charity Eye Hospital, New Delhi, India
[2]Department of Ophthalmology, Dayanand Medical College and Hospital, Ludhiana, India
[3]Department of Ophthalmology, BPS Government Medical College for Women, Sonepat, India
[4]Department of Ophthalmology, NNJS Banke Fateh Bal Eye Hospital, Nepalganj, Nepal
Email: *drsumaganesh@yahoo.com

Abstract

Purpose: Use of appropriate cycloplegic agent is an essential area of management in children with strabismus and refractive error. This study was designed to audit our own department's understanding and practice with respect to cycloplegia. Methods: Children in age group of 0 - 12 years with refractive errors and strabismus were evaluated with respect to four parameters: adherence to cycloplegic refraction (group-I), choice of cycloplegic agent (group-II), dosage of cycloplegia (group-III) and duration of cycloplegia (group-IV). Following the initial audit, the hospital audit committee evaluated the results; thereafter concerned staff was educated and aide-memoires of the dilatation protocol were introduced; a second audit cycle was carried out after 3 months. Results: First and second audit cycle included 334 children (mean age 6.2 ± 2.2 years) and 436 children (mean age 7.25 ± 2.9 years) respectively. A statistically significant improvement was found in all four parameters in the second audit cycle: adherence to dilation protocol (82.3% in first cycle to 94.3% in second cycle; $p = 0.001$), choice of cycloplegic agent (77% in the first cycle to 94.8% in the second cycle; $p = 0.001$), dosage of cycloplegic agent (84% in the first cycle to 96.3% in the second cycle; $p = 0.001$) and duration of cycloplegic agents (65% in the first cycle to 97.5% in the second cycle; $p = 0.001$ for CTC and 71.8% in the first cycle to 98% in the second cycle; $p = 0.001$ for Tropicamide). Conclusions: A complete audit cycle demonstrated a statistically significant improvement in all four parameters related to cycloplegic refraction in children. Regular auditing coupled with targeted interventions aimed to maintain the "best practice guidelines" for determination of refractive errors in children could prove effective in improving standards of clinical practice.

---

*Corresponding author.

Keywords

Cycloplegic Refraction, Audit, Children

1. Introduction

Cycloplegic refraction has been described as an essential part of the paediatric ophthalmic assessment [1] and the cornerstone of strabismus evaluation [2]. An ideal cycloplegic agent removes the detrimental effects of accommodation on measurement repeatability thus revealing the correct and appropriate refractive error. The primary differences in the action of the various cycloplegics used in the clinical practice are the time course for the onset and recovery of cycloplegia and the depth of cycloplegia. In order to obtain reliable measurements following instillation of a particular cycloplegic drug, there is a time limit for maximum cycloplegia to be reached and for refraction to be carried out. However overmedication, when maximum cycloplegia has already been reached increases the probability of systemic absorption and therefore intensifies the side effects. The use of appropriate cycloplegic agent in appropriate dosage and for appropriate duration, for different categories of children with strabismus and refractive error is thus an important and a challenging area of paediatric ophthalmology.

Refractive errors and strabismus are the major causes of ocular morbidity amongst children and appropriate refractive correction is vital to attain optimal vision and binocularity. However in literature, there is no specific mention regarding evidence based standards of refraction practices in children. In order to maintain the "best practice" guidelines for determination of refractive errors according to different categories of patients, we planned a complete audit cycle at our centre with the following aims:

1) To evaluate our own department's understanding and practice with respect to cycloplegia.

2) To ensure that all optometrists and doctors in the practice team carry out examinations to the same standard; so as to improve clinical effectiveness.

2. Materials and Methods

The study was planned and carried out at the department of Paediatric Ophthalmology and Strabismology of Dr. Shroff's charitable eye hospital after approval from the institutional review board. A full audit cycle was planned in 2 cycles; in the first cycle data was collected over a 4-week period, following which a 3 month period was allowed to incorporate implemented changes and a second audit cycle was planned.

1) Subjects: All children younger than 12 years of age requiring cycloplegic refraction for refractive error or strabismus were included in the study after taking informed consent from parents. Patients were excluded if they were emmetropic or were older than 12 years of age.

2) Methodology: It has been our department's policy to place stickers for details of cycloplegic refraction on all the case sheets of children younger than 12 years of age; notes were audited using these stickers. Variables collected included the age of the patient, type of refractive error (myopia/hyperopia), presence or absence of strabismus, type of strabismus (esotropia/exotropia), cycloplegic agent used, duration of instillation, time gap from instillation of first drop to dilated refraction done and side effects of the drug if any. Results were analysed with respect to four parameters adherence to cycloplegic refraction (group-I), choice of cycloplegic agent (group-II), dosage of cycloplegia (group-III) and duration of cycloplegia (group-IV).

3) Standards: Since there are currently no standardized national guidelines or protocols for dilated refraction in children, we have established our own standard protocols in accordance with the available literature [3]-[5]; details mentioned in **Table 1**.

4) The audit cycle: A standard based audit of the dilatation practices among the pediatric optometrists and ophthalmologists was carried out.

a) First cycle: Case sheets of children in age group of 0 - 12 years with refractive errors and strabismus who visited pediatric ophthalmology outpatient services over a period of 4 weeks in the month of April 2012 were reviewed for the four parameters; this was compared to the hospital's dilatation protocol.

b) Intervention: The results of the first audit were analyzed and presented to the audit committee. All the case sheets where the choice of drug was not appropriate were re-evaluated and reasons for not complying with the protocol were noted. After full analysis of the first cycle, the dilatation protocol of the department was for-

Table 1. Standardized protocol for dilation/cycloplegia[3,4,5].

I	All children younger than 12 years, with refractive error or strabismus should undergo cycloplegic refraction in the first visit		

Choice of cycloplegic agent

	Age	Category	Drug of choice
	<2 years	All children	Atropine (1%) eye ointment
	2 - 5 years	With Esotropia [5]	Atropine (1%) eye ointment
		Without Esotropia [3]	Cyclopentolate (1%)—Tropicacyl (1%)—Cyclopentolate (1%) (CTC)
II		With Esotropia [5]	Atropine (1%) eye ointment
	5 - 8 years	Without Esotropia Myopia [4] Hyperopia [3]	Tropicamide (1%) eye drops CTC*
	8 - 12 years	With esotropia	CTC
		Without Esotropia	Tropicamide (1%) eye drops

III	**Dosage of cycloplegic drugs** • **Atropine sulphate (1%):** eye ointment to be instilled twice a day for 3 days. • **Cyclopentolate (1%) and Tropicamide (1%) (CTC):** 3 drops instilled at an interval of 15 minutes. • **Tropicamide (1%):** 3 drops instilled at an interval of 10 minutes each.

IV	**Duration of cycloplegia** • **Atropine sulphate (1%):** After 3 days of first instillation. • **Cyclopentolate (1%) and Tropicamide (1%) (CTC):** After 60 minutes of first instillation. • **Tropicamide (1%):** Within 30 - 45 minutes of first instillation.

*CTC—Cyclopentolate (1%)—Tropicacyl (1%)—Cyclopentolate (1%)—3 drops instilled at an interval of 15 minutes—refraction done after 60 minutes of first installation.

matted into a poster, laminated and placed in all pediatric OPDs. All team members involved in the dilatation process were also educated about the appropriate drug, its dosage and duration of instillation.

c) Second cycle: All the case sheets of children younger than 12 years visiting pediatric ophthalmology outpatient services over a period of 4 weeks in the month of August 2012 were re-audited by the same therapist, for the same four parameters; results were assessed and published to the team.

5) Statistical analysis: Results of the two audit cycles were recorded and compared using SPSS 16 software. Chi-square test was used for comparison of values in each group in the first and second audit cycle; p-value of ≤0.05 was considered significant.

3. Results

Demographic details of children in each cycle are summarized in **Table 2**. Comparison of values in each group in the first and the second audit cycle is summarized in **Table 3**.

First cycle: Of the 334 case sheets audited, 230 (69%) were plain refractive errors and 104 (31%) had associated strabismus. Cycloplegic refraction was performed in 275 (82.3%) children while in the remaining 59 (17.7%) glasses were prescribed based on dry refraction. Cycloplegic agent appropriate for age and category of patient was used for dilatation in 212 (77%) cases. The duration and dosage of instillation was in accordance to formulated protocol in 231 (84%) cases. Final refraction was done after three days in all the 44 children (100%) of the atropine group; after 60 minutes of first drop in 65 out of 99 (65%) children of the Cyclopentolate-Tropicamide-Cyclopentolate (CTC) group and within 30 - 45 minutes in 94 out of 131 cases of the Tropicamide group (**Table 3**).

In most of the cases where the formulated dilation protocol was not adhered to, no reason was documented on the case sheet for the same. In 16 case sheets, stickers were not available so as collect the data for refraction. Parents were not willing for dilated refraction or refraction with a particular cycloplegic agent in 6 cases. Other reasons included allergy to a particular drug, recent switch in department's protocol in a particular category of patients and an outstation patient where atropine refraction was not practical.

Table 2. Demographic details.

	First cycle	**Second cycle**
Patients (n)	**334**	**436**
Age (years) (mean ± SD)	6.2 ± 2.2	7.0 ± 2.9
<2 years	32 (9.6%)	29 (6.7%)
2 - 5 years	91 (27.2%)	104 (23.8%)
5 - 8 years	120 (40%)	160 (36.7%)
8 - 12 years	91 (27.2%)	143 (32.8%)
Boys: Girls, Boys (%)	174/160, 52%	235/201, 54%

Table 3. Comparison of the various protocols in first and second audit cycle.

S no.	Criteria	First cycle n (%)	Second cycle n (%)	p-value
1	Children included for audit	334 (43.9%)	436 (51.9%)	
2	Dilated/Cycloplegic refraction done	275/334 (82.3%)	411/436 (94.3%)	0.001
3	Appropriate Cycloplegia used	212/275 (77%)	390/411 (94.8%)	0.001
4	Cycloplegia used in appropriate dosage	231/275 (84%)	396/411 (96.3%)	0.001
5	Refraction done after appropriate duration • Atropine • CTC* • Tropicamide	44/44 (100%) 65/100 (65%) 94/131 (71.8%)	42/42 (100%) 158/162 (97.5%) 203/207 (98%)	Not applicable 0.001 0.001

*CTC—Cyclopentolate (1%)—Tropicacyl (1%)—Cyclopentolate (1%)—3 drops instilled at an interval of 15 minutes—refraction done after 60 minutes of first installation.

Second cycle: Of the 436 case sheets audited, 310 (71%) were plain refractive errors and 126 (29%) had associated strabismus. Cycloplegic refraction was performed in 411 (94.3%) children while in the remaining 25 (5.7%) glasses were prescribed based on dry refraction. Cycloplegic agent appropriate for age and category of patient was used for dilatation in 390 (94.8%) cases. The duration and dosage of instillation was in accordance to formulated protocol in 396 (96.3%) cases. Final refraction was done after 3 days in all the 36 children (100%) of the atropine group, after 60 minutes of first drop in 158 out of 162 (97.5%) cases of the CTC group and within 30 - 45 minutes in 203 out of 207 (98%) children in the Tropicamide group.

4. Discussion

Evidence-based clinical guidelines, aiming to improve the effectiveness and efficiency of care delivery, have become a major feature of patient care [6] [7]. Non-adherence to guidelines may lead to unnecessary diagnostics, suboptimal treatment, or even adverse events [8] [9]. Owing to lack of knowledge of these standards or due a resistance in change of behaviour; some health care professionals and the technical staff may not adhere to the guidelines perfectly [10]. Active implementation through communication and education may improve adherence to guidelines and reduce sub-optimal care for patients [11].

In our study, each audit cycle provided demographically comparable populations of children with refractive error and strabismus. In the first audit cycle, poor adherence was observed in all the four study parameters. It was interesting to observe a statistically significant improvement in all these parameters in the second audit cycle. The parameters included were adherence to the dilatation protocol which improved markedly (82.3% in first cycle to 94.3% in second cycle; p = 0.001), choice of cycloplegic agent (77% in the first cycle to 94.8% in the second cycle, p = 0.001), dosage of cycloplegic agent (84% in the first cycle to 96.3% in the second cycle, p = 0.001) and duration of cycloplegic agents (65% in the first cycle to 97.5% in the second cycle; p = 0.001 for CTC and 71.8% in the first cycle to 98% in the second cycle; p = 0.001 for Tropicamide) (**Table 3**).

The results of our study have several practical implications. Firstly, it indicates that despite availability of well defined standards, a greater number of children were prescribed inappropriate glasses. There is a possible explanation to this; junior medical staff might not understand the importance of appropriate drug, dosage and duration of cycloplegia and could have been frequently unaware of the standard guidelines. Ours is a training institute with a huge turnover of optometrists performing pediatric refraction and fellow trainees in pediatric ophthalmology; this could account for the variations in practice. The second implication was finding a significant improvement in the practices following certain criteria aimed at increasing the awareness of the junior staff in the department. This included simple exercise like educating the staff and placing the aide memoires of the protocol at various places in the outpatient services.

Accurate prescription of glasses is the responsibility of the pediatric ophthalmology team. It was clear that compliance with guidelines was poor in all respects in the first audit cycle. This audit therefore targeted the practice patterns for cycloplegic refraction in children and the improvement clearly represents how simple measures can result in better adherence to protocols and uniformity in prescribing glasses. Though our results were encouraging, total compliance was not achieved with this audit. Achieving this must be the aim and re-auditing these results in the future after further re-enforcement of the guidelines would assess this.

Our study has certain limitations. The audit was dependent on clear documentation. Patients may have been assessed without documentation and therefore missed during data collection. However, the authors maintain that failing to document assessments is unsafe. Without documentation, the staff is left to pass on instructions, often causing confusion, and deteriorating examination findings. Another limitation was a relatively small number of children in either group; however statistical analysis demonstrated significant differences.

5. Conclusion

To conclude, our study demonstrated that a complete audit cycle with targeted interventions could be effective in improving compliance with evidence-based best clinical practice. Although predefined audit standard was not reached, the strategy used showed promise and further audit cycles would be needed to improve clinical practice further.

References

[1] Shah, P., Jacks, A.S. and Adams, G.G. (1997) Paediatric Cycloplegia: A New Approach. *Eye*, **11**, 845-846. http://dx.doi.org/10.1038/eye.1997.216

[2] Mehta, A. (1999) Chief Complaint, History and Physical Examination. In: Santiago, A.P. and Rosenbaum, A.I., Eds., *Clinical Strabismus Management*, Saunders, Philadelphia, 18.

[3] Miranda, M.N. (1972) Residual Accommodation. A Comparison between Cyclopentolate 1 Percent and a Combination of Cyclopentolate 1 Percent and Tropicamide 1 Percent. *Archives of Ophthalmology*, **87**, 515-517. http://dx.doi.org/10.1001/archopht.1972.01000020517004

[4] Manny, R.E., Hussein, M., Scheiman, M., *et al.* (2001) Tropicamide (1%): An Effective Cycloplegic Agent for Myopic children. *Investigative Ophthalmology & Visual Science*, **42**, 1728-1735.

[5] Rosenbaum, A.L., Bateman, J.B., Bremer, D.L., *et al.* (1981) Cycloplegic Refraction in Esotropic Children. Cyclopentolate versus Atropine. *Ophthalmology*, **88**, 1031-1034. http://dx.doi.org/10.1016/S0161-6420(81)80032-2

[6] (1992) Guidelines for Clinical Practice: From Development to Use. In: Lohr, K.N., Field, M.J., Eds., *Institute of Medicine Committee on Clinical Practice Guidelines*, National Academy Press, Washington DC,.

[7] Cabana, M.D., Rand, C.S., Powe, N.R., *et al.* (1999) Why Don't Physicians Follow Clinical Practice Guidelines? A Framework for Improvement. *JAMA*, **282**, 1458-1465. http://dx.doi.org/10.1001/jama.282.15.1458

[8] Foy, R., MacLennan, G., Grimshaw, J., *et al.* (2002) Attributes of Clinical Recommendations That Influence Change in Practice Following Audit and Feedback. *Journal of Clinical Epidemiology*, **55**, 717-722. http://dx.doi.org/10.1016/S0895-4356(02)00403-1

[9] Grol, R. and Grimshaw, J. (2003) From Best Evidence to Best Practice: Effective Implementation of Change in Patients' Care. *The Lancet*, **362**, 1225-30. http://dx.doi.org/10.1016/S0140-6736(03)14546-1

[10] Grol, R. and Buchan, H. (2006) Clinical Guidelines: What Can We Do to Increase Their Use? *Medical Journal of Australia*, **185**, 301-302.

[11] Freemantle, N. (2000) Implementation Strategies. *Family Practice*, **17**, S7-S10. http://dx.doi.org/10.1093/fampra/17.suppl_1.S7

35

A Systematic Review of Clinical Studies Using VEGF Inhibitors in the Treatment of Macular Edema from Diabetic Retinopathy

Karim Diab[1], Swati Chavda[1], Nathan Gorfinkel[1], Francie Si[2], Brad Dishan[3], William Hodge[2*]

[1]Western University, London, Canada
[2]Ivey Eye Institute, Western University, London, Canada
[3]Library Service, St. Joseph's Hospital Health Care, London, Canada
Email: *William.Hodge@sjhc.london.on.ca

Abstract

Purpose: To synthesize the present clinical evidence of efficacy and adverse events of commonly used anti-VEGF drugs for Diabetic Macular Edema. Methods: A systematic review was undertaken from the Medline, Biosis, CINAHL, Cochrane and Web of Science databases. Grey literature that consisted of lectures, seminars and conferences was also retrieved. The cut-off date was January 1 2014. A two-stage screening process was undertaken followed by a data extraction stage using the systematic review software EPPI. These were done by two reviewers. Heterogeneous meta-analysis was performed on the primary outcome which was change in macular thickness from baseline after injection. Side effects were tabulated. Results: From 846 articles that were initially screened, 18 papers were included in the data extraction stage. For all anti-VEGF treatments, the average decrease in macular thickness was 114.4 microns (95% CI: 66.8 - 162 µM). The average decrease in thickness from Lucentis (161.9 µM) was larger than that for Avastin (96.5 µM) but this was not statistically significant (p = 0.23). The most common complications were vitreous hemorrhage, endophthalmitis and retinal detachment. Vision threatening complications were rare but were reported regularly. Conclusions: The synthesized clinical evidence to date supports both of these treatments as efficacious and safe for diabetic macular edema (DME). There is a trend toward greater efficacy for Lucentis over Avastin but this is not statistically significant and will need a head-to-head RCT to assess accurately.

Keywords

Diabetic Retinopathy, VEGF Inhibitors, Macular Edema, Intraocular Injections, Systematic Review

*Corresponding author.

1. Introduction

There is a major rise in the percentage of individuals with diabetes in the global population. This growing number is expected to reach 366 million individuals by 2030 compared to 171 million individuals with the condition in the year 2000 [1]. Most of these cases in the western world are attributed to a change in lifestyle and an increase in obesity and longevity [1]. Patients with diabetes have a diverse set of complications that range from microvascular to macrovascular complications. Microvascular complications are retinopathies, nephropathies and neuropathies while macrovascular complications include myocardial infarctions, hypertension and peripheral arterial diseases [2]. In this paper, we focus on damages caused to the retina by the complications associated with diabetes mellitus; the leading cause of vision loss in working-age individuals worldwide [3].

Vascular Endothelial Growth Factor (VEGF) is a hormone normally liberated by cells in the body in case of a wound or an infection in order to form new blood vessels and restore oxygen levels in the damaged tissue. Symptoms caused by diabetes such as hyperglycemia, oxidative stress, hypoxia and inflammatory reactions increase the expression of VEGF [4]. Also, retinal endothelial cells have a high number of VEGF receptors that increase in patients with diabetes [4]. VEGF contribute significantly to the development of Diabetic macular edema (DME) by affecting the tight junctions of endothelial cells in the retina by increasing leukocyte count and these leukocytes are known to cause leakage [3]. This causes the breakdown of the blood-retinal barrier and the accumulation of fluid in the macula [5] which in turn will result in reduced or distorted vision. In addition, VEGF is at least partly responsible for the formation of new blood vessels in the retina (proliferative diabetic retinopathy).

One of the treatments of DME is the injection of antibodies that specifically target VEGF in patients suffering from DME. Three anti-VEGF agents are currently commercially available: Pegaptanib (Macugen, OSI/Eyetech, Melville, NY, USA), Ranibizumab (Lucentis, Genentech, Inc., South San Francisco, CA, USA) and Bevacizumab (Avastin, Genentech, Inc.)

Lucentis and Avastin are humanized antibodies specific to all isoforms of VEGF that are used commonly clinically for intraocular vascular disorders. Although Lucentis is approved by the FDA, Avastin is still undergoing clinical trials to determine whether it is safe and effective for the treatment of DME and other pathologies of the retina. Avastin is primarily an anti-cancer drug but it is used off-label by physicians to treat DME because of its low cost and availability [3]. One of the reasons that Avastin's safety as a treatment for ophthalmic conditions is still being considered is the drug's side effects when used as an anti-cancer drug. Trials of Avastin for Age-related Macular Degeneration (AMD) patients rather than cancer patient presented hypertension as a side effect though occlusive stroke was also seen [6]. However these trials were made on AMD patients who tend to be of an older age group than patients of DME.

Side effects of these anti-VEGF drugs for intraocular conditions are usually rare and procedure related rather than reactions to the medication [3]. Some procedure related outcomes consist of endophthalmitis, retinal detachment and lens injury. DME patients treated with both Avastin and Lucentis have shown significant improvements in vision [3]. A comparative study of Avastin against Lucentis needs to be done in order to evaluate the best candidate for DME treatment. At that point, we will be able to evaluate all the possible outcomes and side effects of each drug along with their costs.

In this study, we are synthesizing all of clinical research results to date of anti-VEGF drugs for DME via a systematic review and meta-analysis.

2. Methods

The search for relevant literature was conducted based on the research question "How do Avastin and Lucentis compare to each in terms of outcomes and complications for the treatment of diabetic macular edema"? This research question along with the subsequent keywords used in the different databases was defined with the help of clinical content experts and an information specialist. Multiple synonyms were created for VEGF inhibitors and macular edema treatment.

Relevant literature published in English was obtained using an exhaustive search from the Medline, Biosis, CINAHL, Cochrane and Web of Science databases. Grey literature that consisted of lectures, seminars and conferences was also retrieved. These included abstracts from the American Academy of Ophthalmology, Association for Research in Vision and Ophthalmology, Canadian Ophthalmology Society and European Association of Ophthalmology. The cut-off date was January 1, 2014. No beginning date was specified. The monograph results were then inserted into EPPI, a systematic review software program. Duplicates were then removed using EPPI after a bibliographic record was made. Literature was then passed through two levels of screening followed by a data extraction level. Papers had to be included after each level of screening in order for data to be extracted from them. EPPI records whether a publication is included or excluded after each level of screening. The software also records the reason why the paper was excluded.

The first level of screening determined the eligibility of the paper based on the title and the abstract. This level excluded papers that did not focus on patients with diabetic retinopathy. Experimentations on animals were excluded. In addition, research papers that conducted the study on patients under the age of 18 were excluded. Papers that did not examine the effects of Avastin or Lucentis as a treatment were also excluded. Finally, the study had to be conducted in an industrialized country for reasons of generalizability.

The second level of screening involved reviewing the full paper in EPPI in order to determine its eligibility. In this level, papers that were not primary research studies were excluded. Hence, surveys, editorial comments, small case studies, conferences, meetings and systematic reviews were excluded. A sample size of 20 patients or more was necessary in order for the paper to be included. Also, the paper needed to examine the effect of one of the two anti-VEGF drugs on patients with diabetic retinopathy to be included. Both the first and the second level of screening were conducted by multiple reviewers but at least two had to review each paper. Disagreements in the decision to include or exclude a paper were noted and a conclusion was reached by consensus if possible and if not by a third party adjudicator (WGH).

During data extraction, the quality of included articles and risk of bias was assessed by multiple reviewers using the Downs and Black instrument. Both randomized controlled trials and observational studies were assessed using this instrument.

Data was extracted from the included articles and organized using the EPPI software. This data included demographic data, treatment data, outcome data and side effect data. All data was collected on a premade data collection sheet in EPPI. For statistical analysis, the final data was imported into the statistical software STATA (v 14 College Station Texas) for analysis. For outcomes where the data was sufficiently homogenous, a meta-analysis was performed for the defined outcomes. A pooled weighted mean difference was used as the primary outcome. Due to study heterogeneity, the pooled effects were assumed to follow a random effects model (DerSimonian-Laird). Formal meta-analysis was performed for the outcome of macular thickness change from baseline after anti-VEGF injection but was not possible for adverse events.

The Begg test was used to check for publication bias after graphing the potential bias via Funnel plots. Meta-regressions were performed for study level and clinical level variables to see if confounders had influenced the outcomes studied. Multiple comparisons in the meta-regression were adjusted by using a Monte Carlo simulation of 20,000 trials.

3. Results

The PRISMA diagram for this study is shown in **Figure 1**. 846 articles were sent through level I abstract screening followed by 402 that went through full text level II screening. Data extraction occurred on a final sample of 18 articles [7]-[24] that met all inclusion criteria. All of these 18 articles reported on either macular thickness change after injection, adverse events or both. Of the 18 articles included, 11 were randomized clinical trials, 1 was an observational study and 6 were case series. The Downs and Black checklist is a 27 point checklist that assesses study quality. The average score in studies used for this review was 20.6. The range was 13 to 27.

Table 1 provides the baseline data from the studies. The average sample size from the studies was 188 with a little under 50% being female. **Table 2** reveals the treatment characteristics. There were on average 2.66 anti VEGF injections per treatment over an average span of 86 days and patients were followed an average of 317 days from onset of macular edema.

Figure 2 and **Figure 3** provide the weighted mean differences Forest Plots from all studies. **Figure 2** is the Forest plot of all anti-VEGF drug treatment on macular thickness. As can be seen all but one study demonstrated a significant decrease in macular thickness after treatment compared to before treatment. The average decrease in macular thickness was 114.4 microns (95% CI: 66.8 - 162 μM). **Figure 3** is the Forest plot of anti VEGF treatment stratified by type of VEGF inhibitor. As can be seen from the Forest plot, the average decrease in thickness from Lucentis (161.9 μM) was larger than that for Avastin (96.5 μM) but this was not statistically

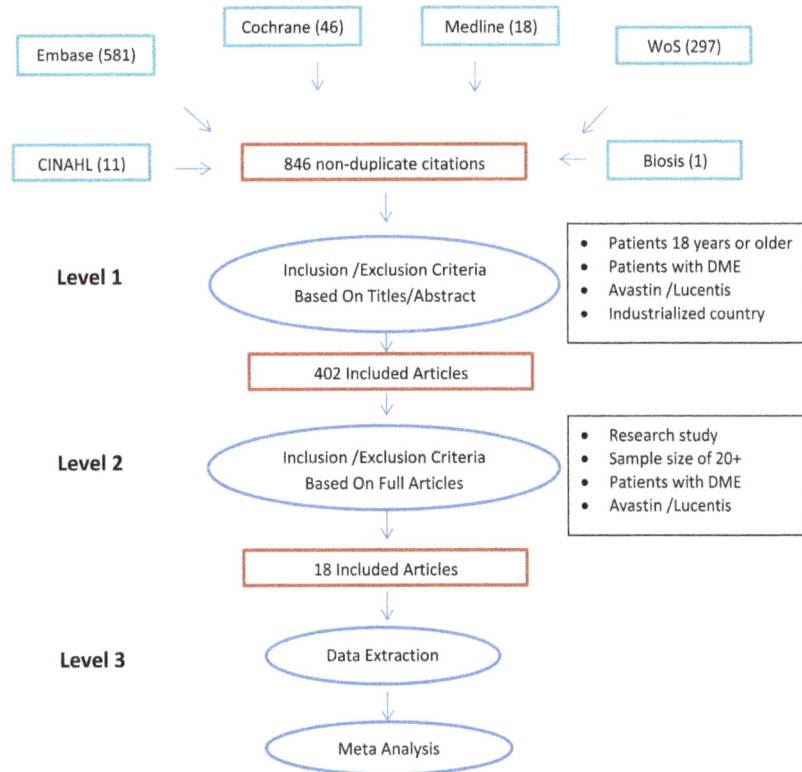

Figure 1. The PRISMA diagram.

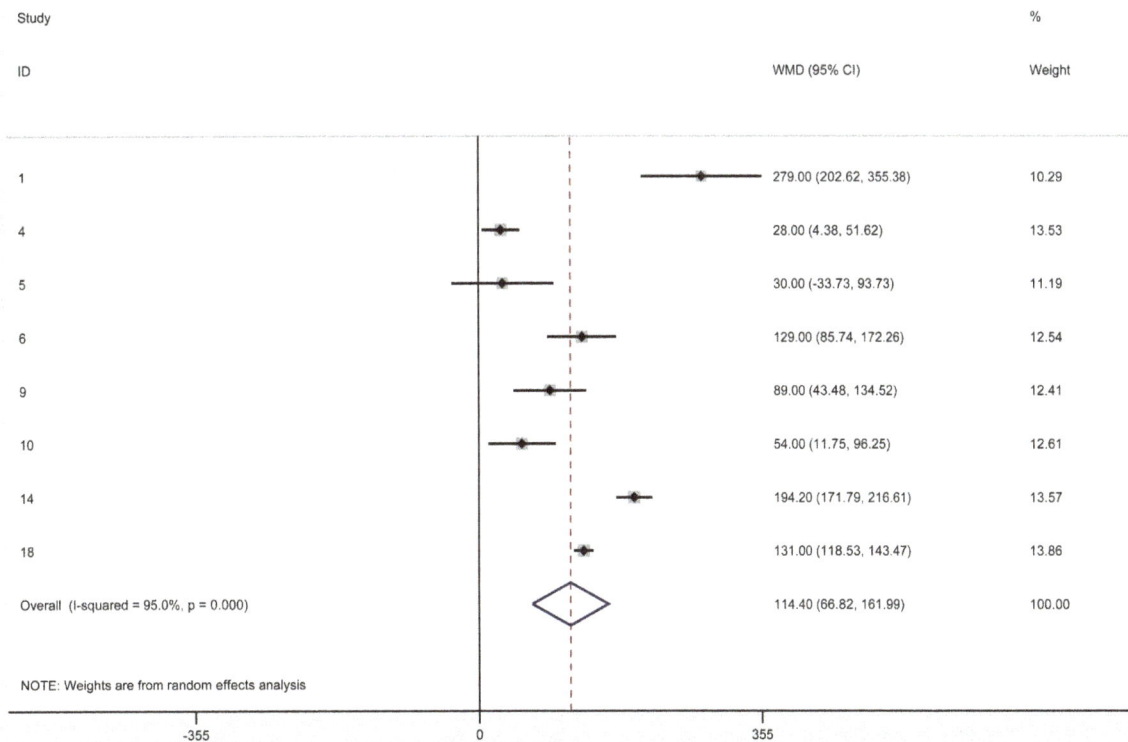

Figure 2. Forest Plot-macular thickness change post anti-VEGF for DR.

significant (p = 0.23).

Table 3 reveals the compilation of most commonly reported complications from all studies. The most common complications were vitreous hemorrhage, endophthalmitis and retinal detachment. Vision threatening complications were rare but were reported regularly.

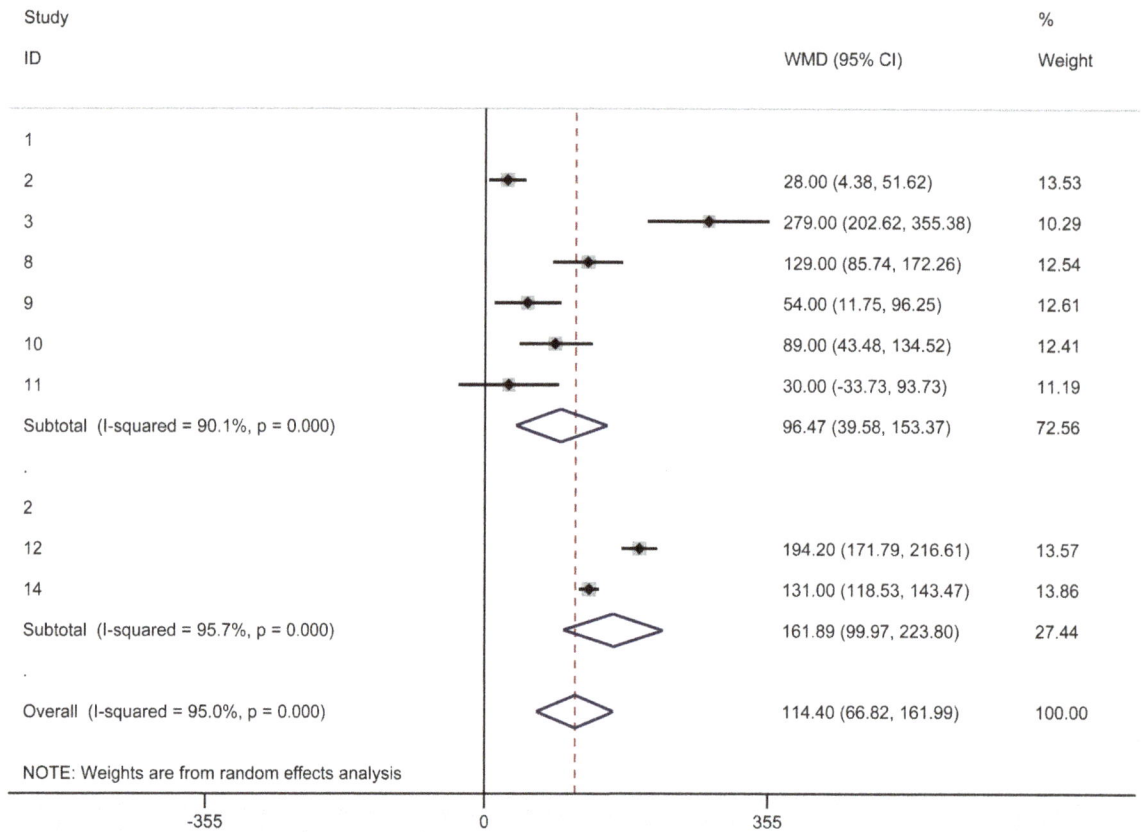

Upper Forest Plot=Bevacizumab, Lower=Ranibizumab

Figure 3. Macular thickness change by VEGF inhibitor.

Table 1. Baseline data.

	Number of Studies	Mean	Standard Deviation	Minimum Value	Maximum Value
Studies	18				
Patients	17	187.5	213.5	26	691
% Female	15	45.1	9.5	31	58.7
HbA1c	8	7.6	0.50	6.95	8.48

Table 2. Treatment characteristics.

	Number of Studies	Mean	Standard Deviation	Minimum Value	Maximum Value
Number of Eyes	17	207.9	262.0	26	854
Treatment Duration (days)	15	85.9	126.5	1	365
Number of Injections	14	2.66	2.51	1	10
Follow-Up (days)	17	317.1	259.6	7	730

Table 3. Most commonly reported complications.

	Number of Studies Reporting Complication	Mean Number of Patients with Complication	Standard Deviation	Minimum	Maximum
Vitreous Hemorrhage	7	15	18.8	1	54
Retinal Detachment	6	5.2	9.2	1	24
Endophthalmitis	5	3	2.3	1	6

Meta-regression was performed to assess the impact of age, gender, type of diabetes, study type and study quality (via Downs and Black instrument) on the outcome of macular thickness after VEGF injections. For age, gender, type of diabetes and study quality, there was no significant effect on the main outcome. For study type, the stratified sample sizes were too small to make any type of robust assessment.

4. Conclusions

Diabetic Retinopathy can be classified into several stages based on the level of disease severity. Non proliferative retinopathy consists of background microvascular dot hemorrhages and exudative changes termed "hard exudates". Preproliferative retinopathy consists of microvascular beading abnormalities and retinal infarcts (cotton wool spots). Proliferative retinopathy consists of fragile new vessels that can bleed into the vitreous and result in tractional retinal detachment. Broadly speaking, the main vision threatening complications are macular edema; this can occur at any stage but involves exudative thickening of the macula and neovascular bleeding which can only occur in the proliferative stage [25].

While the molecular pathogenesis of DME is not fully understood, Vascular Endothelial Growth Factor plays an important role. VEGF has a molecular weight of 46 kDa and is a homodimer. It mediates many important physiologic processes including the development and maintenance of the vasculature, regulation of hematologic coagulation and vascular integrity through the production of nitric oxide [26] [27].

The human VEGF family comprises five related glycoproteins: the most important of which clinically is VEGF-A. VEGF-A is the best characterized, and is mainly responsible for angiogenic and vasopermeability [28] [29]. All VEGF family members signal through three tyrosine kinase receptors but most of the vascular-hyperpermeability responses to VEGF-A are mediated through VEGFR-2, which is expressed by the vascular endothelium [27].

In patients with diabetic retinopathy, chronic hyperglycemia leads to the upregulation of VEGF, resulting in angiogenesis, increased vascular permeability, and the production of pro-inflammatory cytokines [29] [30]. Thickening of the basement membrane and pericyte drop out, which are key hallmarks of retinopathy will further cascade stimulation of VEGF production and result in an increased severity of diabetic retinopathy clinically [29].

Hence anti-VEGF intraocular injections have gained widespread use in retina-choroidal vascular diseases such as age related macular degeneration and diabetic retinopathy. The synthesized evidence to date from this paper reveals that both commonly used anti VEGF treatments are effective for diabetic related clinically significant macular edema. Our results do not distinguish efficacy differences amongst the two anti-VEGF treatments studied but there is a trend toward Lucentis being superior to Avastin based on macular thickness measurements. Hence, it is possible that a homogenous randomized clinical trial for diabetic macular edema could find differences amongst the two treatments for this condition.

Complications were not common and serious vision threatening complications were especially rare amongst reported papers. Less than half the papers analyzed revealed any vision threatening complications and they were rare when reported. Hence it can be concluded that the synthesis of evidence to date favors these treatments as being safe given the overall synthesized sample size was so large.

Acknowledgements

We acknowledge the funding support from AMOSO AFP Innovation Fund (Ontario, Canada) (INN12-010) for making the project possible.

References

[1]   Lutty, G.A. (2013) Effects of Diabetes on the Eye. *Investigative Ophthalmology and Visual Sciences*, **54**, 81-87. http://dx.doi.org/10.1167/iovs.13-12979

[2]   Heydari, I., Radi, V., Razmjou, S. and Amiri, A. (2010) Chronic Complications of Diabetes Mellitus in Newly Diagnosed Patients. *International Journal of Diabetes Mellitus*, **2**, 61-63. http://dx.doi.org/10.1016/j.ijdm.2009.08.001

[3]   Nicholson, B.P. and Schachat, A.P. (2010) A Review of Clinical Trials of Anti-VEGF Agents for Diabetic Retinopathy. *Graefe's Archive for Clinical and Experimental Ophthalmology*, **248**, 915-930. http://dx.doi.org/10.1007/s00417-010-1315-z

[4]   Caldwell, R.B., Bartoli, M., Behzadian, M.A., El-Remessey, A.E.B., Al-Shabrawey, M., Platt, D.H. and Caldwell, R.W. (2003) Vascular Endothelial Growth Factor and Diabetic Retinopathy: Pathophysiologic Mechanisms and Treatment Perspectives. *Diabetes/Metabolism Research and Reviews*, **19**, 442-455. http://dx.doi.org/10.1002/dmrr.415

[5]   Lang, G.E. (2012) Diabetic Macular Edema. *Ophthalmologica*, **227**, 21. http://dx.doi.org/10.1159/000337156

[6]   Michels, S., Rosenfeld, P.J., Puliafito, C.A., Marcus, E.N. and Venkatraman, A.S. (2005) Systemic Bevacizumab (Avastin) Therapy for Neovascular Age Related Macular Degeneration: Twelve-Week Results of an Uncontrolled Open-Label Clinical Study. *Ophthalmology*, **112**, 1035-1047. http://dx.doi.org/10.1016/j.ophtha.2005.02.007

[7]   Aiello, L.P., Beck, R.W., Bressler, N.M., Browning, D.J., Chalam, K.V., Davis, M., Ferris, F.L., *et al.* (2011) Rationale for the Diabetic Retinopathy Clinical Research Network Treatment Protocol for Center-Involved Diabetic Macular Edema. *Ophthalmology*, **118**, 5-14. http://dx.doi.org/10.1016/j.ophtha.2011.09.058

[8]   Campochiaro, P.A., Heier, J.S., Feiner, L., Gray, S., Saroj, N., Rundle, A.C., Murahasi, W.Y., *et al.* (2010) Ranibizumab for Macular Edema Following Branch Retinal Vein Occlusion: Six-Month Primary End Point Results of a Phase III Study. *Ophthalmology*, **117**, 1102-1112. http://dx.doi.org/10.1016/j.ophtha.2010.02.021

[9]   di Lauro, R., De Ruggiero, P., di Lauro, R., di Lauro, M.T. and Romano, M.R. (2010) Intravitrealbevacizumab for Surgical Treatment of Severe Proliferative Diabetic Retinopathy. *Graefe's Archive for Clinical and Experimental Ophthalmology*, **248**, 785-791. http://dx.doi.org/10.1007/s00417-010-1303-3

[10]   Elman, M.J., Aiello, L.P., Beck, R.W., Bressler, N.M., Bressler, S.B., Edwards, A.R., Ferris, F.L., *et al.*(2010) Randomized Trial Evaluating Ranibizumab plus Prompt or Deferred Laser or Triamcinolone plus Prompt Laser for Diabetic Macular Edema. *Ophthalmology*, **117**, 1064-1077. http://dx.doi.org/10.1016/j.ophtha.2010.02.031

[11]   Elman, M.J., Qin, H., Aiello, L.P., Beck, R.W., Bressler, N.M., Ferris, F.L., Glassman, A.R., *et al.* (2012) Intravitreal Ranibizumab for Diabetic Macular Edema with Prompt versus Deferred Laser Treatment. *Ophthalmology*, **119**, 2312-2318. http://dx.doi.org/10.1016/j.ophtha.2012.08.022

[12]   Googe, J., Brucker, A.J., Bressler, N.M., Qin, H., Aiello, L.P., Antoszyk, A., Beck, R.W., *et al.* (2011) Randomized Trial Evaluating Short-Term Effects of Intravitreal Ranibizumab or Triamcinolone Acetonide on Macular Edema after Focal/Grid Laser for Diabetic Macular Edema in Eyes Also Receiving Panretinal Photocoagulation. *Retina*, **31**, 1009-1027. http://dx.doi.org/10.1097/IAE.0b013e318217d739

[13]   Kook, D., Wolf, A., Kreutzer, T., Neubauer, A., Strauss, R., Ulbig, M., Kampik, A., *et al.* (2008) Long-Term Effect of Intravitreal Bevacizumab (Avastin) in Patients with Chronic Diffuse Diabetic Macular Edema. *Retina*, **28**, 1053-1060. http://dx.doi.org/10.1097/IAE.0b013e318176de48

[14]   Kook, P.E., Maier, M., Schuster, T., Feucht, N. and Lohmann, C.P. (2011) Nine-Month Results of Intravitreal Bevacizumab versus Triamcinolone for the Treatment of Diffuse Diabetic Macular Oedema: A Retrospective Analysis. *Acta Ophthalmologica*, **89**, 769-773. http://dx.doi.org/10.1111/j.1755-3768.2009.01823.x

[15]   Massin, P., Bandello, F., Garweg, J., Hansen, L., Harding, S.P., Larsen, M., Mitchell, P., *et al.* (2010) Safety and Efficacy of Ranibizumab in Diabetic Macular Edema (RESOLVE Study). A 12-Month, Randomized, Controlled, Double-Masked, Multicenter Phase II Study. *Diabetes Care*, **33**, 2399-2405. http://dx.doi.org/10.2337/dc10-0493

[16]   Mehta, S., Blinder, K.J., Shah, G.K., Kymes, S.M., Schlief, S.L. and Grand, M.G. (2009) Intravitreal Bevacizumab for the Treatment of Refractory Diabetic Macular Edema. *Ophthalmic Surgery Lasers and Imaging*, **41**, 323-329.

[17]   Michaelides, M., Fraser-Bell, S., Hamilton, R., Kaines, A., Egan, C., Bunce, C., Peto, T., *et al.* (2010) Macular Perfusion Determined by Fundus Fluorescein Angiography at the 4-Month Time Point in a Prospective Randomized Trial of Intravitreal Bevacizumab or Laser Therapy in the Management of Diabetic Macular Edema (Bolt Study): Report 1. *Retina*, **30**, 781-786. http://dx.doi.org/10.1097/IAE.0b013e3181d2f145

[18]   Michaelides, M., Kaines, A., Hamilton, R.D., Fraser-Bell, S., Rajendram, R., Quhill, F., Boos, C.J., *et al.* (2010) A Prospective Randomized Trial of Intravitreal Bevacizumab or Laser Therapy in the Management of Diabetic Macular Edema (BOLT Study): 12-Month Data: Report 2. *Ophthalmology*, **117**, 1078-1086.e2. http://dx.doi.org/10.1016/j.ophtha.2010.03.045

[19]   Nguyen, Q.D., Shah, S.M., Heier, J.S., Do, D.V., Lim, J., Boyer, D., Abraham, P., *et al.* (2009) Primary End Point (Six

Months) Results of the Ranibizumab for Edema of the mAcula in Diabetes (READ-2) Study. *Ophthalmology*, **116**, 2175-2181. http://dx.doi.org/10.1016/j.ophtha.2009.04.023

[20] Nguyen, Q.D., Shah, S.M., Khwaja, A.A., Channa, R., Hatef, E., Do, D.V., Boyer, D., *et al.* (2010) Two-Year Outcomes of the Ranibizumab for Edema of the mAcula in Diabetes (READ-2) Study. *Ophthalmology*, **117**, 2146-2151. http://dx.doi.org/10.1016/j.ophtha.2010.08.016

[21] Oshima, Y., Shima, C., Wakabayashi, T., Kusaka, S., Shiraga, F., Ohji, M. and Tano, Y. (2009) Microincision Vitrectomy Surgery and Intravitreal Bevacizumab as a Surgical Adjunct to Treat Diabetic Traction Retinal Detachment. *Ophthalmology*, **116**, 927-938. http://dx.doi.org/10.1016/j.ophtha.2008.11.005

[22] Robaszkiewicz, J., Chmielewska, K., Figurska, M., Wierzbowska, J. and Stankiewicz, A. (2012) Triple Therapy: Phaco-Vitrectomy with ILM Peeling, Retinal Endophotocoagulation, and Intraoperative Use of Bevacizumab for Diffuse Diabetic Macular Edema. *Medical Science Monitor*, **18**, 241-251. http://dx.doi.org/10.12659/MSM.882624

[23] Scott, I. and Flynn Jr., H.W. (2007) Reducing the Risk of Endophthalmitis Following Intravitreal Injections. *Retina*, **27**, 10-12. http://dx.doi.org/10.1097/IAE.0b013e3180307271

[24] Takamura, Y., Kubo, E. and Akagi, Y. (2009) Analysis of the Effect of Intravitreal Bevacizumab Injection on Diabetic Macular Edema after Cataract Surgery. *Ophthalmology*, **116**, 1151-1157. http://dx.doi.org/10.1016/j.ophtha.2009.01.014

[25] Ulbig, M.W., Kampik, A. and Hamilton, A.M. (1993) Diabetic Retinopathy. Epidemiology, Risk Factors and Staging. *Ophthalmology*, **90**, 197-209.

[26] He, H., Venema, V.J., Gu, X., Venema, R.C., Marrero, M.B. and Caldwell, R.B. (1999) Vascular Endothelial Growth Factor Signals Endothelial Cell Production of Nitric Oxide and Prostacyclin through flk-1/KDR Activation of c-Src. *The Journal of Biological Chemistry*, **274**, 25130-25135. http://dx.doi.org/10.1074/jbc.274.35.25130

[27] Foy, K.C., Miller, M.J., Moldovan, N., Carson III, W.E. and Kaumaya, P.T. (2012) Combined Vaccination with HER-2 Peptide Followed by Therapy with VEGF Peptide Mimics Exerts Effective Anti-Tumor and Anti-Angiogenic Effects *in Vitro* and *in Vivo*. *Oncoimmunology*, **1**, 1048-1060. http://dx.doi.org/10.4161/onci.20708

[28] Papadopoulos, N., Martin, J., Ruan, Q., Rafique, A., Rosconi, M.P., Shi, E., Pyles, E.A., Yancopoulos, G.D., Stahl, N. and Wiegand, S.J. (2012) Binding and Neutralization of Vascular Endothelial Growth Factor (VEGF) and Related Ligands by VEGF Trap, Ranibizumab and Bevacizumab. *Angiogenesis*, **15**, 171-185. http://dx.doi.org/10.1007/s10456-011-9249-6

[29] Stewart, M.W. (2012) Anti-Vascular Endothelial Growth Factor Drug Treatment of Diabetic Macular Edema: The Evolution Continues. *Current Diabetes Reviews*, **8**, 237-246. http://dx.doi.org/10.2174/157339912800840488

[30] Bhagat, N., Grigorian, R.A., Tutela, A. and Zarbin, M.A. (2009) Dibetic Macular Edema: Pathogenesis and Treatment. *Survey of Ophthalmology*, **54**, 1-32. http://dx.doi.org/10.1016/j.survophthal.2008.10.001

36

Prevalence and Associations of Hepatitis B Seropositivity in a Rural African Ophthalmic Surgical Population

Obiekwe Okoye[1]*, Boniface Eze[1], Chimdia Ogbonnaya[2], Chinyelu Ezisi[2], Olughu Obasi[3]

[1]Department of Ophthalmology, University of Nigeria, Enugu, Nigeria
[2]Department of Ophthalmology, Federal Teaching Hospital, Abakiliki, Nigeria
[3]Eye Unit, Presbyterian Joint Hospital, Uburu, Nigeria
Email: *obiekwe.okoye@unn.edu.ng

Abstract

Objective: Globally, Hepatitis B virus (HBV) infection remains a public health issue. It is a major cause of morbidity and mortality, especially in developing countries. Working in a healthcare setting particularly in low resource area is a major risk factor for contracting HBV infection. Despite this, routine pre-operative screening for HBV infection has not yet practiced in many Nigerian hospitals. This study assessed the prevalence and associations of hepatitis B seropositivity in a rural south-eastern Nigerian population of ophthalmic surgical patients. Methods: This was a prospective cross-sectional survey of ophthalmic surgical patients at the Presbyterian Joint Hospital—a rural missionary eye care facility in south-eastern Nigeria, conducted between December 2012 and June 2013. Participant's socio-demographic and clinical data and result of screening for hepatitis B surface antigen (HbSAg) were collected. Results: The participants (n = 100; males, 40; females, 50) were aged 52.9 SD ± 15.4 (range 1 - 88 years). They were predominantly farmers—45% and traders—26% who had cataract—58% and glaucoma—16% as their leading clinical diagnosis indicating ophthalmic surgical intervention. Of them only 2 (2.0%) were sero-positive for HbSAg. HBV seropositivity was not associated with age, gender or occupation. Conclusion: Though the prevalence of hepatitis B viral infection is low in this study, universal measures to prevent cross infection of the healthcare worker is indicated.

Keywords

HBV, Prevalence, Associations, Ophthalmic Surgical Patients

---

*Corresponding author.

1. Introduction

Hepatitis B is an infectious inflammatory disease of the liver caused by the hepatitis B virus (HBV) that affects hominoidea (primates), including humans. Originally known as "serum hepatitis" [1], the disease has caused epidemics in parts of Asia and Africa, and it is endemic in China [2]. About a third of the world's population has been infected at one point in their lives [3], including about 400 million who are chronic carriers [4] [5].

The virus is transmitted by exposure to infected blood, blood products, and other body fluids like semen and vaginal fluids. Additional risk factors for contracting HBV infection include perinatal and transplacental transmission, working in a healthcare settings, peritoneal and hemo-dialysis, acupuncture, tattooing, intravenous drug abuse, unprotected surgical procedures, sharing razors or toothbrushes with an infected person and travel to countries where it is endemic [6]-[9].

Prior reports suggest a prevalence of 10% - 15% in the average risk Nigerian population [10]. Chronic disease or carrier state, which follows recovery from acute phase, is usually asymptomatic; however carriers remain sero-positive and potentially transmit the infection.

The reported prevalence of HBV infection ranges from 2.0% in developed countries to 8.0% in developing countries. In developing countries, HBV infection is often endemic with male gender, older age and lower socio-economic status as important risk factors for infection [11]-[13]. Despite the availability of a safe and effective vaccine, Nigeria has remained hyper-endemic for HBV infection, with an estimated 12.0% of the population being chronic carriers [14]. Globally HBV infection remains a major public health issue, with new cases still being reported annually [15] [16]. Globally, ophthalmic surgical interventions are among the most frequently performed surgical procedures. The indications include visual restoration, preservation of vision, patients comfort and cosmesis. During these procedures, surgeons and other operating room personnel are exposed to the risk of potential transmission of infection from surgical patients. Despite the high sero-prevalence of HBV infection in the general public and the risk of its peri-operative transmission, currently, in the study center and most other eye care facilities in Nigeria, routine hepatitits B serology is not performed on patients undergoing eye surgeries. Consequently, in Nigeria, HBV sero-prevalence data on ophthalmic surgical patients is scarce. This study is aimed to assess HBV sero-prevalence, and its associations, in a rural ophthalmic surgical patient population in south-eastern Nigeria. The findings will assist ophthalmic surgical care providers and public health workers in preventing peri-operative HBV transmission.

2. Methods

2.1. Background

Ebonyi state, created on October 1st, 1996 is one of the five component states of Nigeria's south-east geo-political zone. The state is made up of 13 administrative sub-units or Local Government Areas (LGA). The state is located in the tropical rain forest climatic belt. The state's inhabitants are predominantly farmers; however, there are an appreciable number of traders, artisans and civil servants.

There are numerous public and privately-owned eye care centers in Ebonyi state. Of this Presbyterian Joint Hospital-the study center is a rural mission hospital established in 1912 and located in Uburu, Ohaozara LGA. In addition to general medical care, the center provides medical, surgical and refractive eye care to the inhabitants of the LGA and the neighboring eight rural LGAs of Ebonyi State. The hospital's eye care unit is a 20-bed facility manned by one visiting consultant ophthalmologist, one diplomate ophthalmologist, one optometrist, one trained ophthalmic nurse, and six auxiliary nurses.

The study was a prospective descriptive cross-sectional survey of all the patients who accessed ophthalmic surgical care at Presbyterian Joint Hospital between December 1, 2012 and June 1, 2013.

2.2. Sample Size and Sampling

Based on the previously reported HBsAg seroprevalence of 1.7% in a cohort of ophthalmic surgical patients [17] and an error margin of 5%, a sample size of 26 was envisaged. However all the consecutively presenting, and eligible participants seen at the study center during the study period were recruited to obtain an adjusted sample size of 100.

Baseline socio-demographic (age, sex, occupation) and clinical (ophthalmic diagnosis and type of surgery) were collected from each participant. Subsequently, each participant was screened for HbSAg seropositivity using Wondfo onestep HBsAg serum/plasma test strip, (Worldbridge Inc, Manila, Phillipines). The test was also done based on this principle "Wondfo one step HBsAg serum/Plasma test strip is a rapid Immuno-chromato-graphic test for visual detection of hepatitis B virus surface antigen (HBs Ag) in serum/plasma samples. The membrane is pre-coated with anti-HBV antibodies on the test line region of the strip. During testing, the speci-men reacts with the particle coated with the HBV antibody. The mixture migrates upwards on the membrane chromatographically by capillary action to react with anti-HBV antibodies on the membrane and generate a co-lored line. Presence of colored line on the test region indicates positive result. A procedural colored line on the control line region will always appear to serve as control".

The test was interpreted as per the manufacturer's criteria as follows: *positive test*: if the white line on the test strip changes to red; this indicates serum HBsAg titre of ≥ 1 ng/ml. Negative test; no color change indicates se-rum HBsAg titer of zero or below the detection level of the test.

Data analysis was performed using the Statistical Package for Social Sciences (SPSS) software version 18 (SPSS Inc., Chicago, Illinois, USA). Descriptive statistics yielded percentages, frequencies and proportions; Comparative statistical tests for significance of observed intergroup differences utilized chi square for categori-cal variables and student-t test for continuous variables. For all comparisons, significance level was at $p < 0.05$.

2.3. Eligibility

All consecutively presenting, and consenting, patients who accessed ophthalmic surgical care at the study center during the 6-month study period were included in the study. Non-consenting patients and patients who had non-surgical treatments were excluded from the study.

2.4. Ethics

Ethics approval compliant with the 1964 Helsinki Declaration on research involving human subjects as amended in London 2008 was obtained from the Medical and Health Research Ethics Committee (Institutional Review Board) of the study center. Informed consent was received from the patients.

3. Results

A total of 100 patients comprising 40 (40.0%) males and 60 (60.0%) females (Male: Female, 1:1.5) aged 52.9 ±15.4 SD years (range 1 and 88 years) who had various ophthalmic surgeries at the study center during the study pe-riod constituted the participants. The average annual hospital admission is 226. The participant's socio-demo-graphic profile is shown in **Table 1**. The participants were predominantly farmers—45 (45.0%) and their leading clinical ophthalmic diagnoses necessitating surgical intervention were cataract—58 (58.0%) and glaucoma (16.0%), **Table 2** and **Table 3**. Of the participants, only 2 (2.0%) were seropositive for HbsAg. The two, both females aged between 21 - 40 years, comprised a student and a civil servant. The surgical procedure performed on them was evisceration; in one and cataract extraction in the other.

Table 1. Demographic characteristics of participants.

Age range (years)	Sex		Total (%) n = 100
	Male	Female	
1 - 10	1	1	2 (2.0)
11 - 20	0	1	1 (1.0)
21 - 30	4	2	6 (6.0)
31 - 40	5	4	9 (9.0)
41 - 50	5	21	26 (26.0)
51 - 60	10	15	25 (25.0)
61 - 70	12	12	24 (24.0)
71 - 80	3	3	6 (6.0)
81 - 90	0	1	1 (1.0)
Total	40	60	100 (100.0)

Table 2. Occupational distribution of participants.

Occupation	Number (%) n = 100
Farmers	45 (45.0)
Traders	23 (23.0)
Civil servants	11 (11.0)
Artisan	10 (10.0)
Pensioners	6 (6.0)
Students	5 (5.0)
Total	100 (100)

Table 3. Distribution of surgical procedures performed on the patients.

Surgical procedure	Number (%) n = 100
Cataract surgery	58 (58.0)
Trabeculectomy	16 (16.0)
Evisceration	10 (10.0)
Pterygium excision	7 (7.0)
Combined cataract and trabeculectomy surgery	4 (4.0)
Incision and curettage of chalazia	2 (2.0)
Canthoplasty	1 (1.0)
Corneal repair	1 (1.0)
Conjuctival cyst excision	1 (1.0)
Total	100 (100)

HBV seropositivity did not show any significant association with participant's gender (Fisher's exact test, p = 0.5152), age (student-t test; mean age of HBV positives vs mean age of HBV negatives; 53.4 ± 15.2SD vs 30.0 ± 4.2SD; p = 0.207; CI, $-44.89 - -1.95$) or occupation (p = 0.928).

4. Discussion

During the period under review more females than males who were frequently aged 40 years or older accessed ophthalmic surgical care at the study center. This differs from other similar studies [17] [18] which reported variable degrees of male gender preponderance. The observed gender distribution could be attributed to reported higher prevalence of surgical eye diseases in females [19]. Additionally, this may be partly accounted for by the positive impact of the sustained public health education aimed at eliminating gender bias in the uptake of health care services particularly, in rural areas [20]. Efforts to sustain the campaign for gender equity in access to health services through public health education, pro-female gender economic empowerment and cross-gender affordability of health services are highly indicated.

The observed age characteristic consistent with the findings in related studies [16] [20]-[22] is attributable to the dominance of cataract often an age-related surgical eye disease, among the participants in the present and previous surveys [17] [21]-[23]. The present age data underscores the need for eye-care planners, implementers and eye health policy makers to deploy the necessary resources and logistics for cataract surgical care in the elderly especially in rural areas.

Although the observed 2.0% seroprevalence of HBV infection in this study is low, it is comparable to the 1.7% reported by Alhassan *et al.* [17] in an urban Nigerian survey. The present finding suggests that rural versus urban location probably does not influence HBV sero-prevalence burden. The observed low prevalence however does not downgrade the risk of peri-operative cross-infection to health workers. While standard universal measures for prevention of cross infection from patient to eye care personnel should be observed in all patients irrespective of serology status, pre-operative testing will help the health care personnel to exercise extra caution such as handling of surgical instruments and also enable the patient to seek early medical treatment. A uniform cross socio-economic cadre approach to advocacy for prevention of HBV infection is recommended. Towards this end, health education, immunization of the general public especially at-risk health workers and provision of affordable medical treatment are therefore instructive. The average monthly cost for the various drug treatment regimen of chronic Hepatitis B infection varies from 422 USD to 2940 USD [24]. This is obviously beyond the economic reach of those requiring treatment in this rural populace where majority are peasant farmers.

One hundred percent of those with HBV infection in our cohort are females. This differed from the male gender preponderance of 59.18% reported by Naeem *et al*. [18] Possible cross infection with contaminated instruments used during the widely practiced female genital mutilation in Ebonyi state [25] may account for the observed female dominance. To this end, dangerous social practice tailored intervention targeting the female gender through aggressive public health education and legislation are warranted.

The extrapolation of the conclusions drawn from this study is limited by its one-center design, relatively low study participants, rural setting and reliability of the sensitivity of the test kit used for the study. A multi-center, larger participant survey preferable involving diverse hospitals and care settings is suggested.

5. Conclusion

There is a low sero-prevalence of HBV among ophthalmic surgical patients at PJH Uburu, Ebonyi state, Nigeria. HBV seropositivity was not associated with gender, age or occupation. Standard preventive measures during outpatient and perioperative ophthalmic care to prevent cross infection from patient to eye care personnel, immunisation of surgical eye care providers and mandatory pre-operative HBV screening are hereby advocated.

Conflict of Interest

None declared.

External Source of Funding

The authors declare no external source of funds for this work.

References

[1]   Barker, L.F., Shulman, N.R., Murray, R., *et al*. (1970) Transmission of Serum Hepatitis. *Journal of the American Medical Associations*, **276**, 841-844. http://dx.doi.org/10.1001/jama.1996.03540100085042

[2]   Williams, R. (2006) Global Challenges of Liver Disease. *Hepatology*, **44**, 521-526. http://dx.doi.org/10.1002/hep.21347

[3]   Hepatitis, B. World Health Organization (WHO). http://www.who.int/mediacentre/factsheets/fs204/en/

[4]   Moyer, L.A. and Mast, E.E. (1994) Hepatitis B: Virology, Epidemiology, Disease, and Prevention and an Overview of Viral Hepatitis. *American Journal of Preventive Medicine*, **10**, 45-55.

[5]   Maddrey, W.C. (2000) Hepatitis B: An Important Public Health Issue. *Journal of Medical Virology*, **61**, 362-366. http://dx.doi.org/10.1002/1096-9071(200007)61:3<362::AID-JMV14>3.0.CO;2-I

[6]   Coopstead, L.C. (2010) Pathophysiology. Saunders Press, Missouri, 886-887.

[7]   Sleisenger, M.H., Feldman, M. and Friedman, L.S. (2006) Fordtran's Gastrointestinal and Liver Disease: Pathophysiology, Diagnosis, Management. Saunders Press, Philadelphia.

[8]   Kidd-Ljunggren, K., Holmberg, A., Bläckberg, J. and Lindqvist, B. (2006) High Levels of Hepatitis B Virus DNA in Body Fluids from Chronic Carriers. *Journal of Hospital Infection*, **64**, 352-357. http://dx.doi.org/10.1016/j.jhin.2006.06.029

[9]   Hepatitis B FAQs for the Public-Transmission. United State Centers for Disease Control and Prevention (CDC). http://www.cdc.gov/hepatitis/b/bfaq.htm#transmit

[10]   Emechebe, G.O., Emodi, I.J., Ikemefuna, A.N., Ilechukwu, G.C., Igwe, W.C., Ejiofor, O.S., *et al*. (2009) Hepatitis B Virus Infection in Nigeria—A Review. *Nigerian Medical Journal*, **50**, 18-22.

[11]   Odusanya, O.O., Alufohai, F.E., Meurice, F.P., Wellens, R., Weil, J. and Ahonkhai, V.I. (2005) Prevalence of Hepatitis B Surface Antigen in Vaccinated Children and Controls in Rural Nigeria. *International Journal Infectious Disease*, **9**, 139-143. http://dx.doi.org/10.1016/j.ijid.2004.06.009

[12] Alikor, E.A. and Erhabor, O.N. (2007) Seroprevalence of Hepatitis B Surface Antigenaemia in Children in a Tertiary Health Institution in the Niger Delta of Nigeria. *Nigerian Journal of Medicine*, **16**, 250-251.

[13] Tswana, S., Chetsanga, C., Nystrom, L., Moyo, S., Nzara, M. and Chieza, L. (1996) A Sero-Epidemiological Cross-Sectional Study of Hepatitis B Virus in Zimbabwe. *South African Medical Journal*, **86**, 72-75.

[14] Ugwuja, E.I. (2010) Seroprevalence of Hepatitis B Surface Antigen and Liver Function Tests among Adolescents in Abakaliki, South-Eastern Nigeria. *Internet Journal of Tropical Medicine*, **6**, 1-6.

[15] Shahnaz, S., Reza, B. and Seyed-Moayed, A. (2005) Risk Factors for Chronic Hepatitis B Infection: A Case Controlled Study. *Hepatitis Monthly*, **5**, 109-115.

[16] Seyed-Moayed, A. (2006) Immunization, an Important Strategy to Control Hepatitis. *Hepatitis Monthly*, **6**, 3-5.

[17] Alhasan, M.B., Unung, P. and Adejor, G.O. (2013) HIV and HBsAg Seropositivity amongst Patients Presenting for Ocular Surgery at a Tertiary Eye Care Hospital in Nigeria. *Open Journal of ophthalmology*, **22**, 18-19. http://dx.doi.org/10.2174/1874364101307010018

[18] Naeem, S.S., Siddiqui, E.U., Kazi, A.N., Khan, S.T., Abdullah, F.E. and Adhi, I. (2012) Prevalence of Hepatitis B and Hepatitis C among Preoperative Cataract Patients in Karachi. *BMC Research Notes*, **5**, 492. http://dx.doi.org/10.1186/1756-0500-5-492

[19] Lewallen, S. and Courtright, P. (2002) Gender and Use of Cataract Surgical Services in Developing Countries. *Bulletin of World Health Organization*, **80**, 300-303.

[20] AMURT Starts Work in Nigeria. www.africa.amurt.net/nigeria

[21] Okoye, O., Magulike, N. and Chuka-Okosa, C. (2012) Prevalence of Human Immunodeficiency Virus Seropositivity among Eye Surgical Patients at a Rural Eye Care Facility in South-Eastern Nigeria. *Middle East African Journal of Ophthalmology*, **19**, 93-96. http://dx.doi.org/10.4103/0974-9233.92122

[22] Ezegwui, I.R., Akariwe, N.N. and Onwasigwe, E.N. (2012) HIV Seroprevalence in Ophthalmic Surgery Patients at ESUT Teaching Hospital Enugu. *Nigerian Journal of Medicine*, **21**, 194-195.

[23] Eze, B.I. (2013) Audit of Ophthalmic Surgical Interventions in a Resource-Deficient Tertiary Eye Care Facility in Sub-Saharan Africa. *Journal of Health Care for the Poor and Underserved*, **24**, 197-205. http://dx.doi.org/10.1353/hpu.2013.0013

[24] Approved HBV Antiviral and Interferon Therapy Cost Comparison 2011. Hepatitis B Foundation. www.hepb.org/2011_drug_comparison

[25] Ibekwe, P.C., Onoh, R.C., Onyebuchi, A.K., Ezeonu, P.O. and Ibekwe, R.O. (2012) Female Genital Mutilation in Southeast Nigeria: A Survey on the Current Knowledge and Practice. *Journal of Public Health and Epidemiology*, **4**, 117-122.

37

Ocular Graft versus Host Disease: A Review of Clinical Manifestations, Diagnostic Approaches and Treatment

Sridevi Nair, Murugesan Vanathi*, Anita Ganger, Radhika Tandon

Cornea & Ocular Surface Services, Dr Rajendra Prasad Centre for Ophthalmic Sciences, All India Institute of Medical Sciences, New Delhi, India
Email: *vanathi_g@yahoo.com

Abstract

Allogenic haematological stem cell transplantation (allo-SCT) from a human leukocyte antigen (HLA) matched related or unrelated donor is used as a curative therapy for a large number of malignant and non-malignant haematological diseases. The curative effect of allo-SCT is achieved by graft versus leukaemia effect while the downside of the graft versus patient activity is the graft-versus-host-disease (GVHD), a major reason for mortality and morbidity. The search of articles for this review had been accomplished using Ovid, Medline, Embase, Pubmed and was supplemented by retrieving cross references also. Electronic literature search for English language articles with full text access was performed using graft versus host disease, ocular, management, dry eyes as key words. This review has been intended to explicate the classification, pathogenesis, risk factors and management of ocular graft versus host disease.

Keywords

Stem Cell Transplantation, Ocular, Graft Host Disease

1. Introduction

GVHD is a disease related to allogenic haematological stem cell transplantation. This disease is due to T cell response of donor cells to the proteins of recipient host cells which are genetically defined. These proteins are usually consisting of highly polymorphic HLA which are encoded by the major histocompatibility complex (MHC). HLA class I antigens which includes A, B, C are proteins expressed on nearly all the nucleated cells of

---

*Corresponding author.

the body. Whereas primary expression of class II proteins which includes DR, DQ, DP is mainly on hematopoietic cells like dendritic cells, B cells and monocytes except in the conditions of any inflammation and trauma [1] [2]. Even after giving thorough consideration to HLA matching acute GVHD can develop in significant number of patients due to minor histocompatibility antigen (genetic difference which lie outside the HLA loci) [3] [4]. The search of articles for this review had been accomplished using Ovid, Medline, Embase, Pubmed and was supplemented by retrieving cross references also. Electronic literature search for English language articles with full text access was performed using graft versus host disease, ocular, management, dry eyes as key words. This review has been intended to explicate the classification, pathogenesis, risk factors and management of ocular graft versus host disease.

2. Classification of Systemic GVHD

Currently, the classification of acute or chronic GVHD is based on clinical symptoms, unlike earlier time in which time interval was the deciding factor. In earlier times graft-versus-host-disease (GVHD) was divided on the basis of duration after the transplantation. For example GVHD occurring before and at 100 day after the transplantation was referred as acute GVHD (aGVHD), whereas GVHD occurring more than 100 days was termed as chronic GVHD (cGVHD) [5] [6]. Later the two new terms/categories named persistent/recurrent/late-onset were added for cases of aGVHD persisted for >3 months and overlap syndrome in which features of chronic and acute GVHD appear together without any consideration to time limit. Various categories are shown in **Table 1** [7].

3. Systemic GVHD Clinical Features

The incidence of acute and chronic GVHD is reported to be around 40% and 30% - 70% respectively among the HLA-matched patients [8] [9]. According to a study by Vanathi *et al.* on Indian population the prevalence of chronic systemic GVHD was found to be 33% in post allo-SCT patients [10]. The classical aGVHD presentation includes involvement of mainly three organ systems: skin, gastrointestinal tract and liver. Patients can present with rashes/blisters over skin along with nausea, vomiting, diarrhoea, abdominal bloating, blood in stool and loss of appetite in acute stage. Liver involvement is not uncommon, it manifests as jaundice and dark colour urine in acute stage. Whereas in cGVHD additional organs for example-joints, eyes, lungs and genitals also get involved.

3.1. Pathogenesis of Acute GVHD Proceed in 3 Steps

Step 1: Includes activation of antigen-presenting cells (APCs) due to the damage resulted from the allo-SCT conditioning regimen.

Step 2: Includes activation, proliferation, differentiation and migration of donor T cells due to the host histoincompatible antigens presented by the APCs.

Step 3: Includes local tissue injury, inflammation and target tissue destruction due to the cascade of both cellular mediators such as cytotoxic T lymphocytes and natural killer cells [11].

The chronic GVHD is of autoimmune nature which involves the skin, mouth, GI tract, genitalia, eyes, musculoskeletal system and fibrotic as well as stenotic changes [12]. cGVHD usually starts after aGVHD, though it can start *de novo* with either involvement of one single organ or widespread in several organs. The most commonly documented sites of involvement in systemic GVHD are skin (75%), mouth (51% - 63%) and liver (29% - 51%) along with associated ocular involvement in 40% - 60% of the patients [1].

Table 1. Classification of systemic GVHD.

Category	Time interval between SCT & onset of GVHD	Presence of acute GVHD features	Presence of chronic GVHD features
Acute GVHD			
• Classic	<100 days	Yes	No
• Late-onset	>100 days	Yes	No
Chronic GVHD			
• Classic	No time limit	No	Yes
• Overlap syndrome	No time limit	Yes	Yes

3.2. Pathogenesis of Chronic GVHD

In pathogenesis of cGVHD T cells have been reported to have role whereas detection of auto antibodies support the role of B cells. As cGVHD is of autoimmune nature, it resembles autoimmune diseases like systemic sclerosis [12].

4. Risk Factors for the Development of Systemic GVHD

The risk factors for the development of acute GVHD as documented in past literature are [13]-[20]:
- Disparity in HLA;
- The use of high doses of total body irradiation under conditioning regimens;
- If female is donor for male recipient and female donor is having history of prior pregnancies or transfusions
- Lack of prophylaxis for acute GVHD;
- The recipient's older age;
- The peripheral blood stem cells in unrelated donor transplantation have been found associated with both acute and chronic GVHD;
- Lower incidence of aGVHD is reported in Tacrolimus-based prophylaxis as compared to cyclosporine-based prophylaxis;
- ABO incompatibility, prior herpes virus exposure, racial predilection and antibiotic gut decontamination are among the other risk factors.
  The risk factors for development of cGVHD as documented in past literature are [21]:
- History of prior aGVHD;
- Donor's or recipient's older age;
- In transplants where chronic myeloid leukaemia or aplastic anaemia was the primary diagnosis;
- If female is a donor for male recipient;
- Incomplete HLA matching for related donors and selection of unrelated donors;
- If peripheral blood is accepted as a stem cells source;
- Lack of T-cell depletion.

5. Diagnostic Criteria for Chronic GVHD

According to National Institutes of Health (NIH) working group consensus document, the diagnosis of cGVHD requires distinction from acute GVHD as well as other possible diagnosis. The criterion for diagnosis is either at least one diagnostic clinical sign of cGVHD seen or at least one distinctive manifestation noted which is confirmed by pertinent biopsy/other relevant tests. The diagnosis of cGVHD needs the occurrence of at least one of the diagnostic features in the skin (poikiloderma, lichenoid changes and scleroderma), in gastrointestinal tract (stenosis in the upper or mid-third of the oesophagus or the presence of oesophageal web or strictures), in mouth (restricted mouth opening due to sclerosis , hyperkeratotic patches and lichen-type features), in genitalia (vaginal scarring or stenosis), bronchiolitis obliterans, and in musculoskeletal system manifestations like fasciitis, joint stiffness, or contractures secondary to sclerosis [7].

According to NIH consensus though dry eye is a characteristic sign reported in cGVHD, however it itself is not sufficient to make a diagnosis of cGVHD [22].

6. Ocular GVHD

After allo-SCT, ocular GVHD (oGVHD) develops in 40% - 60% of patients and in already diagnosed GVHD patients, oGVHD develop in 60% - 90% which results in exceedingly severe ocular surface disease [23]-[25]. oGVHD is considered as a poor prognostic sign and develops in about 10% of aGVHD patients [26] [27]. According to study done by Vanathi et al. oGVHD was documented in 30% of post allo-HSCT patients in the Indian population [28].

The keratoconjunctivitis sicca (KCS) is reported to be the most frequent manifestation of chronic oGVHD (40% - 76% of patients) [29] [30]. In previous literature the patients with skin or mouth involvement are documented to be more prone for the development of oGVHD [31]. oGVHD can occur as an early manifestation of systemic GVHD [32]. KCS can also be initiated by total body irradiation and can also occur due to the immune suppression treatment as it can lead to lacrimal deficiency.

6.1. Pathophysiology of Ocular GVHD

The acute oGVHD is essentially a T-cell-mediated process [27]. Whereas chronic oGVHD is characterized by excessive fibrotic changes and destruction of tubule alveolar glands which ultimately cause damage to ocular surface and result in dry eye [33]. In chronic usually there is increase in number of stromal CD34 β fibroblasts as well as infiltration of T cell in periductal areas [27]. High-risk factors for oGVHD:

- In patients with skin or mouth involvement [31].
- Allo-SCT from unmatched related donors [29].

6.2. Diagnosis of Ocular GVHD

1) As per NIH consensus, for diagnosing oGVHD [7] the criteria includes either documentation of new ocular sicca with a low mean value of ≤5 mm at 5 minutes in both eyes with Schirmer's test or documentation of newly onset Keratoconjunctivitis sicca on slit-lamp examination with Schirmer's test mean values of 6 - 10 mm. If above mentioned two criteria are seen along with the presence of distinctive manifestations in at least one other organ, diagnosis of chronic GVHD is confirmed [7].

However Schirmer's score is not sufficient criterion for the diagnosis of chronic oGVHD, as high false positives and negatives are reported if diagnosis is based on Schirmer's test alone [34]. Other factors like patient's symptoms, ocular surface staining and tear film dynamics are also important while evaluating such patients of oGVHD [22].

2) The new diagnostic metrics for chronic oGVHD is defined by the International chronic oGVHD consensus group. As per the consensus group the measurement of following four subjective and objective variables is must in patients of post allogenic hematopoietic stem cell transplantation (HSCT) [22].

- Ocular Surface Disease Index (OSDI);
- Schirmer's score without putting anaesthetic drops;
- Staining of corneal surface (CFS);
- Conjunctival injection.

The variable of conjunctival staining was not taken as parameter due to its high variability in its values. Each variable was scored 0 - 2 or 0 - 3, with a maximum composite score of 11.

The corneal fluorescein staining scores are marked from 0 to 3 points

- Grade 0 = If no staining noted;
- Grade 1 = If minimal staining noted;
- Grade 2 = If mild/moderate staining noted;
- Grade 3 = if severe staining noted.

The slit lamp pictures of corneal fluorescein staining used for grading are shown in **Figure 1**.

The conjunctival hyperaemia score noted in conjunctiva varied from 0 to 2 points

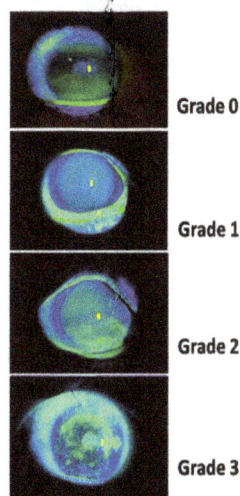

Figure 1. Depicting the corneal fluorescein staining grades.

- Grade 0 = None;
- Grade 1 = Mild/moderate;
- Grade 2 = Severe.

The slit lamp pictures of conjunctival injection used for grading are shown in **Figure 2**.

A score above 1 point is regarded as abnormal. On the basis of their combined score and after consideration of presence or absence of systemic GVHD, patients are divided in to three diagnostic categories: No, Probable and Definite ocular GVHD.

Based on accumulative scores for each parameter disease severity is assessed by grading patients as none, mild/moderate and severe (**Table 2**). Based on the total scores assessed and the assessment of presence or absence of systemic GVHD, the diagnosis of oGVHD is made (**Table 3**).

Severity classification

Total score points are the sum of Schirmer's test score, CFS score, OSDI Score and Conjunctival injection score.

- None = 0 - 4;
- Mild/Moderate = 5 - 8;
- Severe = 9 – 11.

3) Grading Scales for Ocular GVHD

A) NIH consensus criteria

In the NIH consensus, the criteria for diagnosing oGVHD is as mentioned in section 6.2.1.

The NIH eye score has a range of 0 - 3 as shown in **Table 4**.

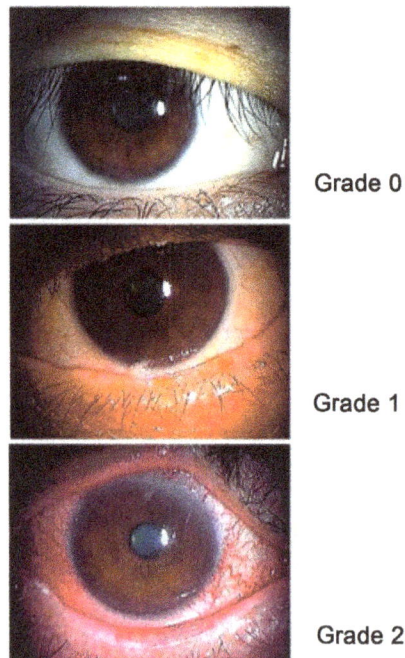

Figure 2. Conjunctival hyperaemia grading.

Table 2. Severity scale used in grading of chronic ocular GVHD.

Severity score	Schirmer's test (mm)	Corneal Fluorescein Staining (points)	Ocular Surface Disease Index (points)	Conjunctival injection (points)
0	>15	0	<13	None
1	11 - 15	<2	13 - 22	Mild/Moderate
2	6 - 10	2 - 3	23 - 32	Severe
3	≤5	≥4	≥33	Severe

Table 3. Diagnosis of chronic ocular GVHD.

Classification	Systemic GVHD (absent)	Systemic GVHD (present)
None (points)	0 - 5	0 - 3
Probable GVHD (points)	6 - 7	4 - 5
Definite GVHD (points)	≥8	≥6

Table 4. NIH consensus criteria: Ocular GVHD staging.

Eyes: Mean tear test (mm)	Score	Definition
>10	0	No symptoms
6 - 10	1	Mild dry eye symptoms without any effect on daily activities, but person needs eye drops >3 times per day or may be signs of KCS can be seen without symptoms.
<5	2	Moderate dry eye symptoms which partially affects daily activities and topical drops are required >3 times a day with or without the need of punctual plugs. In this grade vision does not get affected.
Test not done	3	Severe dry eye symptoms resulting in inability to do person's daily activities and causing significant disability for work due to severe uncomfortable or impaired vision due to KCS

B) Japanese dry eye score

The Japanese dry eye criteria [35] for diagnosis is as follows:

1) Presence of symptoms related to dry eye

2) Abnormality of the tear film to be seen by doing Schirmer's and TBUT test

a) If Schirmer's1 test values ≤5 mm

b) If Tear film breakup time values ≤5 seconds

3) The damage to the conjunctivocorneal epithelial surface to be noted as follows:

c) With Fluorescein staining, score of ≥3 points

d) With Rose Bengal staining score of ≥3 points

e) With Lissamine Green staining score of ≥3 points

The positive result in at least one of the above tests indicates the conjunctivocorneal epithelial surface damage.

Definite dry eye: Diagnosis of definite dry eye is considered if all three above written criteria are fulfilled.

Probable dry eye: Diagnosis of probable dry eye is considered if either one or two out of 3 above mentioned criteria are fulfilled.

Normal eye: If none of the above written criteria is getting fulfilled.

With this Japanese dry eye scoring system the severity of the dry eye is scored with a range of 0 - 2.

- Score of 0 = No dry eye if no manifestations/symptoms seen;
- Score of 1 = Mild dry eye if symptoms present along with Schirmer's test ≤ 5 mm but fluorescein and rose bengal score are <3 points;
- Score of 2 = Severe dry eye is diagnosed if symptoms, Schirmer's test ≤ 5 mm are there along with fluorescein and rose bengal scores are ≥ 3 points.

C) DEWS 2007 score

In DEWS 2007 classification scores of 0 - 4 are given which are determined by evaluating 9 parameters including symptoms of dry eyes, scoring on Schirmer's test, tear film breakup time, and other abnormalities noted in the conjunctiva, cornea, tear, lid, and meibomian glands [36].

0 = No dry eye,

1 = Mild dry eye,

2 = Moderate dry eye,

3 = Severe dry eye,

4 = Very severe dry.

6.3. Clinical Features of oGVHD

The oGVHD disease includes wide range of clinical manifestations which affects almost all layers of the eye like the lids, lacrimal glands, conjunctiva, cornea, the vitreous and the choroids. The involvement of the posterior segment is less likely [37] [38].

6.3.1. The Ocular Surface Manifestations in oGVHD

The outcome of both direct or an indirect conjunctival goblet cell involvement, of lacrimal gland stasis caused by immunosuppression or total body irradiation can give rise to the ocular surface and corneal complications of GVHD [38]. The corneal and conjunctival findings include epithelial thinning, keratinization and squamous metaplasia [39].

Patients of aGVHD can present with both corneal and conjunctival findings and the severity of their ocular signs generally correlates with the severity of systemic disease.

In aGVHD pseudo membranous conjunctivitis has been documented in 12% - 17% of patients and it is marker of systemic involvement associated with a poor prognosis [40]. The pseudo membranous conjunctivitis can arise after conjunctival hyperaemia associated with epithelial sloughing which subsequently leads to scarring. In severe cases corneal epithelial sloughing presents along with the pseudo membranous changes which occurs in up to one third of patients [40]. Documentation of strong correlation of Dry-eye syndrome or kerato conjunctivitis sicca (KCS) with aGHVD is there in literature [25].

Chronic GVHD manifestations include new onset of dry, gritty, or painful eyes, excessive tearing, burning sensation, light sensitivity, blurring of vision, cicatricial conjunctivitis, kerato conjunctivitis sicca, and confluent areas of punctate keratopathy [41].

6.3.2. Dry Eye

In literature dry eye syndrome (DES) is reported as the most frequent complication and documented to be found in 40% to 76% of GVHD patients. The main cause of DES in cGVHD is fibrosis of the acini and ductules proceeded by lymphocytic infiltration of the accessory and major lacrimal glands [29] [30]. However other contributing factors include irradiation, chemotherapy, immunosuppressive therapy, infection and meibomian gland dysfunction [29].

Though the median time of development of dry eyes is around six months, but it can develop any time between few weeks up to 100 months after transplantation. Most of the patients start experiencing dry eye or foreign body sensation with associated ocular fatigue and discharge which later on progress further to severe dry eye like Sjogren's syndrome. Burning, stinging, itching, soreness and heaviness sensations in eyelids, and photophobia are among the other symptoms [38].

6.3.3. Conjunctiva

Conjunctival involvement is found to be rare in aGVHD, though if present, it is a poor prognostic factor and marker for severe systemic involvement. The manifestations of conjunctival involvement vary from mild erythema to pseudo membranous and cicatrizing conjunctivitis similar to Ocular cicatricial pemphigoid.

In aGVHD ulcerative and haemorrhagic conjunctivitis are the more common manifestations, which subsequently progress to scarring and symblepharon formation. These cicatricial changes progress further during chronic phase of GVHD [39] [40].

Conjunctival Grading in Acute and Chronic GVHD

A) Classification of Conjunctivitis in Acute GVHD [40]

Grade 0—None.

Grade 1—Hyperaemia.

Grade 2—Hyperaemia associated with serosanguinous discharge.

Grade 3—Pseudo membranous conjunctivitis.

Grade 4—Pseudo membranous conjunctivitis with associated corneal epithelial sloughing.

B) Classification of Conjunctivitis in Chronic GVHD [42]

Grade 0—None.

Grade 1—Hyperaemia.

Grade 2—If fibro vascular changes in palpebral conjunctiva seen with or without epithelial sloughing.

Grade 3—If fibro vascular changes in palpebral conjunctiva involve 25% - 75% of total surface area.

Grade 4—If more than 75% of total surface area involved with or without cicatricial entropion.

6.3.4. Corneal Involvement

Corneal involvement is more commonly seen in cGVHD than in aGVHD. In aGVHD features like filamentary keratitis and corneal epithelial keratitis are common. Chronic GVHD mostly shows features of keratoconjunctivitis sicca. Severe dry eyes may present which in turn can cause filamentary keratitis, corneal ulceration, corneal neovascularization, and ultimately corneal perforation if not treated [43] [44].

6.3.5. Lacrimal Gland Involvement

Lacrimal gland dysfunction is found to be the most common ocular manifestation of ocular GVHD in past literature. In cGVHD disease there is documented tear dysfunction due to infiltration of mononuclear cell into major as well as accessory lacrimal of Kraus and Wolfring [30].

6.3.6. Cataract

Even though cataract formation is the most common cause of visual acuity loss in these patients, its incidence increase further because of side effects of corticosteroid or total body irradiation therapy [44].

6.3.7. Other Findings

Anterior uveitis is not very commonly seen during exacerbations of systemic GVHD. It is important to distinguish infectious aetiology or neoplastic masquerade syndrome from non-infectious uveitis [45] [46].

Posterior segment complications are seen in around 12% of patients. The common vitreoretinal complications seen in GVHD are retinal microvasculopathy including features like intraretinal or vitreous haemorrhage and cotton wool spots [47].

Central serous chorioretinopathy (CSCR) is not commonly seen in HSCT patients. GVHD itself has been reported to affect the choroidal vasculature leading to choroidal hyper permeability and the development of CSCR.

Association of acute ocular GVHD with posterior scleritis has also been documented in past [48]-[50]. Posterior segment infections such as infectious retinitis due to cytomegalovirus (CMV), herpes simplex virus and varicella zoster virus had also been reported as complications in literature [38]. The manifestation of disc oedema although irreversible is reported to be due to the toxic effects of treating drugs like chemotherapeutic agents for example cyclosporine A and due to coexisting medical conditions [47].

6.4. Patient Workup

The following parameters should be checked while doing work up of patients suspected of having chronic ocular GVHD [20].

- Vision assessment.
- Slit lamp examination for tear-film break-up time and Schirmer's test.
- Intraocular pressure measurement (IOP).
- Staining the conjunctival surface with lissamine green and cornea with fluorescein dye and then grading of corneal fluorescein staining by using either the National Eye Institute scale or the modified Oxford grading scale.
- Perform conjunctival or corneal swabs or scrapes for microbiological evaluation in cases of questionable aetiology.
- Tear film osmolarity and confocal microscopy to help in deciding the treatment modality and follow-up assessment.
- A dilated fundus examination to rule out posterior segment manifestations of chronic GVHD or cytomegalovirus.
- Slit lamp examination of Lens, IOP measurement and visual field examination is required to assess any posterior capsular cataract or glaucoma development due to prolonged steroid use or radiation.
- Symptoms evaluation can be performed by using the Ocular Surface Disease Index (OSDI).
- Video keratoscope can be used to see difference of higher aberrations of indices in patients with chronic ocular GVHD as compared to normal counterparts.

6.5. GVHD Management Strategies

1) Systemic GVHD prevention and prophylaxis

To prevent GVHD following strategies should be followed:

- Optimal HLA-matching is must for the prevention of GVHD both MHC class I and II loci between donor and recipient should be matched.
- The use of Calcineurin inhibitors like cyclosporine and tacrolimus have been reported for the prophylaxis of GVHD. Tacrolimus along with the low doses of methotrexate use is documented for the prophylaxis of acute GVHD. Tacrolimus when used was found to have a lower rate of aGVHD occurrence as compared to cyclosporine [18].

6.5.1. Acute GVHD Treatment

Systemic immune suppression is the most important aspect while managing GVHD. Steroid therapy, although considered the gold standard for treatment of GVHD due to its antilymphocytic and anti-inflammatory properties, can help in complete remission in less than 50% of patients only and the severe cases more likely don't respond to steroid therapy alone. Such cases may require a more effective prophylaxis and treatment [51]. 5-year survival rates are also low in the steroid-resistant cases, implying a poorer prognosis. Although MMF, ATG, TNF inhibitors, and other agents are commonly used as second line agent, there is no data to support their use as the same [20].

6.5.2. Chronic GVHD Treatment

Corticosteroids are the mainstay of therapy for chronic GVHD. Even though they are not totally satisfactory, no other agent has been demonstrated to be better than steroids in the treatment of chronic GVHD in a randomized trial [52].

The newer treatment modalities which are under trial include:

- Regulatory T cells modulation using ultra-low dose IL-2 [53].
- ECP (Extracorporeal photopheresis) has been shown to be effective in acute steroid refractory GVHD with better long term survival [54].
- Imatinib meslylate has shown promising results as an adjunctive therapy in sclera dermatous chronic GVHD [55].

The most essential step of GVHD management is to avoid infections by giving supportive care in the form of either prevention, prophylaxis and giving treatment. After transplantation during the first year prescription of Acyclovir for viral prophylaxis and trimethoprim sulfamethoxazole or atovaquone for pneumocystis prophylaxis are advised and can be given later on also, if systemic immune suppression is indicated for chronic GVHD [20].

6.5.3. Ocular GVHD Treatment

The systemic treatments for GVHD help in oGVHD too, but the severity of systemic disease cannot be directly correlated with the ocular manifestations. Therefore increasing the systemic immunosuppression is not the best approach to treat oGVHD. An organ specific approach is more desirable [20].

The treatment modalities in oGVHD target the following: [56]

- Ocular surface lubrication and support for the tear film;
- Control of inflammation;
- Epithelial and mucosal support;
- Prevention of tear evaporation.

1) Ocular Surface Lubrication and Support for the Tear Film

Frequent topical lubrication with artificial non-preserved free tears is usually the mainstay of treatment in ocular GVHD with severe aqueous deficiency dry eye [1]. Lubricating medications assist in the dilution of the inflammatory mediators present at the ocular surface.

- Acetylcysteine (5% - 10%) eye drops can be useful in patients presenting with ocular surface adherent filament [20].
- To preserve tears punctal occlusion can be done either with thermal cauterization or with silicone punctual plugs. These when used with autologous serum were found to increase the retention of the same [57].

Although they haven't been specially studied in GVHD patients systemic selective muscarinic agonists such as cevimeline or pilocarpine may be used to increase aqueous tear flow [58].

2) To Control Inflammation

• Topical steroids

Topical steroids have been shown to be beneficial in aGVHD due to its immunosuppressive action by Kim *et al.* [59]. Topical steroids have also been shown to be beneficial in cGVHD patients with cicatricial changes without having corneal epithelial defects, infiltrate and stromal thinning [42].

• Topical cyclosporine

Topical cyclosporine (CsA) eye drops are useful in patients with chronic ocular GVHD and KCS where other treatment modalities are not successful. Mechanism of action of CsA is to inhibit release of lymphokines from their activated T cells present in the conjunctiva by inhibiting proliferation and production of lymphokines itself. It also increases the conjunctival goblet cell density and decreases the epithelial cell turnover. Topical cyclosporine role in improving corneal fluorescein staining, by improving basal tear secretion in ocular GVHD patients is well documented [60]-[62].

• Tacrolimus (FK506)

Tacrolimus (FK506) is a macrolide antibiotic which is similar to CsA in terms of mechanism of action and its pharmacokinetics. Although Systemic tacrolimus has been shown to have a beneficial effect in some cases of ocular GVHD, not enough data is available for the use of topical tacrolimus in these patients. Tam et al have reported successful treatment of a case of oGVHD using topical tacrolimus [63].

• Topical Tranilast

Topical tranilast is an anti allergic medication which acts by inhibition of production and release of various ocular inflammatory mediators as well as cytokines. It interferes with migration and the proliferation of vascular medial smooth muscle cells along with inhibition of collagen synthesis and TGF-b induced matrix production. A small group of GVHD patients on treatment with topical tranilast were reported to have shown improvement in reflex tearing and Rose Bengal scores [64].

3) For Epithelial Support

• Autologous serum eye drops

In literature autologous serum had been documented to be not only safe but effective modality for the treatment of severe dry eye associated with chronic GVHD. Various factors for example epithelia trophic growth factors, nerve growth factors, cytokines and vitamins present in autologous serum helps in proliferation, differentiation, maturation as well as in maintaining integrity of the both corneal and conjunctival epithelial surfaces [57].

• Contact lenses

Contact lenses can be used in moderate to severe dry by stabilising the tear film and also improve the epithelial cells turn over. Significant improvement in dry eye manifestations in terms of both symptoms and visual acuity has been documented in patients with dry eye due to GVHD with the use of silicon hydrogel contact lenses by Russo *et al.* [65]. Scleral lenses help in relieving the symptoms in dry eye patients by creating a tear filled vault over the cornea [66].

• Surgical interventions like limbal stem cell transplantation, amniotic membrane transplantation and penetrating keratoplasty had also been documented as an option to treat severe dry eye. However one should keep in mind the poor prognosis associated with the allografts in these patients is due to poor ocular surface and tear deficiency [67].

4) For the Prevention of Tear Evaporation

The evaporation of tears may be prevented by maximising the Meibomian gland output by using measures like warm compresses, lid hygiene, topical erythromycin and oral doxycycline therapy. Doxycycline has both antibiotic and anti-inflammatory properties. The latter is due to the inhibition of matrix metalloproteinase and IL-1 activity [68] [69].

Other treatment modalities that could be used include nutritional supplements such as flax seed oil and fish oil (omega-3 fatty acids), moist chamber glasses and retinoic acid [70].

5) Use of Systemic Immunosuppression for Ocular GVHD

To avoid unwanted systemic side effects systemic immunosuppression is not suggested in patients with ocular GVHD alone. It is advised in chronic ocular GVHD patients only if, not getting benefit from topical treatment. In terms of ocular surface improvement extracorporeal photopheresis is one another option in chronic GVHD. Imatinib improved the Schirmer's scores in a small series of patients with chronic GVHD and has shown promise.

7. Conclusion

To summarize, it can be said that transplantation related morbidity has been decreased due to advances in technology used for transplantation these days as well as treatment modality. Though ocular GVHD is contributed mainly by conjunctival and lacrimal gland abnormality but involvement of other ophthalmic structures is also documented especially in chronic GVHD. In chronic ocular surface disorder disease severity can vary from dry eye to severe inflammation and scarring which can lead to sight threatening sequel. In past ocular GVHD was overlooked due to deficiency of exact diagnostic criteria. However, future advances by involving biomarkers for disease identification as well as targeted individual based therapy will lead to focused management protocol and optimal visual outcomes.

References

[1]   Riemens, A., *et al.* (2010) Current Insights into Ocular Graft-versus-Host Disease. *Current Opinion in Ophthalmology*, **21**, 485-494. http://dx.doi.org/10.1097/ICU.0b013e32833eab64

[2]   Chinen, J. and Buckley, R.H. (2010) Transplantation Immunology: Solid Organ and Bone Marrow. *Journal of Allergy and Clinical Immunology*, **125**, 324-335. http://dx.doi.org/10.1016/j.jaci.2009.11.014

[3]   Bleakley, M.R. (2004) Molecules and Mechanisms of the Graft-Versus Leukaemia Effect. *Nature Reviews Cancer*, **4**, 371-380. http://dx.doi.org/10.1038/nrc1365

[4]   Goulmy, E., Schipper, R., Pool, J., Blokland, E., *et al.* (1996) Mismatches of Minor Histocompatibility Antigens between HLA Identical Donors and Recipients and the Development of Graft-Versus Host Disease after Bone Marrow Transplantation. *New England Journal of Medicine*, **334**, 281-285. http://dx.doi.org/10.1056/NEJM199602013340501

[5]   Vigorito, A.C., Campregher, P.V., Storer, B.E., *et al.* (2009) Evaluation of NIH Consensus Criteria for Classification of Late Acute and Chronic GVHD. *Blood*, **114**, 702-708. http://dx.doi.org/10.1182/blood-2009-03-208983

[6]   Shulman, H.M., Sullivan, K.M., Weiden, P.L., *et al.* (1980) Chronic Graft-versus-Hostsyndrome in Men. A Long-Term Clinic Pathologic Study of 20 Seattle Patients. *American Journal of Medicine*, **69**, 204-217. http://dx.doi.org/10.1016/0002-9343(80)90380-0

[7]   Filipovich, A.H., Weisdorf, D., Pavletic, S., *et al.* (2005) National Institutes of Health Development Project on Criteria for Clinical Trials in Chronic Graft Versus-Host Disease: I. Diagnosis and Staging Working Group Report. *Biology of Blood and Marrow Transplantation*, **11**, 945-956. http://dx.doi.org/10.1016/j.bbmt.2005.09.004

[8]   Balaram, M., Rashid, S., Dana, R., *et al.* (2005) Chronic Ocular Surface Disease after Allogeneic Bone Marrow Transplantation. *The Ocular Surface*, **3**, 203-211. http://dx.doi.org/10.1016/S1542-0124(12)70207-0

[9]   Ferrara, J.L., Levine, J.E., Reddy, P., Holler, E., *et al.* (2009) Graft-versus-Host Disease. *Lancet*, **373**, 1550-1561. http://dx.doi.org/10.1016/S0140-6736(09)60237-3

[10]   Vanathi, M., Kashyap, S., Khan, R., Seth, T., *et al.* (2014) Ocular GVHD in Allogeneic Hematopoietic Stem Cell Transplantation. *European Journal of Ophthalmology*, **24**, 656-666. http://dx.doi.org/10.5301/ejo.5000451

[11]   Goker, H., Haznedaroglu, I.C. and Chao, N.J. (2001) Acute Graft versus Host Disease—Pathobiology and Management. *Experimental Hematology*, **29**, 259-277. http://dx.doi.org/10.1016/S0301-472X(00)00677-9

[12]   Shimabukuro-Vornhagen, A., Hallek, M.J., Storb, R.F., von Bergwelt-Baildon, M.S., *et al.* (2009) The Role of B Cells in the Pathogenesis of Graft-versus-Host Disease. *Blood*, **114**, 4919-4927. http://dx.doi.org/10.1182/blood-2008-10-161638

[13]   Beatty, P.G., Clift, R.A., Mickelson, E.M., *et al.* (1985) Marrow Transplantation from Related Donor Other Than HLA-Identical Siblings. *The New England Journal of Medicine*, **313**, 765-771. http://dx.doi.org/10.1056/NEJM198509263131301

[14]   Hale, G., Slavin, S., Goldman, J.M., *et al.* (2002) Alemtuzumab (Campath-1H) for Treatment of Lymphoid Malignancies in the Age of Non Myeloablative Conditioning. *Bone Marrow Transplant*, **30**, 797-804. http://dx.doi.org/10.1038/sj.bmt.1703733

[15]   Gale, R.P., Bortin, M.M., van Bekkum, D.W., *et al.* (1987) Risk Factors for Acute Graft-versus-Host Disease. *British Journal of Haematology*, **67**, 397-406. http://dx.doi.org/10.1111/j.1365-2141.1987.tb06160.x

[16]   Eapen, M., Logan, B.R., Confer, D.L., *et al.* (2007) Peripheral Blood Grafts from Unrelated Donors Are Associated with Increased Acute and Chronic Graft-versus-Host Disease without Improved Survival. *Biology of Blood and Marrow Transplantation*, **13**, 1461-1468. http://dx.doi.org/10.1016/j.bbmt.2007.08.006

[17]   Hahn, T., McCarthy Jr., P.L., Zhang, M.J., *et al.* (2008) Risk Factors for Acute Graft-versus-Host Disease after Human

Leukocyte Antigen-Identical Sibling Transplants for Adults with Leukemia. *Journal of Clinical Oncology*, **26**, 5728-5734. http://dx.doi.org/10.1200/JCO.2008.17.6545

[18] Nash, R.A., Antin, J.H., Karanes, C., *et al.* (2000) Phase 3 Study Comparing Methotrexate and Tacrolimus with Methotrexate and Cyclosporine for Prophylaxis of Acute Graft-versus-Host Disease after Marrow Transplantation from Unrelated Donors. *Blood*, **96**, 2062-2068.

[19] Ratanatharathorn, V., Nash, R.A., Przepiorka, D., *et al.* (1998) Phase III Study Comparing Methotrexate and Tacrolimus (Prograf, FK506) with Methotrexate and Cyclosporine for Graft-versus-Host Disease Prophylaxis after HLA-Identical Sibling Bone Marrow Transplantation. *Blood*, **92**, 2303-2314.

[20] Shikari, H., *et al.* (2013) Ocular Graft-versus-Host Disease: A Review. *Survey of Ophthalmology*, **58**, 233-251. http://dx.doi.org/10.1016/j.survophthal.2012.08.004

[21] Higman, M.A. and Vogelsang, G.B. (2004) Chronic Graft versus Host Disease. *British Journal of Haematology*, **125**, 435-454. http://dx.doi.org/10.1111/j.1365-2141.2004.04945.x

[22] Ogawa, Y., Kim, S.K., Dana, R., Clayton, J., *et al.* (2013) International Chronic Ocular Graft-vs.-Host-Disease (GVHD) Consensus Group: Proposed Diagnostic Criteria for Chronic GVHD (Part I). *Scientific Reports*, **3**, 3419. http://dx.doi.org/10.1038/srep03419

[23] Bray, L.C., Carey, P.J. and Proctor, S.J. (1991) Ocular Complications of Bone Marrow Transplantation. *British Journal of Ophthalmology*, **75**, 611-614. http://dx.doi.org/10.1136/bjo.75.10.611

[24] Franklin, R.M., Kenyon, K.R., Tutschka, P.J., *et al.* (1983) Ocular Manifestations of Graft-vs.-Host Disease. *Ophthalmology*, **90**, 4-13. http://dx.doi.org/10.1016/S0161-6420(83)34604-2

[25] Hirst, L.W., Jabs, D.A., Tutschka, P.J., *et al.* (1983) The Eye in Bone Marrow Transplantation. I. Clinical Study. *Archives of Ophthalmology*, **101**, 580-584. http://dx.doi.org/10.1001/archopht.1983.01040010580010

[26] Holler, E. (2007) Risk Assessment in Haematopoietic Stem Cell Transplantation: GVHD Prevention and Treatment. *Best Practice & Research Clinical Haematology*, **20**, 281-294. http://dx.doi.org/10.1016/j.beha.2006.10.001

[27] Saito, T., Shinagawa, K., Takenaka, K., *et al.* (2002) Ocular Manifestation of Acute Graft versus Host Disease after Allogeneic Peripheral Blood Stem Cell Transplantation. *International Journal of Hematology*, **75**, 332-334. http://dx.doi.org/10.1007/BF02982052

[28] Vanathi, M., Khan, R., Kashyap, S., Tandon, R., *et al.* (2014) Ocular Surface Evaluation in Allogenic Hematopoietic Stem Cell Transplantation Patients. *European Journal of Ophthalmology*, **24**, 655-666. http://dx.doi.org/10.5301/ejo.5000451

[29] Tabbara, K.F., Al Ghamdi, A., Al Mohareb, F., Ayas, M., *et al.* (2009) Ocular Findings Following Allogeneic Hematopoietic Stem Cell Transplantation (HSCT). *Ophthalmology*, **116**, 1624-1629. http://dx.doi.org/10.1016/j.ophtha.2009.04.054

[30] Tuchocka-Piotrowska, A., Puszczewicz, M., Kołczewska, A. and Majewski, D. (2006) Graft-versus-Host Disease as the Cause of Symptoms Mimicking Sjögren's Syndrome. *Annales Academiae Medicae Stetinensis*, **52**, 89-93.

[31] Westeneng, A.C., Hettinga, Y., Lokhorst, H., *et al.* (2010) Ocular Graft-versus-Host Disease after Allogeneic Stem Cell Transplantation. *Cornea*, **7**, 758-763. http://dx.doi.org/10.1097/ico.0b013e3181ca321c

[32] Kim, S.K. (2006) Update on Ocular Graft versus Host Disease. *Current Opinion in Ophthalmology*, **17**, 344-348. http://dx.doi.org/10.1097/01.icu.0000233952.09595.d8

[33] Ogawa, Y. and Kuwana, M. (2003) Dry Eye as a Major Complication Associated with Chronic Graft-versus-Host Disease after Hematopoietic Stem Cell Transplantation. *Cornea*, **22**, 19-27. http://dx.doi.org/10.1097/00003226-200310001-00004

[34] Jacob, R., Tran, U., Chan, H., Kassim, A., *et al.* (2012) Prevalence and Risk Factors Associated with Development of Ocular GVHD Defined by NIH Consensus Criteria. *Bone Marrow Transplant*, **47**, 1470-1473. http://dx.doi.org/10.1038/bmt.2012.56

[35] Shimazaki, J. (2007) Definition and Diagnosis of Dry Eye. *Journal of the Eye*, **24**, 181-184.

[36] Herrero, V.R. and Peral, A. (2007) The Definition and Classification of Dry Eye Disease: Report of the Definition and Classification Subcommittee of the International Dry Eye Workshop. *The Ocular Surface*, **5**, 75-92. http://dx.doi.org/10.1016/S1542-0124(12)70081-2

[37] Kim, S.K. (2004) Ocular Graft versus Host Disease. In: Krachmer, J.H., Mannis, E.J. and Holland, E.J., Eds., *Cornea*, Mosby, St Louis, 879-885.

[38] Hessen, M. and Akpek, E.K. (2012) Ocular Graft-versus-Host Disease. *Current Opinion in Allergy and Clinical Immunology*, **12**, 540-547. http://dx.doi.org/10.1097/aci.0b013e328357b4b9

[39] Jabs, D.A., Hirst, L.W., Green, W.R., *et al.* (1983) The Eye in Bone Marrow Transplantation. II. Histopathology. *Archives of Ophthalmology*, **101**, 585-590. http://dx.doi.org/10.1001/archopht.1983.01040010585011

[40] Jabs, D.A., Wingard, J., Green, W.R., *et al.* (1989) The Eye in Bone Marrow Transplantation. III. Conjunctival Graft-vs.-Host Disease. *Archives of Ophthalmology*, **107**, 1343-1348.
http://dx.doi.org/10.1001/archopht.1989.01070020413046

[41] Townley, J.R., Dana, R. and Jacobs, D.S. (2011) Keratoconjunctivitis Sicca Manifestations in Ocular Graft versus Host Disease: Pathogenesis, Presentation, Prevention, and Treatment. *Seminars in Ophthalmology*, **26**, 251-260.
http://dx.doi.org/10.3109/08820538.2011.588663

[42] Robinson, M.R., Lee, S.S., Rubin, B.I., *et al.* (2004) Topical Corticosteroid Therapy for Cicatricial Conjunctivitis Associated with Chronic Graft-versus-Host Disease. *Bone Marrow Transplant*, **33**, 1031-1035.
http://dx.doi.org/10.1038/sj.bmt.1704453

[43] Yeh, P.T., Hou, Y.C., Lin, W.C., Wang, I.J., *et al.* (2006) Recurrent Corneal Perforation and Acute Calcareous Corneal Degeneration in Chronic Graft-versus-Host Disease. *Journal of the Formosan Medical Association*, **105**, 334-339.
http://dx.doi.org/10.1016/S0929-6646(09)60125-X

[44] Allan, E.J., Flowers, M.E., Lin, M.P., Bensinger, R.E., Martin, P.J. and Wu, M.C. (2011) Visual Acuity and Anterior Segment Findings in Chronic Graft-versus-Host Disease. *Cornea*, **30**, 1392-1397.
http://dx.doi.org/10.1097/ICO.0b013e31820ce6d0

[45] Hettinga, Y.M., Verdonck, L.F., Fijnheer, R., *et al.* (2007) The Anterior Uveitis: A Manifestation of Graft-versus-Host Disease. *Ophthalmology*, **114**, 794-797. http://dx.doi.org/10.1016/j.ophtha.2006.07.049

[46] Wertheim, M. and Rosenbaum, J.T. (2005) The Bilateral Uveitis Manifesting as a Complication of Chronic Graft-versus-Host Disease after Allogeneic Bone Marrow Transplantation. *Ocular Immunology and Inflammation*, **13**, 403-404.
http://dx.doi.org/10.1080/09273940490912470

[47] Coskuncan, N.M., Jabs, D.A., Dunn, J.P., Haller, J.A., *et al.* (1994) The Eye in Bone Marrow Transplantation. VI. Retinal Complications. *Archives of Ophthalmology*, **112**, 372-379.
http://dx.doi.org/10.1001/archopht.1994.01090150102031

[48] Cheng, L.L., Kwok, A.K., Wat, N.M., Neoh, E.L., *et al.* (2002) Graft versus Host Disease Associated Conjunctival Chemosis and Central Serous Chorioretinopathy after Bone Marrow Transplant. *American Journal of Ophthalmology*, **134**, 293-295. http://dx.doi.org/10.1016/S0002-9394(02)01464-2

[49] Kim, R.Y., Anderlini, P., Naderi, A.A., Rivera, P., *et al.* (2002) Scleritis as the Initial Clinical Manifestation of Graft-versus-Host Disease after Allogenic Bone Marrow Transplantation. *American Journal of Ophthalmology*, **133**, 843-845. http://dx.doi.org/10.1016/S0002-9394(02)01425-3

[50] Strouthidis, N.G., Francis, P.J., Stanford, M.R., Graham, E.M., *et al.* (2003) Posterior Segment Complications of Graft versus Host Disease after Bone Marrow Transplantation. *British Journal of Ophthalmology*, **87**, 1421-1423.
http://dx.doi.org/10.1136/bjo.87.11.1421-a

[51] MacMillan, M.L., Weisdorf, D.J., Wagner, J.E., *et al.* (2002) Response of 443 Patients to Steroids as Primary Therapy for Acute Graft versus Host Disease: Comparison of Grading Systems. *Biology of Blood and Marrow Transplantation*, **8**, 387-394. http://dx.doi.org/10.1053/bbmt.2002.v8.pm12171485

[52] Soiffer, R. (2008) Immune Modulation and Chronic Graft versus Host Disease. *Bone Marrow Transplant*, **42**, 66-69.
http://dx.doi.org/10.1038/bmt.2008.119

[53] Koreth, J., Matsuoka, K., Kim, H.T., *et al.* (2011) Interleukin-2 and Regulatory T Cells in Graft-versus-Host Disease. *The New England Journal of Medicine*, **365**, 2055-2066. http://dx.doi.org/10.1056/NEJMoa1108188

[54] Greinix, H.T., Knobler, R.M., Worel, N., *et al.* (2006) The Effect of Intensified Extracorporeal Photochemotherapy on Long-Term Survival in Patients with Severe Acute Graft-versus-Host Disease. *Haematologica*, **91**, 405-408.

[55] Magro, L., Catteau, B., Coiteux, V., *et al.* (2008) Efficacy of Imatinib Mesylate in the Treatment of Refractory Sclerodermatous Chronic GVHD. *Bone Marrow Transplant*, **42**, 757-760. http://dx.doi.org/10.1038/bmt.2008.252

[56] Nassiri, N., *et al.* (2013) Ocular Graft versus Host Disease Following Allogeneic Stem Cell Transplantation: A Review of Current Knowledge and Recommendations. *Journal of Ophthalmic and Vision Research*, **8**, 351-358.

[57] Ogawa, Y., Okamoto, S., Mori, T., *et al.* (2003) Autologous Serum Eye Drops for the Treatment of Severe Dry Eye in Patients with Chronic Graft-versus-Host Disease. *Bone Marrow Transplant*, **31**, 579-583.
http://dx.doi.org/10.1038/sj.bmt.1703862

[58] Couriel, D.R. (2008) Ancillary and Supportive Care in Chronic Graft-versus-Host Disease. *Best Practice & Research Clinical Haematology*, **21**, 291-307. http://dx.doi.org/10.1016/j.beha.2008.02.014

[59] Kim, S.K., Couriel, D., Ghosh, S., *et al.* (2006) Ocular Graft vs. Host Disease Experience from MD Anderson Cancer Center: Newly Described Clinical Spectrum and New Approach to the Management of Stage III and IV Ocular GVHD. *Biology of Blood and Marrow Transplantation*, **12**, 49-50. http://dx.doi.org/10.1016/j.bbmt.2005.11.155

[60] Kiang, E., Tesavibul, N., Yee, R., *et al.* (1998) The Use of Topical Cyclosporin A in Ocular Graft versus Host-Disease.

Bone Marrow Transplant, **22**, 147-151. http://dx.doi.org/10.1038/sj.bmt.1701304

[61] Lelli Jr., G.J., Musch, D.C., Gupta, A., *et al.* (2006) The Ophthalmic Cyclosporine Use in Ocular GVHD. *Cornea*, **25**, 635-638. http://dx.doi.org/10.1097/01.ico.0000208818.47861.1d

[62] Rao, S.N. and Rao, R.D. (2006) Efficacy of Topical Cyclosporine 0.05% in the Treatment of Dry Eye Associated with Graft versus Host Disease. *Cornea*, **25**, 674-678. http://dx.doi.org/10.1097/01.ico.0000208813.17367.0c

[63] Tam, P.M., Young, A.L., Cheng, L.L. and Lam, P.T. (2010) Topical 0.03% Tacrolimus Ointment in the Management of Ocular Surface Inflammation in Chronic GVHD. *Bone Marrow Transplant*, **45**, 957-958. http://dx.doi.org/10.1038/bmt.2009.249

[64] Ogawa, Y., Dogru, M., Uchino, M., *et al.* (2010) Topical Tranilast for Treatment of the Early Stage of Mild Dry Eye Associated with Chronic GVHD. *Bone Marrow Transplant*, **45**, 565-569. http://dx.doi.org/10.1038/bmt.2009.173

[65] Russo, P.A., Bouchard, C.S. and Galasso, J.M. (2007) Extended-Wear Silicone Hydrogel Soft Contact Lenses in the Management of Moderate to Severe Dry Eye Signs and Symptoms Secondary to Graft-versus-Host Disease. *Eye & Contact Lens*, **33**, 144-147. http://dx.doi.org/10.1097/01.icl.0000244154.76214.2d

[66] Takahide, K., Parker, P.M., Wu, M., *et al.* (2007) Use of Fluid-Ventilated, Gas-Permeable Scleral Lens for Management of Severe Keratoconjunctivitis Sicca Secondary to Chronic Graft-versus-Host Disease. *Biology of Blood and Marrow Transplantation*, **13**, 1016-1021. http://dx.doi.org/10.1016/j.bbmt.2007.05.006

[67] Heath, J.D., Acheson, J.F. and Schulenburg, W.E. (1993) Penetrating Keratoplasty in Severe Ocular Graft versus Host Disease. *British Journal of Ophthalmology*, **77**, 525-526. http://dx.doi.org/10.1136/bjo.77.8.525

[68] Smith, V.A. and Cook, S.D. (2004) Doxycycline—A Role in Ocular Surface Repair. *British Journal of Ophthalmology*, **88**, 619-625. http://dx.doi.org/10.1136/bjo.2003.025551

[69] Smith, V.A., Khan-Lim, D., Anderson, L., *et al.* (2008) Does Orally Administered Doxycycline Reach the Tear Film. *British Journal of Ophthalmology*, **92**, 856-859. http://dx.doi.org/10.1136/bjo.2007.125989

[70] Couriel, D., Carpenter, P.A., Cutler, C., Bolanos-Meade, J., *et al.* (2006) Ancillary Therapy and Supportive Care of Chronic Graft-versus-Host Disease: National Institutes of Health Consensus Development Project on Criteria for Clinical Trials in Chronic Graft-versus-Host Disease: V. Ancillary Therapy and Supportive Care Working Group Report. *Biology of Blood and Marrow Transplantation*, **12**, 375-396. http://dx.doi.org/10.1016/j.bbmt.2006.02.003

Permissions

All chapters in this book were first published in OJOPH, by Scientific Research Publishing; hereby published with permission under the Creative Commons Attribution License or equivalent. Every chapter published in this book has been scrutinized by our experts. Their significance has been extensively debated. The topics covered herein carry significant findings which will fuel the growth of the discipline. They may even be implemented as practical applications or may be referred to as a beginning point for another development.

The contributors of this book come from diverse backgrounds, making this book a truly international effort. This book will bring forth new frontiers with its revolutionizing research information and detailed analysis of the nascent developments around the world.

We would like to thank all the contributing authors for lending their expertise to make the book truly unique. They have played a crucial role in the development of this book. Without their invaluable contributions this book wouldn't have been possible. They have made vital efforts to compile up to date information on the varied aspects of this subject to make this book a valuable addition to the collection of many professionals and students.

This book was conceptualized with the vision of imparting up-to-date information and advanced data in this field. To ensure the same, a matchless editorial board was set up. Every individual on the board went through rigorous rounds of assessment to prove their worth. After which they invested a large part of their time researching and compiling the most relevant data for our readers.

The editorial board has been involved in producing this book since its inception. They have spent rigorous hours researching and exploring the diverse topics which have resulted in the successful publishing of this book. They have passed on their knowledge of decades through this book. To expedite this challenging task, the publisher supported the team at every step. A small team of assistant editors was also appointed to further simplify the editing procedure and attain best results for the readers.

Apart from the editorial board, the designing team has also invested a significant amount of their time in understanding the subject and creating the most relevant covers. They scrutinized every image to scout for the most suitable representation of the subject and create an appropriate cover for the book.

The publishing team has been an ardent support to the editorial, designing and production team. Their endless efforts to recruit the best for this project, has resulted in the accomplishment of this book. They are a veteran in the field of academics and their pool of knowledge is as vast as their experience in printing. Their expertise and guidance has proved useful at every step. Their uncompromising quality standards have made this book an exceptional effort. Their encouragement from time to time has been an inspiration for everyone.

The publisher and the editorial board hope that this book will prove to be a valuable piece of knowledge for researchers, students, practitioners and scholars across the globe.

List of Contributors

Valliammai Muthappan and Carlton R. Fenzl
John A. Moran Eye Center, University of Utah, Salt Lake City, USA

Jared G. Smedley
College of Human Medicine, Michigan State University, Lansing, USA

Majid Moshirfar
Department of Ophthalmology, Francis I. Proctor Foundation, University of California San Francisco, San Francisco, USA

Huseyin Gursoy and Hikmet Basmak
Eskisehir Osmangazi University Medical Faculty, Department of Ophthalmology, Eskisehir, Turkey

Hamza Esen and Ferhan Esen
Eskisehir Osmangazi University Medical Faculty, Department of Biophysics, Eskisehir, Turkey

Hans Callø Fledelius
Copenhagen University Eye Clinics, Rigshospitalet and Glostrup Hospital, Capital Region, Denmark

Kirsten Korsholm and Ian Law
Department of Clinical Physiology, Nuclear Medicine and PET, Rigshospitalet, Capital Region, Denmark

O. Pokrovskaya, D. Wallace and C. O'Brien
School of Medicine and Medical Science, University College Dublin, Dublin, Ireland
Department of Ophthalmology, Mater Misericordiae University Hospital, Dublin, Ireland

Miltiadis Papathanassiou and Lamprini Papaioannou
Cornea Clinic, 2nd Ophthalmology Department, Attikon University Hospital, Athens, Greece

John C. Merriam and Lei Zheng
Edward S. Harkness Eye Institute, College of Physicians and Surgeons, Columbia University, New York, NY, USA

Eva Nong
Department of Ophthalmology, University of Maryland, Baltimore, MD, USA

Malka Stohl
New York State Psychiatric Institute, New York, NY, USA

Ewa Porwik, Erita Filipek and Maria Formińska-Kapuścik
Ophthalmology Clinic and Department of Ophthalmology, School of Medicine in Katowice, Medical University of Silesia in Katowice, Katowice, Poland

Riley Sanders and Johnny Gayton
Mercer University School of Medicine, Macon, USA
Eyesight Associates, Warner Robins, USA

Uma Sridhar and Jyoti Batra
Cornea Department, ICARE Eye Hospital, Noida, India

Amil Ausaf Ur Rahman
Training Centre, ICARE Eye Hospital, Noida, India

Neelam Sapra
Microbiology Depatment, Shroff Charity Eye Hospital, New Delhi, India

Tatiana Iureva, Andrey Shchuko and Yulia Pyatova
Irkutsk Branch, S. Fyodorov Eye Microsurgery Federal State Institution, Irkutsk, Russia

Tatiana Iureva
Irkutsk State Medical Academy for Postgraduate Education, Irkutsk, Russia

Derya Buran Kağnici
Department of Ophthalmology, Aydın State Hospital, Aydın, Turkey

Tolga Kocatürk, Harun Çakmak and Sema Oruç Dündar
Department of Ophthalmology, Adnan Menderes University Medical Faculty, Aydın, Turkey

Michal S. Nowak
Department of Ophthalmology and Visual Rehabilitation, Medical University of Lodz, Lodz, Poland

Janusz Smigielski
Department of Geriatrics, Medical University of Lodz, Lodz, Poland

Martin Heur
Department of Ophthalmology, Keck School of Medicine of the University of Southern California, Los Angeles, CA, USA

Samuel Yiu
Department of Ophthalmology, The Wilmer Eye Institute, The John Hopkins University, Baltimore, Maryland, USA

Daniel S. Churgin, Jonathan H. Tzu and Harry W. Flynn
Department of Ophthalmology, Bascom Palmer Eye Institute, University of Miami Miller School of Medicine, Miami, FL, USA

Fusako Fujimura, Nobuyuki Shoji and Kazunori Hirasawa
Department of Rehabilitation, Orthoptics and Visual Science Course, School of Allied Health Sciences, Kitasato University, Tokyo, Japan

Kazuhiro Matsumura, Tetsuya Morita, Kimiya Shimizu and Nobuyuki Shoji
Department of Ophthalmology, School of Medicine, Kitasato University, Tokyo, Japan

Sean M. Gratton
Truman Medical Center, Department of Neurology and Cognitive Neuroscience, University of Missouri— Kansas City School of Medicine, Kansas City, USA

Angela Herro, Jose Antonio Bermudez-Magner and John Guy
Bascom Palmer Eye Institute, University of Miami Miller School of Medicine, Miami, USA

Baixiang Xiao and Jinglin Yi
Affiliated Eye Hospital of Nanchang University, Nanchang City, China

Nathan Congdon and Baixiang Xiao
Zhongshan Ophthalmic Center, Guangzhou City, China

Hans Limburg
London School of Hygiene & Tropical Medicine, London, United Kingdom

Guiseng Zhang
Inner Mongolia Red Cross Chaoju Eye Hospital, Hohhot, China

Beatrice Iezzi and Richard Le Mesurier
The Fred Hollows Foundation, Sydney, Australia

Andreas Müller
World Health Organization, Western Pacific Regional Office, Manila, Philippines

Naser Salihu and Belinda Pustina
Department of Ophthalmology, University Clinical Center of Kosova, Prishtina, Kosova

Brigita Drnovšek-Olup
Eye Clinic, University Medical Center Ljubljana, Ljubljana, Slovenia

George D. Kymionis, Konstantinos I. Tsoulnaras, Stella V. Blazaki and Michael A. Grentzelos
Vardinoyiannion Eye Institute of Crete (VEIC), Faculty of Medicine, University of Crete, Heraklion, Crete, Greece

George D. Kymionis
Department of Ophthalmology, Bascom Palmer Eye Institute, University of Miami, Miami, FL, USA

Olya Pokrovskaya
Department of Ophthalmology, Mater Miscericordiae University Hospital, Dublin, Ireland

Ian Dooley, Salma Babiker, Catherine Croghan, Claire Hartnett and Anthony Cullinane
Department of Ophthalmology, Cork University Hospital, Cork, Ireland

Bassey Fiebai and Chinyere N. Pedro-Egbe
Department of Ophthalmology, University of Port Harcourt Teaching Hospital, Port Harcourt, Nigeria

Suleyman Ciftci and Eyup Dogan
Department of Ophthalmology, Diyarbakır Training and Research Hospital, Diyarbakır, Turkey

Leyla Ciftci
Department of Cardiology, Faculty of Medicine, Dicle University, Diyarbakır, Turkey

Ozlem Demirpence
Department of Biochemistry, Tunceli State Hospital, Tunceli, Turkey

Tanie Natung, Jacqueline Syiem, Avonuo Keditsu, Nilotpal Saikia, Ranendra Hajong and Laura Amanda Lyngdoh
North Eastern Indira Gandhi Regional Institute of Health & Medical Sciences, Shillong, India

Seyed Ali Tabatabaei, Mohammad Soleimani, Mohammad Reza Mansouri
Mohammad Ebrahimi, Parisa Abdi and Mohammad Riazi Esfahani
Eye Research Center, Farabi Eye Hospital, Tehran University of Medical Sciences, Iran

Gysbert van Setten
St Eriks Eye Hospital, Karolinska Institutet, Stockholm, Sweden
Belinda Pustina and Naser Salihu
Department of Ophthalmology, University Clinical Center of Kosovo, Prishtina, Kosovo

Syed S. Hasnain
General Ophthalmology, Porterville, CA, USA

Hongjun Du
Department of Ophthalmology, Xijing Hospital, Xi'an, China

Travis Stiles, Christopher Douglas, Daisy Ho, Peter X. Shaw and Hongjun Du
Department of Ophthalmology and Shiley Eye Institute, University of California San Diego, San Diego, USA

Xu Xiao
Sichuan Provincial People's Hospital, Chengdu, China

Nada Otmani and Oudidi Abdellatif
Hassan II Hospital, Fez, Morocco

Bennani Othmani Mohamed, Serheir Zineb and Housbane Sami
Faculty of Medicine, Casablanca, Morocco

Lamprini Papaioannou and Miltiadis Papathanassiou
Cornea Clinic, 2nd Ophthalmology Department, Attikon University Hospital, Athens, Greece

Tao Li, Xiaodong Zhou
Department of Ophthalmology, Jinshan Hospital of Fudan University, Shanghai, China

Zhi Chen and Xingtao Zhou
Department of Ophthalmology, Eye and ENT Hospital of Fudan University, Shanghai, China

Maria Kazaki, Ilias Georgalas, Alexandros Damanakis, Sergios Taliantzis, Chryssanthi Koutsandrea and Dimitris Papaconstantinou
Department of Glaucoma, University of Athens, Athens, Greece

Georgios Labiris
Department of Ophthalmology, University of Alexandroupolis, Alexandroupolis, Greece

Chandra Gurung
Department of Ophthalmology, NNJS Banke Fateh Bal Eye Hospital, Nepalganj, Nepal
Suma Ganesh
Department of Pediatric Ophthalmology and Strabismus, Dr Shroff's Charity Eye Hospital, New Delhi, India

Priyanka Arora
Department of Ophthalmology, Dayanand Medical College and Hospital, Ludhiana, India

Sumita Sethi
Department of Ophthalmology, BPS Government Medical College for Women, Sonepat, India

Karim Diab, Swati Chavda and Nathan Gorfinkel
Western University, London, Canada

Francie Si and William Hodge
Ivey Eye Institute, Western University, London, Canada

Brad Dishan
Library Service, St. Joseph's Hospital Health Care, London, Canada

Obiekwe Okoye and Boniface Eze
Department of Ophthalmology, University of Nigeria, Enugu, Nigeria

Chimdia Ogbonnaya and Chinyelu Ezisi
Department of Ophthalmology, Federal Teaching Hospital, Abakiliki, Nigeria

Olughu Obasi
Eye Unit, Presbyterian Joint Hospital, Uburu, Nigeria

Sridevi Nair, Murugesan Vanathi, Anita Ganger and Radhika Tandon
Cornea & Ocular Surface Services, Dr Rajendra Prasad Centre for Ophthalmic Sciences, All India Institute of Medical Sciences, New Delhi, India

www.ingramcontent.com/pod-product-compliance
Lightning Source LLC
Chambersburg PA
CBHW080505200326
41458CB00012B/4096